MOTOR SPEECH DISORDERS

Essays for Ray Kent

MOTOR SPEECH DISORDERS

Essays for Ray Kent

Edited by
Gary Weismer, Ph.D.

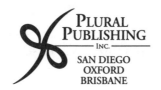

PLURAL
PUBLISHING
INC.
SAN DIEGO
OXFORD
BRISBANE

MW

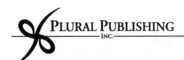

PLURAL PUBLISHING
INC.

5521 Ruffin Road
San Diego, CA 92123

e-mail: info@pluralpublishing.com
Web site: http://www.pluralpublishing.com

49 Bath Street
Abingdon, Oxfordshire OX14 1EA
United Kingdom

Copyright © by Plural Publishing, Inc. 2007

Typeset in 11/12 Garamond by Flanagan's Publishing Services, Inc.
Printed in the United States of America by Bang Printing

Library of Congress Cataloging-in-Publication Data:

Motor speech disorders : essays for Ray Kent / edited by Gary G.
Weismer.
    p. ; cm.
Includes bibliographical references and index.
ISBN-13: 978-1-59756-115-0 (hardcover)
ISBN-10: 1-59756-115-0 (hardcover)
1. Speech therapy.   I. Weismer, Gary. II. Kent, Raymond D.
[DNLM: 1. Kent, Raymond D. 2. Dysarthria–Festschrift.
3. Apraxias–Festschrift. 4. Speech Disorders–Festschrift.
WL 340.2 M919 2006]
RC423.M6844 2006
616.85'506–dc22

                            2006031942

2|8|07

"A man is a bundle of relations, a knot of roots, whose flower and fruitage is the world"
—Ralph Waldo Emerson, *Essays. First Series. History* (1847)

To three roots:
Bette Weismer (1918-2002)
S. Gabriel Weismer
And, of course:
Ray Kent

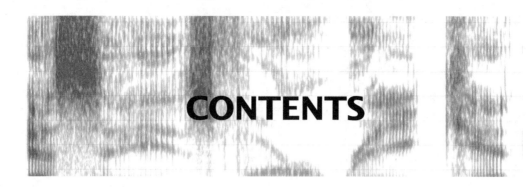

CONTENTS

ABOUT THE EDITOR

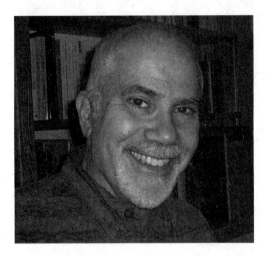

Gary Weismer, Ph.D., is Professor of Communicative Disorders and an investigator at the Waisman Center, University of Wisconsin-Madison. He received his bachelor's and master's degrees from Pennsylvania State University and his doctorate from UW-Madison in 1975. Dr. Weismer's research papers concern normal speech production and various aspects of motor speech disorders. He is currently serving as Associate Editor for Speech, *Journal of Speech, Language, and Hearing Research*, and Associate Editor, Motor Speech Disorders, *Folia Phoniatrica et Logopaedica*. Dr. Weismer is a Fellow of the Acoustical Society of America and his research has been funded by the NIH for the past 25 years.

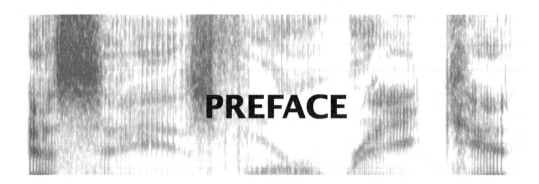

PREFACE

In the late spring of 2005 I contacted Sadanand Singh about an idea I had to honor Ray Kent's remarkable, three-decades-plus contribution to the field of speech-language pathology. I proposed a textbook on motor speech disorders, authored by a group of Ray's former doctoral students and former and current colleagues. In addition, I proposed to Dr. Singh—somewhat naively, I thought at the time, but you never know until you ask—that the editor and author proceeds from sales of the text be dedicated completely to a scholarship fund to be administered through Ray's long-time department here at the University of Wisconsin-Madison. The scholarship fund would be for doctoral students in our program, and would support various aspects of their research training; needless to say, the scholarship would be named for Ray. Imagine my happy surprise when Dr. Singh not only endorsed the proposal, but offered to match the editor and author proceeds and therefore build the scholarship fund that much more quickly. Our agreement, our mutual and deep for respect for Ray, set this project in motion and the book you hold in your hand is truly the product of a joint effort among authors and publisher.

I corresponded with potential authors in the summer of 2005 as I sat in the dining room of the Apollon Hotel in Xylokastro, Greece, where the semi-reliable Internet connections were located. Interest in this project among Ray's former students and his colleagues was very high, and everyone agreed immediately to forego payment for their contributions to provide a lasting tribute to this great mentor, scientist, and colleague. The timely completion of the book became more pressing when Ray announced in the Spring 2006 that he was retiring his faculty position, effective the end of that same semester.

So, the Department of Communicative Disorders at UW-Madison began the post-Kent era this past semester (Fall, 2006) and it will, at first and perhaps for a while, be a strange transition, and especially for me. I came to UW-Madison in 1972 as a doctoral student, a year after Ray arrived, and in 1975 he directed my dissertation which I believe was his first. (He got it more than right with his future students, after allowing me to experiment on him with a truly weird study that has made me say more than once, "What was I thinking?"). I left Madison for 5 years, during which time I was in more or less constant contact with him; and when the chance came to come back, Ray's presence here was a huge factor in the decision to do so. I am forever indebted to him for his ceaseless support and open colleagiality. Oh yes, and for teaching me how to do science and train students. This is all meant to say, things will not be the same without Ray Kent in the hallways of Goodnight Hall and the Waisman Center, without his gentle but pointed questions in doctoral qualifying exams and dissertation defenses, without the brief visits to his office where one wondered how he found anything among the masses of papers, journals, and books stacked on every available level surface.

I believe the book you are holding, the one with chapters written by Ray's ex-students and former and current colleagues, is a pretty good one; I think he and you will like it. It is appropriate for a graduate level course in motor speech disorders and has some features that other books in the area do not. I truly believe that the student who reads this text carefully and with the guidance of a committed instructor will know a lot more about motor speech disorders than when the book was opened for the first time.

There are a lot of people to thank for making this project work. First and foremost, I am very grateful to Dr. Sadanand Singh who took a personal interest in this project right from the start and saw to it that the text would be published prior to the 2006 ASHA convention in Miami. And second on the list would be the contributing authors, who donated their time, literally and financially, to pay tribute to a man who has made such a difference in their professional lives.

Thanks are also due to Susan Ellis Weismer and Yunjung Kim, who read chapters in manuscript form and made valuable comments about them. Nikki Weismer assisted with the development of figures, and my lab staff and doctoral students showed enormous patience with me as I canceled meetings and hid behind doorways (caught, one time) so I could get into my office unseen to write another paragraph. Thanks to all.

Thanks mostly to Ray, without whose influence this text would not have been written. Whatever value it has, the good parts are largely due to you.

Gary Weismer
Madison, WI

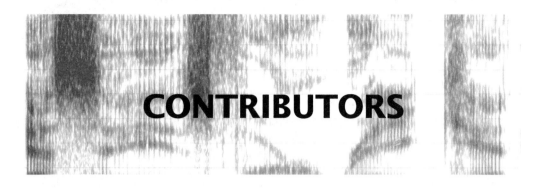

CONTRIBUTORS

Eugene H. Buder, Ph.D.
Associate Professor
School of Audiology and Speech-
   Language Pathology
The University of Memphis
Memphis, Tennessee
Chapter 5

Joseph R. Duffy, Ph.D.
Head, Division of Speech Pathology
Department of Neurology
Mayo Clinic
Professor of Speech Pathology
Mayo Clinic College of Medicine
Rochester, Minnesota
Chapter 2

Katherine C. Hustad, Ph.D.
Assistant Professor
Department of Communicative
   Disorders
University of Wisconsin
Madison, Wisconsin
Chapter 9

Harrison N. Jones, M.A.
Doctoral candidate, Rehabilitation
   Science
Department of Communicative Sciences
University of Florida
Gainesville, Florida
Chapter 8

Julie M. Liss, Ph.D.
Associate Professor
Department of Speech and Hearing
   Sciences
Arizona State University
Tempe, Arizona
Chapter 7

John C. Rosenbek, Ph.D.
Professor and Chair
Department of Communicative
   Disorders
University of Florida
Gainesville, Florida
Chapter 8

Kris Tjaden, Ph.D.
Associate Professor
Department of Communicative
   Disorders and Sciences
University at Buffalo
Buffalo, New York
Chapter 6

Gary Weismer, Ph.D.
Professor
Department of Communicative
   Disorders
Waisman Center
University of Wisconsin
Madison, Wisconsin
Chapters 1, 3, 4, and 9

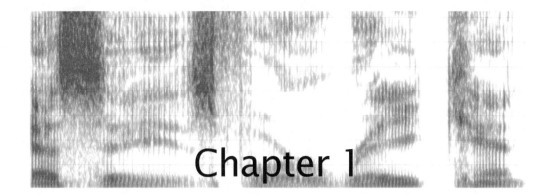

Chapter 1

THE SHAPING OF A FIELD

Kent's Influence on Motor Speech Disorders

Gary Weismer

What does it mean to shape an academic discipline? This question is posed here because it has direct relevance to the area of motor speech disorders—the subject matter of this text—and the man to whom the book is offered as a tribute, a product, and a thank you. In the course of this brief, introductory chapter, we attempt to offer answers to this question and in so doing shed some light on an outstanding academic career.

Ray Kent was born and grew up in Red Lodge, Montana, a small town slightly more than a mile above sea level and originally famed for its coal deposits and bootleg liquor. Ray began his speech-language pathology career at the University of Montana, where he received a B.A., and then earned his masters degree and Ph.D. from the University of Iowa. After a postdoctoral year at MIT, Ray was appointed as an Assistant Professor at the University of Wisconsin-Madison in 1971, and he has been there ever since, with a brief, three-year detour between 1979 to 1982 when he took a leave of absence from UW-Madison and served as a scientist at Boys Town National Institute.

When someone is said to have shaped an academic discipline they have made substantial contributions to defining the discipline, to clarifying what the field can do better and differently than other fields. During Ray's career he has shaped the discipline of speech-language pathology, consistent with the above-stated criteria, in an astonishing number of ways. First, Ray presented a model of scholarship to our discipline that was quite unique. This model placed an emphasis on mastery of literatures and techniques that went well past what the typical speech-language professor regarded as a proper scholarly domain. Early in his career, and indeed throughout his career, Ray was reading extensively in neuroanatomy and neuropathology, general motor control, linguistics, and experimental/cognitive psychology.

The knowledge he absorbed from these different areas found its way into his enormous body of scholarly writings—research papers, book chapters, and textbooks—and pushed other speech-language pathology scholars to broaden their own perspectives. Ray was interdisciplinary long before it was "cool" to be so, long before the term became a buzzword on campuses across the country.

Second, Ray trained a large number of doctoral students who, being exposed to this broad, wise, and unique model of scholarship, presumably incorporated it into their own thinking and work. One hopes these first-generation students, now professors, have passed this ethos along to their own students and colleagues to continue the shaping process. The best legacy a scholar can leave to a field is the people he or she trains, the colleagues he or she influences. That legacy is, hopefully, reflected in the chapters of this text, all written by Ray's students and close colleagues.

Most importantly, Ray showed the field how to marry speech science with speech-language pathology and to make the union happy, productive, and eventually, indispensable. Does the union seem obvious? Is it really so important that a scholar would have provided a model of how the two areas should and could meet? When Ray received his Ph.D. in 1970, there was still a kind of conceptual fault line between those who were interested in "normal" speech production and speech perception and those who were interested in speech disorders. The pursuit of answers to questions concerning normal speech production was not seen as particularly relevant to the "clinical" questions regarding the speech production deficit in cleft palate, motor speech disorders, phonologic disorders, and stuttering, among other disorders. It was not so much that people in the field did not understand the relevance of a speech science outlook on speech disorders—one of Ray's mentors at Iowa, James Hardy, certainly saw the potential in applications to speakers with cerebral palsy and dysarthria—but that they lacked an organizing framework for how to join the two.

This brings us to the topic of this text, motor speech disorders, and how Ray shaped this particular aspect of the field by demonstrating the power of the speech science–speech disorders link. For his dissertation, Ray performed an extensive and painstaking analysis of cinefluographic films (x-ray motion pictures) of normal speakers producing connected utterances. This *speech movement* approach to understanding normal speech production had a limited history before Ray's work, but no one had considered the data the way Ray had, and perhaps no one but Ray had also looked at so many cine films of disordered speakers, these being available at Iowa as part of clinical procedures. Armed with what he had learned formally from his dissertation work on normal speakers and from his observations of disordered speakers, Ray and his colleague Ron Netsell secured funding to study speech movements in persons with cerebral palsy and in a series of publications (Kent & Netsell, 1975, 1978; Kent, Netsell, & Bauer, 1975; Netsell & Kent, 1976) introduced the field to one aspect of the speech science–speech disorders union noted above.

Simultaneously with the exploration of speech movements in normal speakers and speakers with neurologic disease, Ray was turning himself into a top-notch speech acoustician. Like speech movements, speech acoustics had been seen as a tool of the speech scientist who was most likely completely focused on issues in normal speech production. There were scattered studies of acoustic phonetics in persons with speech disorders prior to 1970, but nothing approaching a sustained research program, one with a theoretical viewpoint. Ray demonstrated the potential of acoustic phonetics to reveal interesting phenomena in speakers with motor speech disorders with a series of publications that began in 1979 with a paper on ataxic dysarthria (Kent, Netsell, & Abbs, 1979), and continued in 1982 and 1983 with acoustic analyses of prosody in several different motor speech disorders (Kent & Rosenbek, 1982), and an extensive acoustic analysis of patients with apraxia of speech (Kent & Rosenbek, 1983). This style of acoustic-phonetic work in motor speech disorders, with careful attention to detail and discussions of data from both clinical and theoretical perspectives, has continued unabated to the present day. Ray's contributions to acoustic analysis of motor speech disorders is so pervasive, of so much breadth and depth, that the reader is challenged to find a publication

in this area post-1985 that does *not* cite at least one of his papers. More than anything else, Ray's introduction of the techniques and interpretations of acoustic phonetic analysis for understanding speech disorders, and especially motor speech disorders, is an accomplishment without parallel in our field.

A little more should be said about acoustic phonetics and speech disorders, and Ray's introduction of the methods and thinking surrounding the union. Figure 1–1 is a familiar sight to speech-language pathologists; it is a spectrogram, much like the ones students were introduced to in their undergraduate speech science training and possibly as graduate students, too. We can tell you that the frequency scale (*y*-axis) on this spectrogram extends almost up to 9.0 kHz, and the interval between each of the hash marks on the time (*x*-axis) axis equals 100 milliseconds. We will tell you that the utterance is a well-formed statement in the English language, produced by a 56-year-old healthy male. We will *not* tell you what the spectrogram says, but leave that as an exercise for the closet spectrogram readers among you.

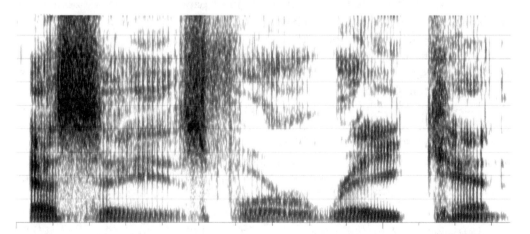

Figure 1–1. Spectrogram of unidentified utterance spoken by 56-year-old healthy male.

The spectrogram in Figure 1-1, and indeed any spectrogram, has a particular power among the various tools used to study communication processes, because it is a record of a signal that reflects not only what happened in the speech mechanism but also what is likely to happen in the listener's ear. The speech acoustic signal serves double-duty, as it were, looking both up- and downstream in the speech chain and, therefore, is capable of providing insight to both processes, and especially when the signal contains disturbances associated with motor speech disorders. In the mid-1980s Ray recognized the potential of combining perceptual analyses with acoustic analyses to gain even more comprehensive information about the speaker-listener interface in motor speech disorders. An extensive program of speech intelligibility studies in dysarthria was planned and funded, and that work has been ongoing for the past 20 years. Ray's idea was that speech intelligibility scores had always been used as a severity index—the worse the score, the worse the inferred speech production deficit— but this said almost nothing about the contributing factors to a particular patient's intelligibility problem. Stated in another way, and as a research question: was it the case that two patients with motor speech disorders, having equivalent speech intelligibility scores, had the same underlying speech production deficit? Ray approached this question by designing a speech intelligibility test structured around speech acoustic measures, so that a sort of co-analysis of speech acoustic and intelligibility data could be performed for individual speakers with dysarthria (Kent et al., 1989). These studies showed conclusively that two patients with (for example) a 60% speech intelligibility score could have very different reasons for the deficit. One patient may have primary problems with the role of the larynx in phonetic contrasts (the voiced-voiceless distinction for stops, fricatives, and affricates, plus the null-glottal fricative contrast in word pairs such as *ate-hate*), whereas the primary reason for the other patient's intelligibility problem may be the failure to control phonetic contrasts requiring good velopharyngeal control. The implications of this finding for management of motor speech disorders were clear: the primary reasons for an intelligibility deficit could be exposed by this kind of analysis, and point to the focus of therapy efforts to improve speech intelligibility (the two patients referred to above would have very different therapy plans, at least at the phonetic level). Thus Ray's joining of the acoustic and perceptual sides of speech intelligibility problems in motor speech disorders provided clinicians with a highly structured plan for attacking the phonetic component of an *individual* patient's communication needs.

Something should also be said about another way in which Ray has shaped the field, that of writing the scholarly review as a kind of progress report and program for future research. Ray revolutionized this kind of paper, and especially because he chose to publish them in peer-reviewed journals. Scientists often do this sort of thing in edited books, but as we all know those vehicles are lightly peer-reviewed and edited; the editor is typically just happy to get a contribution from an author! But Ray, beginning in 1976 and 1977 with review papers published on speech development (Kent, 1976) and coarticulation (Kent & Minifie, 1977), and later with papers on various aspects of motor speech disorders and brain mechanisms for speech (Kent, 1996; Kent et al., 1998, 1999, 2000) instructed us by example in the art of a review-paper style in which the careful assembly of what was known, to date, was made to illuminate the way for what should be known in the future. Review papers such as these—and especially when they are peer-reviewed and published in high-quality journals—are hard to do, still harder to get accepted, and when successful, are a major influence on scientists and clinicians in the field. Any of Ray's former students who have written and published these kinds of papers will tell you how indebted they are to the model of scholarship he presented in this remarkable series of reviews.

When a student comes to you and says, "I'd like an overview of motor speech disorders, what should I read?" you have several options. There are several very good textbooks available, and it would be entirely proper to refer the student to one of these. But you also have another option, a rare one in the communication sciences: you could tell the student to do a search for Ray Kent's publications on motor speech disorders and read them from 1975 to the present. Just about anything contained in one of those good textbooks would be covered in a complete reading of Ray's works, and as a bonus the student would get a sense of how this discipline evolved and flowered over the past 30 years.

We hope the current book is up to the task of representing what the field currently knows about motor speech disorders (This text is about motor speech disorders, and so we have tried to confine our comments in this chapter largely to this area; what we have not noted is that Ray has also made major contributions to the understanding of speech development and stuttering.) The height of the bar set by Ray is impossibly high, but it certainly is fun trying to reach it. We close this chapter by asking, "How do you get a

book written for you as a tribute, a product, a thank you?" The answer is obvious once you have thought about Ray Kent's shaping of the area of motor speech disorders. You ask the right questions and do the right things to push your discipline in the right direction; you give the discipline a shape, and continue to refine its outlines by the example of your work. And you influence many other people in the field by direct mentoring of doctoral students and aspiring clinicians, by congenial and productive collaboration with colleagues, and by maintaining and modeling the highest standards of scholarship. In this regard, Ray is without parallel in our field.

References

Kent, R. D. (1976). Anatomical and neuromuscular maturation of the speech mechanism: Evidence from acoustic studies. *Journal of Speech and Hearing Research*, 19, 421-447.

Kent, R. D. (1996). Hearing and believing: Some limits to the auditory-perceptual assessment of speech and voice disorders. *American Journal of Speech-Language Pathology*, 7, 7-23.

Kent, R. D., Kent, J. F., Duffy, J., & Weismer, G. (1998). The dysarthrias: Speech-voice profiles, related dysfunctions, and neuropathology. *Journal of Medical Speech-Language Pathology*, 6, 165-211.

Kent, R. D., Kent, J. F., Weismer, G., & Duffy, J. R. (2000). What dysarthrias can tell us about the neural control of speech. *Journal of Phonetics*, 28, 273-302.

Kent, R. D., & Minifie, F, D, (1977). Coarticulation in recent speech production models. *Journal of Phonetics*, 5, 115-117.

Kent, R. D., & Netsell, R. (1975). A case study of an ataxic dysarthric: Cineradiographic and spectrographic observations. *Journal of Speech and Hearing Disorders*, 40, 115-134.

Kent, R. D., & Netsell, R. (1978). Articulatory abnormalities in athetoid cerebral palsy. *Journal of Speech and Hearing Disorders, 43*, 353-373.

Kent, R. D., Netsell, R., & Abbs, J. H. (1979). Acoustic characteristics of dysarthria associated with cerebellar disease. *Journal of Speech and Hearing Research, 22,* 627-648.

Kent, R. D., Netsell, R., & Bauer L. L. (1975). Cineradiographic assessment of articulatory mobility in the dysarthrias. *Journal of Speech and Hearing Disorders, 40,* 467-480.

Kent, R. D., & Rosenbek, J. C. (1982). Prosodic disturbance and neurologic lesion. *Brain and Language, 15,* 259-291.

Kent, R. D., & Rosenbek, J. C. (1983). Acoustic patterns of apraxia of speech. *Journal of Speech and Hearing Research, 26,* 231-249.

Kent, R. D., Weismer, G., Kent, J. F., & Rosenbek, J. C. (1989). Toward phonetic intelligibility testing in dysarthria. *Journal of Speech and Hearing Research, 54,* 482-499.

Kent, R. D., Weismer, G., Kent, J. F., Vorperian, H. K., & Duffy, J. R. (1999). Acoustic studies of dysarthric speech: Methods, progress, and potential. *Journal of Communication Disorders, 32,* 141-186.

Netsell, R., & Kent, R. D. (1976). Paroxysmal ataxic dysarthria. *Journal of Speech and Hearing Disorders, 41,* 93-109.

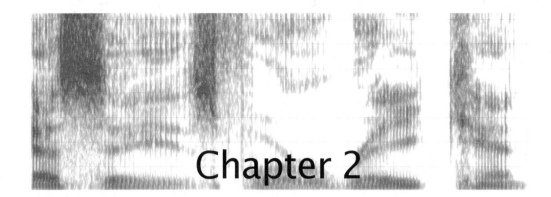

Chapter 2

HISTORY, CURRENT PRACTICE, AND FUTURE TRENDS AND GOALS

Joseph R. Duffy

Neurologic disease can rob our ability to communicate normally. Often the underlying disease is already known, but sometimes the speech deficit is the first or only sign that something is wrong with the nervous system. In either case, life will be different, often marked by efforts to establish the underlying cause of disease and ways to be rid of it, or efforts to reduce or compensate for the impairment knowing that the problem may be chronic or progressive. Frequently, the communication disorder reflects impairment of speech motor control. These difficulties, known as motor speech disorders, are the subject of this book. The intent of this chapter is to provide a broad overview of the topic.

This chapter has several goals. First, it provides some basic definitions essential to understanding motor speech disorders. Second, it summarizes some of the history behind our current understanding of them. Third, it describes and discusses current practice associated with their evaluation,

diagnosis, and management. This information will help the reader think about motor speech disorders from the perspective that a conceptual knowledge base and an understanding of clinical application are of equal importance. Subsequent chapters provide depth to the framework presented here. The final goal of this chapter is to identify some of the gaps in our current knowledge and practice and discuss some short- and long-term research goals that might address them.

The Boundaries of Motor Speech Disorders

The term, motor speech disorders (MSDs), is a generic designation for a variety of speech problems that reflect impairment in the sensorimotor planning, programming, control, or execution of speech. MSDs do not include deficits caused by peripheral structural abnormalities (e.g., craniofacial anomalies such as cleft palate, laryngectomy, glossectomy, missing teeth), nor do they include speech abnormalities that can result from sensorineural hearing loss. They also do not include neurologically based verbal expression deficits from higher level cognitive problems that affect the linguistic formulation, content, or form of spoken messages.

MSDs can be congenital/developmental or acquired; chronic, improving, or worsening in their course; and associated with numerous diseases that affect various portions of the central or peripheral sensorimotor nervous system (Duffy, 2005a, 2005b). They can be subcategorized into the *dysarthrias* and *apraxia of speech* (Table 2-1 summarizes their neurologic correlates and prominent/distinctive features). Dysarthria can be defined as:

> a collective name for a group of neurologic speech disorders resulting from abnormalities in the strength, speed, range, steadiness, tone, or accuracy of movements required for control of the respiratory, phonatory, resonatory, articulatory, and prosodic aspects of speech production. The responsible pathophysiologic disturbances are due to central or peripheral nervous system abnormalities and most often reflect weakness; spasticity; incoordination; involuntary movements; or excessive, reduced, or variable muscle tone (Duffy 2005a, p. 5).

There are several types of dysarthria, each characterized by distinguishable perceptual characteristics that presumably reflect different localization and underlying pathophysiology (Table 2-1). They all share a neurologic cause and reflect disorders of movement or movement control.

Apraxia of speech (AOS), the second broad category of MSDs, can be defined as:

> a neurologic speech disorder reflecting an impaired capacity to plan or program sensorimotor commands necessary for directing movements that result in phonetically and prosodically normal speech (Duffy, 2005a, p. 5).

AOS can occur in the absence of dysarthria and in the absence of disturbances in any component of language. Conceptually, AOS straddles the boundaries between impairment of language functions (aphasia) and problems of neuromotor control and execution (dysarthria).

There are several neurologic speech disturbances that traditionally have not been captured under the subcategories of dysarthria or AOS. Some of them can be considered disorders of speech motor control, including, for example, neurologic stutteringlike behavior, palilalia, certain forms of mutism, pseudoforeign dialect, aprosodia associated with right hemisphere dysfunction, and developmental stuttering and cluttering (Duffy, 2005a; Kent, 2000). They are not addressed in this chapter, but the reader should be aware of their existence because at least some may someday be considered variants of dysarthria or AOS, or as additional major subcategories under MSDs.

Distant History

Knowledge evolves. Even its first glimmers do not spring from "out of the blue." This has certainly been the case for MSDs. Just as understanding who we are as individuals is enhanced by knowing something about where we come from, our current understanding of MSDs is enriched by knowing something about how it evolved.

Table 2–1. Motor Speech Disorders, Their Neurologic Correlates, and Some of Their Distinguishing Auditory-Perceptual Features

Type	Lesion Locus	Presumed Distinguishing Neurophysiologic Impairment	Common Associated Neurologic Signs*	Prominent/Distinctive Auditory-Perceptual Features**
Dysarthrias				
Flaccid	Lower motor neuron One or more of the following: Cranial nerves V, VII, IX, X, XI, XII Cervical and thoracic spinal nerves	Weakness	Atrophy Fasciculations Weakness Hypotonia Reduced reflexes	Dependent on specific cranial and spinal nerves involved, but most often: Continuous breathy-hoarse voice quality Diplophonia Reduced loudness Short phrases Stridor/audible inspiration Hypernasality Nasal emission Imprecise consonants
Spastic	Upper motor neuron (usually bilateral)	Spasticity	Hyperactive reflexes Pathologic reflexes Pseudobulbar affect Dysphagia Limb spasticity and weakness	Strained-harsh voice Monopitch and monoloudness Slow rate Slow, regular speech AMRs
Ataxic	Cerebellar control circuit	Incoordination	Ataxia Dysmetria Hypotonia Intention tremor	Irregular articulatory breakdowns Irregular speech AMRs Excess and equal stress Excess loudness variation Distorted vowels

continues

Table 2–1. *continued*

Type	Lesion Locus	Presumed Distinguishing Neurophysiologic Impairment	Common Associated Neurologic Signs*	Prominent/Distinctive Auditory-Perceptual Features**
Hypokinetic	Basal ganglia control circuit	Rigidity Reduced range of motion	Rigidity Bradykinesia Akinesia Resting tremor Postural abnormalities	Reduced loudness Monopitch and monoloudness Reduced stress Accelerated rate, short rushes of speech Rapid, blurred speech AMRs Repeated sounds Inappropriate silences
Hyperkinetic	Basal ganglia control circuit	Quick-to-slow, regular or irregular involuntary movements	One or more of: Chorea Dystonia Athetosis Dyskinesia Myoclonus Action myoclonus Tics Tremor	Highly variable, affecting one or more of the components of speech production, but often with significant rate and prosodic abnormalities. Speech features consistent with nature of involuntary movements (e.g., voice tremor, spasmodic dysphonia, jaw/face dystonias, palatal-pharyngeal-laryngeal myoclonus).

Type	Lesion Locus	Presumed Distinguishing Neurophysiologic Impairment	Common Associated Neurologic Signs*	Prominent/Distinctive Auditory-Perceptual Features**
Unilateral upper motor neuron	Upper motor neuron (unilateral)	Weakness, spasticity, incoordination, singly or in combination	Hemiparesis/hemiplegia Unilateral central face and tongue weakness	Usually not worse than mild-moderate: Imprecise articulation Irregular articulatory breakdowns Slow rate Harsh-strained or hoarse-breathy voice Reduced loudness
Mixed	Two or more of above	Combinations of above	Combinations of above	Combinations of above
Apraxia of speech	Left cerebral hemisphere	Impaired motor planning/programming	Aphasia Dysarthria Nonverbal oral apraxia Hemiparesis/hemiplegia	Slow rate with syllable segregation Distorted sound substitutions Errors of stress assignment with tendency to equalize stress False starts and restarts Trial-error groping for articulatory postures

*Listed signs may or may not be present. No listed sign is required for dysarthria type diagnosis.

**Other deviant speech characteristics may be present but they tend not to be distinctive of a specific MSD type. All features listed need not be present for diagnosis.

In this section, some history is reviewed, primarily by selectively highlighting important contributions and illustrative examples.

Pre-1900s

MSDs have been observable since humans could speak and sustain brain damage. References to neurologic speech disorders can be found in Egyptian hieroglyphics and the work of Hippocrates, although it is difficult to know if the disorders they referred to are those of aphasia or MSDs (Wertz, LaPointe, & Rosenbek, 1984).

Little in the way of specific information about MSDs emerged across the Middle Ages, Renaissance, and 17th and 18th centuries (Rosenbek & LaPointe, 1985), although progress was made in understanding the neuroanatomy of some of the speech pathways. For example, the branches of the vagus nerve and the spinal nerves to the diaphragm were described by Willis in the 1600s (Feindel, 1999). Willis also provided what was probably the first description of speech impairment in myasthenia gravis, saying, in part, " . . . but after she has spoke long, or hastily, or eagerly, she is not able to speak a word, but becomes mute as a fish . . . " (Darley, 1983, p. xiv). We can only wonder if the analogy to mute fish was necessary or helpful at the time!

In the 19th century, discussion of MSDs was primarily descriptive and conceptual. In the absence of necessary technology, acoustic and physiologic studies were nonexistent, and their perceptual description and localization were crude. Nonetheless, recognition of speech abnormalities as

signs of neurologic disease and clues for localization and neurologic diagnosis was clearly evident.[1] For example, in 1817, Parkinson noted the speech impairment in "shaking palsy," the disease that came to bear his name. In 1887, Charcot described a pattern of "scanning speech" that was associated with what would become known as multiple sclerosis, a pattern now recognized as a possible manifestation of ataxic dysarthria (Darley, 1983).

In 1825, Bouillaud identified the crucial role of the frontal lobes in speech control. He also recognized the fundamental conceptual and diagnostic distinction between language and the ability to convey language through speech (Wertz, LaPointe, & Rosenbek, 1984). The latter notion was reflected later in the writings of Jackson (1878), who clearly separated problems of voice and articulation secondary to vocal fold, facial, lingual, or palatal weakness from loss of speech due to aphasia, in which movements for speech could be preserved.

The seeds for how we would eventually think about dysarthria are clearly tied to increasing knowledge about how the nervous system was organized for movement. For example, in the early 1800s, Bell may have been the first to recognize that "definite nerves have a definite course from some part of the brain to a certain part of the periphery, and further, that different nerves have quite distinct functions" (Rose, 1999, p. 125). In 1867, Jackson observed that the striatum (the caudate nucleus and putamen) is a governing link between each cerebral hemisphere and muscles on the opposite side of the body. He also recognized somatotopic representation within the striatum, saying "there are points

---

[1]More detailed but still brief histories can be found in Darley (1983); Rosenbek and LaPointe (1985), and Wertz, La Pointe, and Rosenbek (1984).

where particular movements are specially represented" (York, 1999, p. 156). And, so classification of the dysarthrias is not mistaken as a 20th century phenomenon, Kussmaul, in 1881, was probably the first to attempt to classify the dysarthrias into distinct groups (Darley, 1983; Grewel, 1957).

In 1843, Little was among the first to describe the condition now labeled cerebral palsy, and the term, cerebral palsy (CP), came into use by the late 1800s. In 1897, Freud argued that there was more than one type of CP (Workinger & Kent, 1991), with the implication that there could be more than one type of dysarthria associated with it.

The conceptual, localization, and behavioral distinctions between aphasia and AOS also were initially drawn in the 1800s. In fact, debate during the mid-1800s about the underlying nature of neurologic speech and language signs helped give birth to behavioral neurology. The most famous cases, in 1861, were two of Broca's patients, LeBorgne and LeLong (patient confidentiality did not seem to be an issue at the time), whose left hemisphere lesions included damage to the third frontal convolution that impaired their ability to articulate words, in the absence of paralysis. Broca called the problem *aphemia*. It is very possible his patients had what today would be called AOS, although debate about whether aphemia (or AOS) represents a problem of language or speech has persisted from the time of Broca to the present.

Finally, in 1891, Hadden, a British physician, described an 11-year-old boy with longstanding severely compromised speech that seemed analogous to the aphemia described by Broca. This may have been the first description of developmental AOS.

1900 to 1960

Dysarthria

The origin of the term dysarthria is obscure (*dys* = abnormal or impaired; *arth* = joint). For a long time it was used to refer to abnormal articulation (Darley, 1983), but by the early 1900s at least some writers recognized that it could reflect more than articulatory problems. Liepman, for example, discussed the speech sensorimotor apparatus "which moves the larynx, palate, mouth, and tongue, with its sensory regulations. If this executive apparatus is injured, we then have *anarthria* or *dysarthria*" (Head, 1926, p. 99, quoting Liepmann, 1913). The distinction between dysarthria and aphasia was drawn more explicitly by Head who stated "These two forms of defective speech are profoundly different in origin and can be distinguished pathologically and clinically" (1926, p. 81). And, the seeds of the important distinction between dysarthria and AOS were implicitly drawn by Henschen (1920–1922) when he noted that left precentral gyrus lesions, near the third frontal convolution, produce both dysarthria *and* aphemia (Head, 1926).

The study of aphasia captured considerably more attention than dysarthria in the first half of the century. However, in spite of the holistic, antilocalization approach to higher level functions popular at the time (Catani & ffytche, 2005), the association of dysarthria with specific diseases or damage to specific areas of the nervous system was increasingly recognized. For example, in 1929 Hiller noted the dysarthria associated with Freidreich's ataxia, and in 1937 Zentay used the term "ataxic" to describe the speech problems associated with cerebellar damage.

Several attempts to classify the dysarthrias were evident in the United States and Europe by the mid-1900s. For example, in 1943, Froeschels suggested that the term "dysarthric" be used rather than "spastic"[2] to refer to people with dysarthria associated with cerebral palsy (CP), at least in part because people with CP were not always spastic. He described speech characteristics associated with lesions to the pyramidal and extrapyramidal tracts, the frontal lobes and their projections, pallidum-projectional pathways, the cerebellum, and the peripheral nerves (see Chapter 3, Neural Perspectives on Motor Speech Disorders: Current Understanding). He also addressed methods for evaluating some of the distinctive speech deficits that could result from respiratory, laryngeal, and articulatory involvement. His contributions had a significant impact on research and treatment of congenital and acquired dysarthrias.

Not much later, Peacher (1950) proposed a neuroanatomically based classification system and attempted to correlate neurophysiology with disrupted speech processes. He urged that dysarthria be studied from neurophysiology, psychology, experimental phonetics, and speech pathology perspectives. In 1955, Morley discussed speech signs associated with several neurologic conditions (e.g., Parkinson's disease, multiple sclerosis, traumatic brain injury) and tied them to recommendations about examination and treatment strategies (Rosenbek & LaPointe, 1985).

In Amsterdam, Grewel (1957) recognized that the dysarthrias reflect neuroanatomy and physiology, and he predicted today's accepted tenet of clinical practice by suggesting that distinctions among dysarthrias can provide "a tentative diagnosis to the phonetically trained ear, when neurological examination still shows no convincing neurological symptoms" (p. 329). His classification system included 14 types of dysarthria (with subtypes), but it lacked a clear description of the speech characteristics that distinguished among the types and did not have a cohesive organizational basis (Rosenbek & LaPointe, 1985). That is, the dysarthria types included a mix of neuroanatomic types (e.g., cortical, subcortical, cerebellar), types of etiology (e.g., diffuse CNS disease, severe epilepsy, myasthenia gravis), and associated-disorder types (e.g., dysarthria associated with subcortical expressive aphasia).

In Zurich and Vienna, the collaborative work of Luchsinger and Arnold led to the publication in 1949 of a book whose second edition was translated into English, with additions, in 1965. Robert West, a founder of American speech pathology, called it "the most detailed of any book issued in any language up to the middle of the twentieth century" (p. v). In it, Luchsinger and Arnold noted that the auditory perceptual features of the various dysarthrias are largely a function of localization, and much less a function of etiology. This principle is largely embraced today. They also recognized six dysarthria types—based on anatomic localization—that included what they called cortical, pyramidal, extrapyramidal, frontopontine, cerebellar, and bulbar dysarthrias.

Dysarthria Associated with Cerebral Palsy

Before the 1960s—when the discipline of speech-language pathology was just

---

[2]At the time, people with cerebral palsy were sometimes referred to as "spastics" (Froeschels, 1943).

emerging—there was little focus on MSDs except for some attention to "cerebral-palsied speech" (LaPointe, 1986; Yorkston, Beukelman, Strand, & Bell, 1999). The attention to CP was reflected in the contributions of a number of individuals from the 1930s to early 1960s.

Several investigators during this time documented problems at the respiratory, phonatory, and resonatory levels, as well as in articulation (e.g., Achilles, 1955; Blumberg, 1955; Hardy, 1964; Ingram & Barn, 1961; Irwin, 1955; Rutherford, 1944; Wolfe, 1950). Different types of speech impairments were also recognized, with some references to athetotic, ataxic, and spastic dysarthria (e.g., Berry & Eisenson, 1956; Clement & Twitchell, 1959; Mecham, Berko & Berko, 1966; West, Ansberry, & Carr, 1957). All of these contributions influenced subsequent concepts for describing, examining, and treating developmental dysarthria.

There was no obvious concerted effort during this time to develop a coherent description and understanding of the commonalities and differences between the developmental and acquired dysarthrias. This was reflected in texts (texts addressing CP outnumbered those on acquired dysarthrias at the time) and in training programs. For example, Netsell (1984) observed that university course work covered dysarthria in children and adults in separate courses, with a consequence that "many students may have missed the phylo-ontogenetic information of the former and the speech physiology data of the latter" (p. 4). This separation seems to persist today. It may be partly fed by ongoing uncertainty about whether Darley, Aronson, and Brown's approach to classification of the acquired dysarthrias is or is not applicable to developmental or acquired dysarthria in children (e.g., Cahill,

Murdoch, & Theodoros, 2002; Caruso & Strand, 1999; van Mourik, Catsman-Berrevoets, Paquier, Yousef-Bak, & van Dongen, 1997; Workinger & Kent, 1991).

Apraxia of Speech

Current notions about apraxia and its types, particularly as it affects the limbs, were strongly, although not exclusively, influenced by several papers by Liepmann in the early decades of the 20th century. Liepmann (1913) believed "motor aphasia" might actually be a speech variant of limb kinetic apraxia, a disturbance of the motor engrams that underlie motor acts.

Developmental Apraxia of Speech

In England in the early 1950s, Morely and her colleagues (e.g., Morley, Court, & Miller, 1954) described a subgroup of children with neurologic speech deficits in whom movements of the articulators appeared normal but became clumsy and awkward during complex, rapid speech movements. She called this problem an "articulatory dyspraxia" (Morley, Court, Miller, & Garside, 1955). This probably marked the birth of the modern concept of developmental AOS.

Management

Although drills for speech sounds and phrases were published in the late 1920s and 1930s, approaches to managing MSDs were vaguely described and generally without explicit rationale. Little attention was paid to variations in treatment based on presumed underlying pathophysiology. Reports of behavioral treatment efficacy or effectiveness, and systematic data-based case reports were essentially nonexistent.

A number of recommended techniques at the time contained the seeds of current controversies about the use of nonspeech oromotor exercise for treating MSDs. For example, Froeschels (1943) advocated "training of the muscles involved" (p. 313) before working on speech itself. He also believed "almost every case needs training of the breathing," and that "training of rhythm" is almost always essential (p. 320). Some of his techniques (e.g., the chewing method, jaw shaking, pushing exercises) are still in use today by some clinicians for some patients. Similarly, Morley (1955) felt the speech musculature should be the focus of rehabilitation and that "the therapist often has to begin the rehabilitation of motor function on an involuntary reflex level" (p. 63) (e.g., gag, cough, swallow). Morley also felt that exercise could be valuable, that management sometimes needed to address compensation (as opposed to reducing impairment), and that treatment could be provided individually or in group settings.

The Modern Era: Late 1960s to the Present

General Overview

Contributions during the 1960s and 1970s set the course for subsequent research and clinical work during the last decades of the century. They are the primary focus of this section. The work of the last quarter century will be integrated within subsequent sections that address current practice.

Prior to the late 1960s, the understanding of MSDs was limited and unsystematic. LaPointe (1986) observed that "the realm of speech motor control and neurologic impairment of speech was practically *terra incognita* in the world of human communication" and that "a systematic science was excruciatingly slow to develop, and application of the meager knowledge that had evolved was infrequent" (p. vii). Even the term, *motor speech disorders,* was not popularized until the 1960s and 1970s when Darley, Aronson, and Brown (1969a, 1969b, 1975) consistently used it and others followed suit.

There is usually a lag between new contributions to knowledge and palpable signs of their influence. During the 1970s and 1980s, efforts in both the laboratory and clinic generated an accumulating empirical data base (LaPointe, 1986). The study of MSDs was coming into its own, enough so that a number of publications began to influence training, research, and practice. Some of the most influential during those decades include Darley, Aronson, and Brown (1975), McNeil, Rosenbek, and Aronson (1984), Netsell, (1984), Perkins (1983), Rosenbek, McNeil, and Aronson (1984), Rosenbek and LaPointe (1985), Wertz, LaPointe, and Rosenbek (1984), and Yorkston, Beukelman, and Bell (1988). These publications remain valuable today for their perspectives on the past, their place in the history of MSDs, and their enduring impact on research and clinical practice. In addition, in 1982 Yorkston, Beukelman, and Berry spearheaded the Clinical Dysarthria Conference, which has been held every other year since (but now called the Conference on Motor Speech), with subsequent publications stemming from it, in book form initially, and now as refereed articles in the *Journal of Medical Speech-Language Pathology*.

The growth of interest in MSDs during the 1960s to 1980s was fueled by many factors, including, but not limited to, growth in the disciplines of speech science and speech-language pathology; relatively good levels of governmental funding for research and training; population growth, increasing life span, and improved survival rates from neurologic disease; and technologic advances that permitted acoustic and physiologic study of speech motor control and MSDs. Research at the time was carried out in relatively few institutions, many in the Midwest. Today, contributions come from institutions throughout the United States and around the world.

The Dysarthrias

Until the late 1960s there were few systematic studies of dysarthria, and it was still considered a singular disorder in most clinical practices. An important advance that emerged in the 1960s was the attempt to quantify the intelligibility of dysarthric speech (e.g., Tikofsky, 1964, 1970), although measuring intelligibility remains problematic in clinical and research settings today.

The Darley, Aronson, and Brown Contribution

In 1965, at an NIH-sponsored conference addressing brain mechanisms underlying speech and language, Darley asked "What shall we let the term dysarthria encompass?" (1967, p. 237). He pointed out that it can be studied as a function of speech system level (e.g., phonatory, articulatory) and as a function of nervous system level of involvement (e.g., lower motor neuron, cerebellar). He also identified the need for modifiers to identify the behavioral phenomena that typify involvement of each

system. Thus, he set the stage for the soon-to-be-published seminal studies (Darley, Aronson, & Brown, 1969a, 1969b) that would introduce an approach to classifying the dysarthrias (now often called the "Mayo approach") that continues its dominance in research and clinical practice today.

By 1975, dysarthria was finally recognized as more than an articulatory disorder; respiratory, phonatory, resonance, and prosodic impairments were included among its features. But the influence of the Darley, Aronson, and Brown studies was not yet pervasive. As late as 1985, for example, in their important and influential chapter titled "The Dysarthrias: Description, Diagnosis, and Treatment," Rosenbek and LaPointe stated that "the definition of dysarthria is being refined" to include the notion of different dysarthria types. Nonetheless, they noted the influence on contemporary thinking of Darley, Aronson, and Brown's work, stating that it "will probably achieve a prominent place as historic milestones on the topic" (p. 99). Today that prediction has been confirmed. Although Darley, Aronson, and Brown did not introduce the notion of dysarthria types, their systematic analysis of the perceptual features of each type and their relationship to lesion loci, "gave method and procedure to an area of neurology and speech-language pathology that had languished from a lack of order and systematicity" (McNeil, 1997, p. xi). Their contributions facilitated numerous studies over subsequent decades that described the speech characteristics of a variety of neurologic diseases, and provided a conceptual framework for acoustic and physiologic studies that have improved our understanding of the neurophysiologic underpinnings of the dysarthrias.

Physiologic Approaches

Kent and Rosen (2004) referred to the two faces of dysarthria. One is the description of speech abnormalities through perceptual and acoustic analyses; the other is physiologic, either by inference or by direct observation. The physiologic face began to mature at about the same time as Darley, Aronson, and Brown's contribution. Netsell (1984), who recorded the history of the approach and has been a leader within it, observed that the call for physiologic research in the 1960s by Hardy (1967) and Darley, Aronson, and Brown (1969a, 1969b) were logical extensions of work in the preceding half-century.

The physiologic approach basically views dysarthrias as neurologic problems in the regulation of movements (Netsell, 1984), thus requiring study of the abnormal speech movements and their underpinnings. It involves measurement of "movements of speech structures and air, the muscle contractions that generate movement, the relationships among movements at different levels of the musculoskeletal speech mechanism, the temporal parameters and relationships among central and peripheral neural activity and biomechanical activity, and the temporal relationships among activities in central nervous system structures during the planning and execution of speech" (Duffy, 2005a, p. 10). Physiologic approaches can provide insight into pathophysiologic features such as weakness, rigidity, slowness, or dyscoordination (Kent, 2000).

One of the primary goals of physiologic approaches—one crucial to basic research and clinical practice—is to discover the relationships between pathophysiology and the signs identified by perceptual studies (Rosenbek & LaPointe, 1985). It is both historically and currently important to recognize that physiologic approaches and the perceptually oriented Mayo approach are not, or at least need not be viewed as, competitive. Since the 1970s, the longstanding and continuing contributions of clinically oriented speech scientists, such as Kent, Netsell, and Hixon, and numerous others in recent years, have helped to bridge the gap between laboratory and clinic.

Physiologic research in the early 1970s was marked by qualitative studies of the "moment to moment" changes in muscle contractions and vocal tract movements during speech (Netsell, 1984). This work was facilitated in the late 1970s by an NIH-supported Clinical Research Center at the University of Wisconsin that supported interdisciplinary basic and clinical investigations of neurogenic speech disorders. By the mid-1980s these efforts (e.g., Abbs, Hunker, & Barlow, 1983; Hunker & Abbs, 1984) were "responsible, in large part, for the marked increase in our current understanding of the dysarthrias" (Netsell, 1984, p. 5). Many of these studies identified gaps in our understanding of the relationships between auditory-perceptual features and the movements that produce them, suggesting they are much more complex than initially thought (Netsell, 1986). These gaps in understanding persist today.

In the 1970s and 1980s, physiologic studies most often employed electromyographic, cineradiographic, kinematic, and aerodynamic measures, many which have become increasingly sophisticated in recent years (e.g., electropalatography). Today, some studies use highly sophisticated neuroimaging techniques such as positron emission tomography, magnetoencephalography, functional magnetic resonance imaging, and transcranial magnetic stimulation. In combination with careful perceptual and acoustic analyses of speech, and other physiologic measures, these imaging techniques have the potential to rapidly increase our understanding of the dysarthrias (Kent, 2000). In addition, the last decade has seen the refinement of computational models of brain activity and the motor, biomechanical, and sensory processes involved in speech production (e.g., Guenther, 1994; Guenther & Perkell, 2004). Such models can be validated with brain imaging, psychophysical, physiologic, anatomic, and acoustic data. They may help address challenges to understanding speech motor control (e.g., contextual variability, motor equivalence, and coarticulation) and likely will have implications for our understanding of the dysarthrias and other MSDs.

It is noteworthy that physiologic and clinical research since the 1970s has largely focused on acquired dysarthria in adults. Nonetheless, acoustic, physiologic, and perceptual studies during and since the 1960s and 1970s of children or adults with CP, as well as children with acquired dysarthria, have yielded insight into their phonatory, velopharyngeal, and articulatory problems, and to some of the perceptual distinctions (or lack thereof) between dysarthrias associated with different types of CP (e.g., Ansel & Kent, 1992; Cahill, Murdoch, & Theodoros, 2002; Hardy, 1964; Ingram & Barn, 1961; Kent & Netsell, 1978; Netsell, 1969; Platt, Andrews, Young, & Quinn, 1980; van Mourik, Catsman-Berrevoets, Paquier, Yousef-Bak, & van Dongen, 1997; Workinger & Kent, 1991). Dysarthrias in children represents a clear, ongoing research need.

Apraxia of Speech

An important milestone in the modern conception of AOS occurred in 1965 at the NIH conference referred to in the previous section. In a presentation titled *"Lacunae and Research Approaches to Them,"* Darley argued that Broca's or motor aphasia should go by another name because it is not fundamentally a language problem (he credited Wepman and colleagues [1955, 1960] as recent authors who had pointed this out). Darley said, "The gropings of the motor aphasic patient for correct positioning of his articulators, his clumsiness in finding the correct pattern of movement to produce a polysyllabic word, his near misses phonemically, and his retrials are predominant . . . his performance represents no cross-modality impairment in the use of language symbols but a specific modality-bound deficit, an oral verbal apraxia" (p. 236). This represented a challenge to a long-embraced two-part model of neurologic speech problems (i.e., aphasia and dysarthria) (McNeil, Pratt, & Fossett, 2004).

At about the same time, in the Soviet Union, Luria (1966) also recognized a speech movement disorder that he felt was distinguishable from aphasia and dysarthria. Noting that "Motor aphasia . . . has always been one of the most complex problems in neurology" (pp. 183–184), he felt the phenomenon could be classed among the apraxias and observed that "The tendency to bring the analysis of motor aphasia closer to the analysis of other motor disorders, and thus include motor aphasia among the apraxias, is undoubtedly one of the progressive tendencies in modern neurology" (p. 186).

Over the next several decades, mostly in the United States, the attention Darley called to AOS spawned a large number of perceptual, psycholinguistic, acoustic, and physiologic (kinematic, aerodynamic, electromyographic) studies that described the disorder's clinical characteristics and associated deficits, clarified some of its differences from dysarthria and aphasia, and identified the conditions that could elicit and modify it (Duffy, 2003; McNeil, Pratt, & Fossett, 2004). By the 1980s the disorder had been studied sufficiently to justify a comprehensive text, and an influential one, *Apraxia of Speech in Adults: The Disorder and Its Management*, by Wertz, LaPointe, and Rosenbek (1984).

Clinical and theoretical notions about AOS have not been without controversy; many would say they have been riddled by it. The "cognitive dissonance"—evident in retrospect—created by definitions of AOS as a phonologic (as opposed to phonetic) disorder, helped to create uncertainty and dispute about diagnostic criteria and the nature of the disorder (McNeil, Pratt, & Fossett, 2004). Opposition to the term AOS and its presumed underpinnings was important because it helped focus debate and research. The basic argument, perhaps best expressed in a 1974 paper by Martin, was that the clinical features that defined AOS at the time could lend themselves equally well to linguistic as opposed to motor explanations. This spawned research that pitted acoustic, physiologic, and narrow transcription perceptual studies against phonologic or distinctive feature analyses in an effort to distinguish the motor from the linguistic attributes of the speech of people with left hemisphere lesions.

Recent critical reviews by McNeil and colleagues (e.g., McNeil, Doyle, & Wambaugh, 2000; McNeil, Pratt, & Fossett, 2004; McNeil, Robin, & Schmidt, 1997) of studies conducted from the 1970s into the 1990s, identified two barriers to progress in understanding the disorder. These include a previous lack of well-specified, testable speech production models that could distinguish phonologic from motoric deficits, and a lack of explicit classification criteria for identifying the disorder. The latter shortcoming raises the possibility that the database for many studies of AOS has been confounded by the inclusion of people with phonologic paraphasias who may or may not also have had AOS.

The last decade has seen the development of more refined models of speech production (e.g., van der Merwe, 1997) and refined definitions of AOS as a phonetic, motor planning/programming disorder, as well as more explicit AOS-specific clinical criteria for its identification (e.g., Duffy, 2005a; McNeil, Pratt, & Fossett, 2004; McNeil, Robin, & Schmidt, 1997). The pared down list of defining characteristics reflects deletion of some that are probably linguistic, or that cannot be clearly separated from linguistic processes, and retention of characteristics that are specifically compatible with motor planning or programming problems. McNeil, Pratt, and Fossett (2004) have predicted that, within the context of current explanatory models of speech production, "a clear and consistent set of diagnostic criteria should allow our research and understanding of AOS to proceed in a manner more straightforward than has previously been observed" (p. 409).

Developmental AOS[3]

During the 1970s, developmental or childhood AOS (CAS) attracted increased attention in rough synchrony with what was

---

[3]The published proceedings (Shriberg & Campbell, 2003) of a research symposium on childhood apraxia of speech, held in 2002, contain a number of papers that, as a group, represent a good summary of current clinical and research thinking and debate on the topic.

happening in acquired AOS. Some of the work at that time came from people who also studied acquired AOS and so brought a combination of bias and valuable insight to their efforts (Duffy, 2003).

Several early studies focused on finding neurologic correlates because there was no obvious neurologic event or lesion that could explain the speech disturbance. In general, they established that both hard and soft neurologic signs occur in children with CAS with higher than expected frequency (e.g., Ferry, Hall, & Hicks, 1975; Rosenbek & Wertz, 1972). Darley's influence was again felt when he and Yoss (1974) published an influential prospective descriptive and comparative study of CAS in children without language impairment. They found that their apraxic children were distinguished from a subgroup of nonapraxic speech-impaired children on the basis of a relatively small number of speech features (e.g., distortions, prolongations, voicing errors). This and other studies at the time (e.g., Rosenbek & Wertz, 1972) began to generate a list of characteristics of the disorder and the clinical milieu in which it tended to occur. The speech characteristics were very similar to those listed for acquired AOS at the time (Duffy, 2003).

Seeds of debate about whether CAS represents a motor versus language problem were sown in the late 1970s and early 1980s by Aram and colleagues (e.g., Aram & Nation, 1982). Their work put forth a still persistent question about whether CAS is an entity unto itself that can co-occur with language disorders or is part of a syndrome in which a core deficit explains both the speech and language characteristics. Uncertainty about the nature of the disorder extended to questions about its very existence. In 1981, Guyette and Dietrich concluded that the vague characterization of the problem made it impossible to distinguish it from other speech disorders and that " . . . no pathognomonic symptoms or necessary and sufficient conditions were found for the diagnosis . . . " (p. 8). Their criticism did not bury the concept of CAS, but over the last two decades there have been frequent pleas for the development of clear diagnostic criteria (e.g., Rosenbek, Kent, & LaPointe, 1984; Strand, 2001). Whether CAS can be reliably distinguished from more general speech impairment in children remains a central problem (Kent, 2000).

To further complicate issues of diagnosis, the idea that subtypes of the disorder might exist has been raised (Crary, 1993; Shriberg, Aram, & Kwiatkowski, 1997). The notion of subtypes mostly reflects attempts to parse the gray areas among phonologic and motor planning and programming deficits. A call to refocus efforts on the motor speech difficulties of children presumed to have the disorder was made in a paper by Robin in 1992, in which he argued that "apraxia, by definition, is a movement disturbance and, as such, any notions of linguistic basis for the disorder are misguided" (p. 19). He argued that the diagnosis should be based on "the speech and motor problems manifested by these children, and not language or cognitive symptoms . . . " (p. 21).

In recent years, efforts have been made to establish diagnostic markers for CAS, with candidates for them extending beyond speech characteristics to include, for example, performance on visuomotor tracking tasks (Ballard, Granier, & Robin, 2000) and measures of nonspeech oral apraxia (Love, 1992). Probably the most programmatic effort to identify a speech marker is evident in the work of Shriberg, Aram, and Kwiatkowski (e.g., 1997) who found that inappropriate stress in the form of reduced prosodic contrast was the only characteristic that differentiated some children with suspected AOS from those with other speech disorders. This work suggested that inappropriate stress may be a diagnostic marker for at least one subtype of the disorder.

Finally, beginning with the observations of Morley and colleagues, significant family histories of speech and language disturbances in children with suspected AOS have been reported by a number of investigators; reports of strong male predominance suggest a sex-linked pattern of genetic transmission in some cases. Recently, the FOXP2 gene has received attention because a mutation associated with it has been linked to speech, language, and nonspeech oromotor deficits. Over the past 15 years, a family, known as the KE family, has been studied because many of its members have significant speech-language impairments, including what has been called "severe developmental verbal dyspraxia." Static and dynamic neuroimaging in some cases have identified abnormalities in cortical and subcortical motor control areas (e.g., Hurst, Baraister, Auger, Graham, & Norell, 1990; Vargha-Khadem et al., 1998; Vargha-Khadem 2003; Watkins, Dronkers, & Vargha-Khadem, 2002). Although problems of definition and description of CAS in these studies create uncertainty about the specific nature of the disorders, the identification of a genetic basis, in some cases with neuroimaging correlates, introduces the possibility of significant progress in our understanding of CAS and related developmental speech and language disorders. Additional reports of non-KE family members with FOXP2 abnormalities (e.g., Shriberg, Ballard, Tomblin, Duffy, & O'Dell, 2006) will likely refine and expand phenotype description and improve criteria for clinical diagnostic and genomic classification.

Management of MSDs

Early references to treatment of dysarthria focused mostly on children, and treatment approaches for acquired dysarthria often failed to distinguish among techniques for managing aphasia, dysarthria, and AOS. Agranowitz and McKeown (1964), for example, noted that "exercises for the motor aphasic are also helpful for the dysarthric" (p. 101).

Little systematic attention was given to the behavioral management of dysarthrias, particularly acquired dysarthrias, until Rosenbek and LaPointe (1985) provided a broad, comprehensive overview of treatment philosophy, goals, approaches, and techniques. They observed that American speech pathology had spent comparatively little energy on developing treatments for the dysarthrias but that efforts at description and explanation "spawned a general, clinical interest in the dysarthrias and have created a basis for an expanding treatment literature" (Rosenbek & LaPointe, 1985, p. 101). They acknowledged that much of their discussion about dysarthria treatment was without the support of data, but their chapter had an enduring influence on concepts and approaches to management. Subsequent research and clinical efforts provided sufficient new information to lead to the publication of entire books largely devoted to management of the dysarthrias, and MSDs in general (e.g., Caruso & Strand, 1999; Yorkston, Beukelman, & Bell, 1988; Yorkston, Beukelman, Strand, & Bell, 1999). Well-designed studies that demonstrate efficacy have been increasing, and the recent development of practice guidelines and systematic reviews developed through the Academy of Neurologic Communication Disorders and Sciences (ANCDS), reflect an increased commitment to evidence-based practice for the dysarthrias and AOS.

Over the last several decades, a large number of treatment programs and techniques have also emerged for AOS and CAS. Many of those recommended for AOS and CAS are strikingly similar to one another; most are well-summarized in recent texts (e.g., Caruso & Strand, 1999; Chapey, 2001; Duffy, 2005a; McNeil, Doyle, & Wambaugh, 2000; Yorkston, Beukelman, Strand, & Bell, 1999). Treatment studies are increasingly theoretically motivated and based on an assumption that AOS is a motor problem. Many rely on principles of motor learning in their structure.

Current Practice

This section reviews some data regarding the prevalence of MSDs and provides a broad overview of current approaches to their evaluation, diagnosis, and management.

Prevalence of MSDs

MSDs occur in a wide variety of neurologic diseases and are frequently present in some of the most common of them. For example, at some point about 90% of people with autopsy-confirmed Parkinson's disease will be dysarthric (PD) (Müller et al., 2001), as will 50% of people with multiple sclerosis (Sandyk, 1995), 50% of people with closed head injuries in rehabilitation settings (Yorkston, Honsinger, Mitsuda, & Hammen, 1989), and 29% of people with stroke associated with hemi-paresis (Melo, Bogousslavsky, van Melle, & Regli, 1992). Dysarthria is one of the first symptoms in about 25% of people with amyotrophic lateral sclerosis (ALS) (Traynor, Codd, Corr, Forde, Frost, & Hardiman, 2000). Estimates of the frequency of dysarthria in CP range from about 30% to nearly 90% (Yorkston, Beukelman, Strand, & Bell, 1999).

Some report that dysarthria ranks second only to aphasia among the most frequent neurologic communication disorders (Yorkston, Beukelman, & Bell, 1988), and others suggest that it is the most common acquired speech disorder (Enderby, 1983b). MSDs are certainly very common in some speech pathology practices. For example, combined inpatient and outpatient data from the Speech Pathology practice at the Mayo Clinic show that dysarthrias accounted for 54% of all acquired neurologic communication disorders (Duffy, 2005a).

AOS is almost certainly much less prevalent than dysarthria; in the Mayo Clinic practice data it represented 4% of the primary communication disorder diagnoses in patients with acquired neurologic communication disorders, and 8% of those with MSDs. The prevalence of developmental AOS is less certain, although one report found that 3 to 4% of children with speech delay of unknown origin evaluated in a large hospital-based practice had CAS (Delaney & Kent, 2004).

Evaluation

The clinical examination of MSDs should reflect its purposes. Common purposes include description; specifying severity; establishing diagnosis; specifying implications for localization and disease diagnosis; consideration of prognosis; and determining the need for and focus of management.

Description and specification of severity are derived directly from the examination. The remaining purposes are achieved through inference, experience, and integration of examination findings with evidence-based information from the literature.

The essential components of the motor speech examination include the (1) history, (2) examination of speech to identify salient clinical features, and (3) identification of nonspeech signs that may help to confirm inferences drawn about the meaning of salient features.[4] This discussion focuses on the examination typically conducted in clinical practice for the purpose of diagnosis and management planning. Acoustic and instrumental physiologic assessments are not widely used in clinical practice at this time (Gerratt, Till, Rosenbek, Wertz, & Boysen, 1991).

An essential principle of diagnostic examination is that *auditory-perceptual judgments are the gold standard for the clinical diagnosis of MSDs*, sometimes supplemented by visual-perceptual judgments of movements during speech. *If the auditory-perceptual characteristics of speech are normal, a clinical diagnosis of dysarthria or AOS cannot be made, even if acoustic and physiologic abnormalities are detected within the speech system on speech and or nonspeech tasks.*[5]

The History

The history reveals the disorder's time course and the patient's observations about its nature and impact on daily functioning.

The value of the history is often underestimated. Patients' description of their difficulties often provide clues to diagnosis (e.g., ataxic dysarthria, more than any other dysarthria type, is described by patients as sounding intoxicated). The patient-provided history also puts their speech on display in a way that probably has greater face and ecologic validity than performance on structured tasks. By the time the history has been completed experienced clinicians often know the diagnosis and can estimate severity.

Speech Examination

The only published test for the diagnosis of dysarthria is the *Frenchay Dysarthria Assessment* (FDA, Enderby, 1983a). The FDA suggests that distinctions among the dysarthrias can be quantified and that the distinctions correlate with neurologic diagnosis, but it relies heavily on patient report and ratings of nonspeech activities and does not yield a rich description of deviant speech characteristics. Several published measures for the assessment of AOS and CAS are available (e.g., Blakely, 2001; Dabul, 2000; Hickman, 1997; Kaufman, 1995). However, considering evolving criteria for the diagnosis of acquired AOS, and uncertainty about the core features of CAS, the measures are currently best considered as organized tasks that elicit speech behaviors or profiles of response that may reflect AOS, rather than as standardized measures that can provide a definitive diagnosis.

---

[4]More detailed discussion of the clinical examination of MSDs can be found in Duffy (2005a) and Yorkston, Beukelman, Strand, and Bell (1999).

[5]This does not mean that acoustic and physiologic data do not help to confirm, support, modify or explain MSDs, nor that they might, in some cases, be more sensitive than auditory-perceptual judgments to the presence of neurologic abnormalities in speech structures or movements.

In most clinical practices today, the conventional method of assessment relies on description rather than standardized testing. The most useful method for describing deviant perceptual characteristics of the dysarthrias derives from the work of Darley, Aronson, and Brown (1969a, 1969b). A review of the details of their work is not possible here but clinicians and researchers who take the study of MSDs seriously should carefully read their classic studies. In the context of this chapter, it is sufficient to know that the conclusions drawn by Darley, Aronson, and Brown were based on examination of 212 dysarthric people with a variety of diseases and dysarthria types, for whom ratings were compiled for 38 deviant speech features that experience had taught them were relevant to the spectrum of dysarthrias. Those features, plus some more recently suggested, mostly task-specific features (Duffy, 2005a), seem to capture the range of possible abnormalities that can occur in dysarthria.[6] The deviant speech characteristics that may be encountered in the dysarthrias and AOS are summarized in Table 2–2.

A small number of tasks can elicit the necessary information for description and diagnosis of MSDs. They often include:

1. *Conversational, narrative, reading, and imitative speech*: Conversational or narrative speech are the most important, valid, and useful basis for evaluating the integrated function of all components of speech (respiration, phonation, resonance, articulation, and prosody) and each of the primary speech valves (i.e., laryngeal, velopharyngeal, articulatory), and for describing most of the possible deviant speech characteristics. Reading of a standard paragraph is also useful (it can be timed for comparison to normative rates, or across-time comparison), but there is great variability in basic reading ability among adults, and reading may help pace rate and provide articulatory and prosodic cues that are not present in discourse. Continuous, repeated reading of a standard paragraph may be helpful for assessing the effects of fatigue on speech, especially when myasthenia gravis is suspected. Repetition of multisyllabic words (e.g. catastrophe, stethoscope) or sentences containing multisyllabic words (e.g., "the municipal judge sentenced the criminal") can help elicit irregular articulatory breakdowns associated with ataxic dysarthria, as well as the prosodic, rate, and articulatory abnormalities associated with AOS.

2. *Vowel prolongation*: Prolongation of the vowel "ah," (or any other vowel) is an effective task for isolating respiratory and laryngeal functions. Assessment of maximum duration (for which normative data are available), and vocal pitch, loudness, and steadiness can be made. This is a commonly used task for the acoustic analysis of voice, for which automated analyses are available (Kay Elemetrics, 1993; Kent, Vorperian, Kent, & Duffy, 2003).

3. *Alternating motion rates (AMRs)*: Also known as diadochokinetic (DDK) rates, speech AMRs (most commonly requiring rapid and steady repetition of "puh," "tuh," and "kuh"; as in "puhpuhpuhpuh . . . ") are useful for assessing the speed and regularity of reciprocal articulatory movements of the jaw, lips, and tongue.

---

[6]It is important to recognize that the classic studies by Darley, Aronson, and Brown did not represent a formal, standardized, clinical test that yields a quantitative score and diagnosis. What their method did was provide a guide for description and diagnosis.

Table 2–2. Deviant Speech Characteristics That May Be Associated with Dysarthrias and Apraxia of Speech*

Respiratory-Phonatory	Resonance	Articulation	Rate	Fluency	Prosody and Other
High pitch	Hypernasality	Imprecise consonants	Slow	Prolonged phonemes	Excess & equal stress
Low pitch	Nasal emission	Weak pressure consonants	Fast	Palilalia	Reduced stress
Monopitch	Hyponasality	Distorted vowels	Increasing	Repeated phonemes	Short rushes of speech
Pitch breaks		Irregular articulatory breakdowns	Variable	False starts and restarts	Inappropriate silences
Elevated loudness		Distorted substitutions	Slow AMRs	Delayed initiation	Vocal tics
Reduced loudness			Fast AMRs		Coprolalia
Loudness decay			Irregular AMRs		Prolonged inter-segment durations between sounds, syllables, words, phrases
Monoloudness					
Excess loudness variation					
Vocal flutter					
Diplophonia					
Voice tremor					
Laryngeal myoclonus					
Strained-strangled					
Voice stoppages					
Harsh					
Hoarse					
Breathy, continuous					
Breathy, transient					
Forced inspiration or expiration					
Audible inspiration					
Stridor					
Grunt at end of expiration					

Source: Adapted and modified from Darley, Aronson, and Brown (1969a, 1969b, 1975), Duffy (2005a), and McNeil, Doyle, and Wambaugh (2000).

*Note that the placement of a number of characteristics under respiratory-phonatory, articulation, rate, fluency, and prosody is somewhat arbitrary because of the interactions that exist among them.

Labeled *quasi-speech tasks* by some (Weismer, 2006), speech AMRs (as well as vowel prolongation and sequential motion rates/SMRs) are often useful in distinguishing among certain dysarthria types.

4. *Sequential motion rates*: SMRs most commonly require the rapid repetitive production of "puhtuhkuh" to assess the ability to move quickly and in accurate sequence to and from several articulatory positions. Compared to AMRs, the sequencing demand is heavy and, for that reason, the task can be sensitive to the presence of AOS. Patients with dysarthria usually do not have difficulty meeting the sequencing demands of SMRs.

Intelligibility and Comprehensibility

In recent years, explicit attention has been given to the important differences between intelligibility and comprehensibility as distinct ways to describe dysarthria severity (Yorkston, Strand, & Kennedy, 1996). Intelligibility—the degree to which a listener understands the auditory signal produced by a speaker—can index the functional impairment imposed by an MSD. Comprehensibility—the degree to which a listener understands the auditory signal plus all other information that contributes to understanding what has been said (topic knowledge, semantic and syntactic context, gestures and signs, orthographic cues, etc.)—can index the disability imposed by an MSD in social, communicative contexts. A third construct is efficiency, or the rate at which intelligible or comprehensible information is conveyed. It contributes to the perception of normalcy of speech in social contexts; efficiency can be quite abnormal, even in the absence of reduced intelligibility. These constructs—intelligibility, comprehensibility, and efficiency—

are also relevant to treatment goals. That is, if treatment aims to reduce impairment associated with an MSD, then intelligibility and its efficiency are logical outcome measures. In contrast, if treatment aims to reduce disability—by manipulating variables independent of the speech signal—then comprehensibility and its efficiency become valid outcome measures (Duffy, 2005a).

Intelligibility Tests

Measures of intelligibility are important because they can quantify the effect of an MSD on a listener, quantify change over time, and provide an index of MSD severity (Ansel & Kent, 1992). Only a few structured measures have been developed for assessing intelligibility in dysarthria. They presumably could be adapted for people with AOS, but there is little evidence that they have been used for that purpose.

For a number of years, the most widely used standardized measure was the *Assessment of Intelligibility in Dysarthric Speakers* (AIDS; Yorkston & Beukelman, 1981), a test that quantifies intelligibility in words and sentences, and can estimate efficiency by examining the rate of intelligible words per minute in sentences. The *Sentence Intelligibility Test* (SIT; Yorkston & Beukelman, 1996), an updated Windows version of the sentence portion of the AIDS, represents a considerable improvement over its predecessor in stimulus selection, speed of scoring, and data storage. The *Word Intelligibility Test* (Kent, Weismer, Kent, & Rosenbek, 1989), although not published as a standardized test, is a measure of single-word intelligibility—in multiple choice or paired-word forms—that provides scores for percentage of intelligible words. It also is designed to permit, through phonetic contrast analysis, the identification of features of abnormal speech (and, by inference, their locus within the speech system) that are associated with decreased intelligibility.

The AIDS, SIT, and Word Intelligibility Test have been very useful in descriptive and treatment studies to quantify intelligibility, to describe phonetic difficulties associated with a number of dysarthria types and neurologic diseases, and to examine the relationship between intelligibility and acoustic variables. Their disadvantage as tools for everyday clinical practice is that they are time demanding and require at least two individuals to accomplish administration and scoring. As a result, many clinicians elect to estimate intelligibility or comprehensibility with less objective rating scales (e.g. Duffy, 2005a; Enderby, 1983a; the Motor Speech component of the ASHA-developed Functional Communication Measures, 1995).

Nonspeech Examination of Speech Structures and Functions

The oral mechanism examination is often overemphasized during clinical evaluation —frequently at the expense of careful speech assessment—especially because there is uncertainty about whether the examination of nonspeech movements can contribute to our understanding of the neurophysiologic underpinnings of MSDs. Nonetheless, for some types of MSDs, observations of speech structures at rest and during sustained postures and movement can provide useful clinical diagnostic information. When compatible with speech observations, such information can support conclusions drawn about speech. For example, lingual atrophy and fasciculations are signs of lower motor neuron involvement of the hypoglossal nerve; together

with weakness of the tongue during non-speech anterior and lateral tongue movements, they are supportive of a diagnosis of flaccid dysarthria in someone with imprecise articulation of lingual sounds.

This part of the examination essentially involves observations of (1) the jaw, lower face, and tongue at rest, during sustained postures, and during movement to make judgments about symmetry, size, steadiness (e.g., adventitious movements), and range, speed, and accuracy of movement; (2) the velopharynx at rest and during movement to make judgments of symmetry, steadiness (e.g., palatal myoclonus), and range of movement; and (3) the integrity of the cough and glottal coup, and the possible presence of stridor, primarily for inferences about strength. Respiration can be crudely assessed through observations of quiet breathing and performance on a few nonspeech tasks (e.g., postural abnormalities that might restrict respiratory movement; rate, regularity and depth of breathing; strength of cough; hiccups). A water glass manometer can be used to assess the degree to which respiratory driving pressure is sufficient for speech (Hixon, Hawley, & Wilson, 1982). Hixon and Hoit (1998, 1999, 2000, 2005) have described comprehensive noninstrumental protocols for examining the diaphragm, abdominal wall, and rib cage, as well as observations from them that are suggestive of neurologic weakness, incoordination, and hyperkinesias. Such extensive assessment is probably not necessary for many people with MSDs; it is estimated that about 15% or more of people with speech disorders have speech breathing difficulty and that their major cause is neurologic disease (Hixon & Hoit, 2005). Nonetheless, the protocols may be particularly valuable for speakers with prominent or predominant respiratory difficulty.

Assessment of normal oral reflexes (e.g., gag) and pathologic (or primitive) oral reflexes (e.g., jaw jerk, sucking, snout) can provide clues to the gross localization of disease in the central or peripheral nervous system. However, because the gag reflex is highly variable among normal individuals, and because primitive oral reflexes can be present in normal individuals, especially the elderly, reflex findings should be interpreted cautiously as confirmatory signs of MSDs.

The comparison of volitional versus vegetative oromotor movements helps identify nonverbal oral apraxia. Some common tasks include coughing, clicking the tongue, or smacking the lips on command or imitatively. Off-target errors, groping, or vocalization, in the presence of ability to make the movement spontaneously or vegetatively, reflect the disorder, which is a sign that localizes to the left hemisphere in most individuals. It is present much more frequently in people with AOS than dysarthria so it can be considered a confirmatory sign of AOS when that is the distinction to be made. However, because it is present in many patients with aphasia, including those with phonemic paraphasias, it cannot be considered confirmatory of AOS when the distinction to be made is between AOS and aphasia.

Diagnosis and Classification

There are many ways to categorize MSDs. Broad classifications sometimes reflect time of onset (childhood versus adult; developmental versus acquired); the course of the condition (e.g., acute, chronic, improving, progressive); neurologic diagnosis (e.g., CP, Parkinson's disease, ALS); or, simply, severity (e.g., mild, severe). These variables are important to patient description in clinical work and research. However, they are often known on the basis of history or basic examination, and they can be independent of the specific distinguishing perceptual, acoustic, and physiologic features of the disorder. The focus here is on the perceptual method of classification as developed by Darley, Aronson, and Brown (with some minor modifications) because of its implications for localization and neurologic diagnosis and management, as well as its heuristic value for clinical research and shaping of hypotheses that can be assessed through acoustic and physiologic study. As Kent (1996, p. 12) noted, "the perceptual rating scales central to the Mayo Clinic system for assessing the dysarthrias are perhaps the most comprehensive set of rating dimensions in speech-language pathology."

The ability to distinguish among the dysarthrias (and between dysarthria and AOS) requires training, experience, and a good working knowledge of neuroanatomy, neurophysiology, and signs of neuromotor abnormality (e.g., weakness, spasticity, rigidity, involuntary movements). These needs obviously cannot be met here. Rather, it may be useful to summarize why the Mayo system represents a useful paradigm, and to assess some of its weakness and shortcomings.

The Mayo approach to classifying the dysarthrias is valuable for the following reasons:

1. Because each dysarthria type is linked to a different component of the motor system (see Table 2–1), establishing type of dysarthria can contribute to the localization of neurologic disease. This is no small matter, especially for degenerative diseases for which abnormalities may not be apparent on standard neuroimaging, or when dysarthria (or AOS) is the prominent, primary, or only sign of neurologic disease. In the hands of experienced clinicians, the ability to distinguish among types of MSDs makes it one of the clinical tests that can be done when clinical neurologic diagnosis is uncertain.

2. The Mayo approach has facilitated substantial research in the salient perceptual, acoustic, and physiologic characteristics of dysarthria associated with a number of neurologic diseases. As a result, clinicians now have data that permit them to indicate the degree to which particular dysarthria types—or speech characteristics—are compatible with a given neurologic diagnosis. In some instances, such indications may raise questions about an established neurologic diagnosis or provide confirmatory evidence for diagnoses which are in doubt. Table 2-3 provides examples of some neurologic diseases that can be associated with MSDs, although MSDs have not been studied systematically in many of them.

3. Because the Mayo system infers underlying neurologic deficits (e.g., weakness, incoordination), establishing dysarthria type has implications for impairment-focused treatments. For example, efforts to improve muscle strength in the face or tongue should be based on evidence or the assumption that those muscles are weak and that weakness bears a relationship to speech deficits. Muscle strengthening might be relevant for flaccid dysarthria, but has no obvious relevance for ataxic or hyperkinetic dysarthria. Knowing dysarthria type also has implications for selection of prosthetic or pharmacologic treatments. For example, people with flaccid dysarthria and significant velopharyngeal weakness are the best candidates for a palatal lift prosthesis (Yorkston et al., 2001a); people with adductor spasmodic dysphonia associated

with dystonia are the best candidates for laryngeal Botox injection (Duffy & Yorkston, 2003).

4. The approach—with some additions—has provided a vocabulary for concisely describing and communicating about the abnormal perceptual speech characteristics of the dysarthrias. Assuming a common understanding of the auditory-perceptual attributes to which the vocabulary refers, this is of great benefit to clinical practice and research.

No classification system is perfect, if for no other reason than a single system cannot capture all variables encompassed by the many possible purposes of evaluation and diagnosis. The Mayo approach is no exception. Some of its current shortcomings include:

1. Several studies have raised questions about the reliability of perceptual judgments and diagnosis of dysarthria type (e.g. Kearns & Simmons, 1988; Sheard, Adams, & Davis, 1991; Southwood & Weismer, 1993; Zeplin & Kent, 1996; Zyski & Weisiger, 1987). This problem may be partly real and partly artifactual. That is, some researchers and clinicians have confused the research methods of Darley, Aronson, and Brown with procedures for clinical diagnosis. Their research method was highly analytic and exhaustive, whereas the clinical process of differential diagnosis may involve pattern recognition and/or reliance on only a few key perceptual features rather than ratings of each of them (Duffy & Kent, 2001). It is clear that systematic efforts to train reliability are necessary, but it is also essential that such efforts use procedures that are compatible with what clinicians actually do in clinical practice (Duffy & Kent, 2001; Kent, Kent, Duffy, & Weismer, 1998). This issue needs to be addressed by clinicians, educators, and researchers.

Table 2–3. A Sampling of Neurologic Diseases in Which Various MSDs Have Been Observed and Their Relationship to Each MSD Type

Etiology	Dysarthria						Apraxia of speech
	Flaccid	Spastic	Ataxic	Hypo-kinetic	Hyper-kinetic	Unilat UMN	
Vascular							
Aneurysm rupture	+	++	+	+	+	++	++
Hypoxic encephalopathy	–	+	+	+	–	+	+
Stroke	+	++	+	+	+	++	++
Degenerative							
ALS/motor neuron disease	++	++	++	++	+	+	+
Corticobasal degeneration	++	++	–	–	–	+	–
Freidreich's ataxia	–	+	+	+	+	–	+
Huntington's chorea	–	+	–	+	+	–	–
Leukoencephalopathy	–	+	+	+	+	–	+
Lewy body disease	–	–	–	+	–	–	–
Multiple system atrophy	+	+	+	+	+	+	+
Parkinson's disease	–	–	–	++	–	–	–
Parkinsonism	–	+	–	++	+	–	–
Primary lateral sclerosis	–	+	–	–	–	–	–
Primary progressive aphasia	–	++	–	–	–	–	++
Progressive bulbar palsy	+	–	–	+	–	+	–
Progressive supranuclear palsy	–	+	–	+	+	–	+
Spinal muscle atrophies	+	+	+	+	+	+	–
Spinocerebellar ataxias	–	–	+	+	–	–	–
Traumatic							
Closed head injury	+	+	+	+	+	+	+
Neck trauma	+	+	+	+	+	+	+
Penetrating head injury	–	–	+	+	–	+	–
Skull fracture	+	–	–	–	–	–	+

continues

Table 2-3. *continued*

Etiology	Dysarthria						Apraxia of speech
	Flaccid	Spastic	Ataxic	Hypo-kinetic	Hyper-kinetic	Unilat UMN	
Surgical Trauma							
Chest/cardiac	++	+	+	-	+	+	+
ENT	++	-	-	-	-	-	-
Neurosurgical	+	+	+	-	+	+	+
Neoplastic							
Paraneoplastic cerebellar degeneration	+	+	++	+	-	+	+
Primary or metastatic tumors	+	+	+	+	+	+	+
Toxic/Metabolic							
Carbon monoxide poisoning	-	+	+	+	++	-	-
Drug toxicity/abuse	+	+	+	+	+	-	-
Heavy metal or chemical toxicity	-	-	+	+	+	-	+
Hepatic encephalopathy	-	+	-	-	+	-	-
Hypothyroidism	-	-	+	-	-	-	-
Wilson's disease	-	+	+	+	+	-	-
Infectious							
AIDS	+	+	+	+	+	-	+
Creutzfeldt–Jacob disease	+	+	+	-	+	-	-
Infectious encephalopathy	-	+	+	+	+	+	+
Polio	+	-	-	-	-	-	-
Sydenham's chorea	-	-	-	-	+	-	-
Inflammatory							
Encephalitis	-	+	+	-	-	-	+
Meningitis	+	+	+	+	-	-	+
Multifocal leukoencephalopathy	-	+	+	+	-	-	-

Dysarthria

Etiology	Flaccid	Spastic	Ataxic	Hypo-kinetic	Hyper-kinetic	Unilat UMN	Apraxia of speech
Demyelinating Disease							
Guillain–Barré syndrome	+	−	−	−	−	−	−
Multiple sclerosis	+	+	+	+	+	+	+
Anatomic Malformation							
Arnold–Chiari	+	+	+	−	+	−	−
Syringobulbia	+	+	+	−	−	−	−
Syringomyelia	+	−	−	−	−	−	−
Neuromuscular Junction Disease							
Lambert–Eaton syndrome	+	−	−	−	−	−	−
Myasthenia gravis	+	−	−	−	−	−	−
Muscle Disease							
Muscular dystrophy	+	−	−	−	−	−	−
Myotonic dystrophy	+	−	−	−	−	−	−
Other							
Hydrocephalus	+	+	+	++	+	+	+
Meige's syndrome	−	+	+	+	+	+	−
Myoclonic epilepsy	−	−	−	−	++	−	−
Radiation necrosis	+	−	+	+	+	+	−
Seizure disorder	−	−	−	−	−	−	+
Tourette's syndrome	−	−	−	−	+	−	−
Undetermined Cause (Idiopathic)	+	+	+	+	++	+	+

Key: ++ = Very frequent cause, + = Possible cause, − = Rare, never, or uncertain cause

Source: Based on reviews of Mayo Clinic cases (Duffy, 2005) and the published literature. The neurologic diseases listed are incomplete; only the more commonly occurring diseases associated with MSDs are included. MSDs associated with many of these conditions have not been studied systematically. (Adapted and abbreviated from Duffy [2005a], with permission).

2. The classification system's accuracy in localizing lesions has never been explicitly studied. It has certainly been indirectly supported in many studies in which dysarthria type is compatible with the known locus of pathology (e.g., as in Parkinson's disease), but more rigorous, blinded assessment of its localization value is necessary. "Such cross-validation would likely contribute to refinements in the classification system as it relates to localization, our understanding of underlying pathophysiology, and to the possibility of additional dysarthria types or subtypes" (Duffy & Kent, 2001, p. 280).

3. The system does not capture all relevant information for research or clinical practice. For example, it does not intend nor does it provide an index of dysarthria severity. It is also independent of disease course (e.g., chronic, degenerative), a variable that has important implications for clinical decision-making. And, sometimes what the Mayo system has inferred about pathophysiology has not been supported by physiologic data. Systematic research that includes thorough perceptual assessment accompanied by thorough acoustic and physiologic assessment is necessary to resolve these discrepancies (Duffy & Kent, 2001). It is clear that acoustic and physiologic analysis can add to the understanding and description of auditory-perceptual features, and they are probably essential to our understanding of their physiologic substrates.

4. Its applicability to dysarthria in children has not been well established and has been questioned (van Mourik, Catsman-Berrevoets, Paquier, Yousef-Bak, & van Dongen, 1997).

In spite of its assumed widespread and dominant influence, observations of clinical practice and the research literature suggest the Mayo approach is not necessarily widely, or at least explicitly, used. For example, many published studies of the dysarthrias do not indicate dysarthria type, and, even more disconcerting, do not offer an adequate description of the speech characteristics of subjects under study. Such omissions place significant limitations on professional communication and the clinical applicability and theoretical value of acoustic and physiologic studies that purport to increase our understanding of MSDs.

Management

This section reviews general issues, decisions, and approaches to managing MSDs and provides an overview of principles and guidelines for their behavioral management. Variations in management as a function of specific MSDs are also addressed. Emphasis is placed on acquired MSDs because they have received more attention than developmental MSDs; note, however, that there is considerable overlap between them in treatment strategies and techniques.[7]

General Issues and Decision Making

The crucial question when addressing management is "What, if anything, can be done to help this person communicate as effectively as possible?" The answer sometimes rests on improving speech produc-

---

[7]Comprehensive reviews of management for MSDs in adults and children can be found in several recent texts (e.g., Caruso & Strand, 1999; Duffy, 2005a; McNeil, 1997; Yorkston, Beukelman, Strand, & Bell, 1999).

tion and its intelligibility, efficiency, or naturalness. Sometimes it requires a strong focus on nonspoken language or extralinguistic and nonverbal activities that will take the place of or supplement speech. Sometimes the answer requires a combination of both approaches, either simultaneously or sequentially. The theme reflected in all of these answers is that management of MSDs often focuses broadly on communication and not simply speech.

Not everyone with an MSD is a candidate for speech therapy. There is no clear formula for how this determination is made but a number of important factors influence the decision. The most relevant factors include patient motivation and needs; medical diagnosis and prognosis; presence and degree of disability and handicap; the environment in which communication takes place, and with whom; co-occurring motor, sensory, and cognitive difficulties; and limitations imposed by the health care system.

Management can take several non-mutually exclusive directions. It may focus on efforts to *restore lost functions* through direct work on the speech impairment. Speech exercise or drill to improve strength, power, endurance, or control is an example of this. It might also focus on *compensation* for lost abilities by, for example, modifying rate and prosody; use of prosthetic devices (e.g., palatal lift, voice amplifier); augmenting speech (gestures, written alphabet, or semantic cues); alternative means of communication (e.g., computer-based systems); or modifying the physical environment (e.g., reducing noise or distance). It might also address temporary or permanent *adjustment* to the loss of normal speech by, for example, changes in work responsibilities, lifestyle, and conditions for social-communicative interaction.

Approaches to Management

Speech therapy is often thought of as a behavioral enterprise. Behavioral modification of speech is certainly at the core of management for many people, but multiple approaches to management are appropriate and necessary for many people with MSDs. These include medical interventions, prosthetic management, alternative and augmentative communication (AAC), and counseling and support. Counseling and support are part of care for any communication disorder and are not discussed here.

Medical interventions for MSDs include pharmacologic and surgical management. When appropriate, they often should be provided prior to or simultaneously with behavioral management because they tend to maximize physiologic functioning and sometimes have a rapid or significant effect on speech. Drug interventions may be directed at the underlying disease (e.g., antibiotics for infection, steroids to reduce inflammatory effects of tumors; anticonvulsants to prevent seizures), with secondary benefits to speech. Other drugs (e.g., dopaminergic agents for PD, Mestinon for myasthenia gravis) are specifically aimed at reducing signs and symptoms of neurologic disease, among which are MSDs. And, a few substances can be used specifically to treat a MSD (e.g., botulinum toxin to treat dystonic spasmodic dysphonia, or orofacial dystonias).

Surgical management can also have indirect and direct effects on speech. For example, neurosurgery for tumors, aneurysms, and occluded arteries may address the causes of the speech impairment and may stabilize, improve, or resolve some MSDs. Other surgeries may be performed solely to improve speech. Pharyngeal flap or sphincter pharyngoplasty to improve velopharyngeal weakness and thyroplasty for vocal fold paralysis are prime examples.

Permanent or temporary mechanical or electronic prosthetic or assistive devices are available to improve speech. Some, such as palatal lift prostheses, modify the vocal tract. Others, such as voice amplifiers, alter speech after it is produced. Others, such as pacing boards, metronomes, delayed auditory feedback, and vocal intensity monitors, improve speech by influencing how it is produced (i.e., more slowly, more loudly).

When an MSD is severe and intelligibility is significantly compromised, AAC may be necessary to augment or substitute for speech. AAC reflects a combination of behavioral strategies and low or high-tech prosthetic aids to facilitate message transmission. Its tools range from gestural strategies (e.g., eye gaze; face, head, and hand gestures), to nonvocal symbols (e.g., pictures; icons; printed words or letters), to electronic devices or computer-based systems with synthesized speech and switching devices for message assembly and activation. The development of AAC systems has undergone dramatic refinement in recent years and AAC has become a subspecialty area of practice in speech-language pathology. For some people with MSDs who need alternatives to speech, particularly those with co-occurring sensory deficits or limb motor deficits, consultation with an AAC expert is often necessary to develop the most appropriate AAC system.

Behavioral Management

Behavioral approaches can be speech-oriented or communication-oriented. They often are used in combination with prosthetic, surgical, and pharmacologic treatments.

Speech-oriented approaches focus on improving physiologic support for speech or on developing compensations that make use of residual physiologic support. Both may focus on respiration, phonation, resonance, articulation, rate, or prosody. Both aim to improve intelligibility or, secondarily, efficiency and naturalness. Both require effort and motor learning. Compensation is usually achieved more rapidly than reduction of physiologic impairment; it seems to be the treatment strategy most often elected, especially if therapy will be short term.

Efforts to reduce impairment focus on deficits that presumably underlie the MSD (e.g., strength, speed, coordination, programming). Activities with the greatest face validity involve speech but some approaches use sensory stimulation and nonspeech motor activities. Some compensatory strategies work to modify aspects of speech (e.g., breathing, phonation, or rate) for which physiologic capacity exists but is not being used. For example, inhaling more deeply before initiating speech or modifying speech rate can affect intelligibility. Other compensatory strategies may include altering language content or style or stress patterns to enhance intelligibility or efficiency. Finally, some speech-oriented treatments focus on altering maladaptive behaviors that sometimes persist beyond their period of usefulness (e.g., speaking on inhalation, producing fewer words per breath group than necessary). Examples of behavioral, prosthetic, and medical/surgical speech-oriented treatments, and their relationship to dysarthria type are provided in Table 2–4.

Communication-oriented approaches work to modify things beyond speech to improve comprehensibility and communication. Some are accomplished by the affected person, others by their listeners.

Table 2–4. Examples of Behavioral, Prosthetic, and Medical-Surgical Speech-Oriented Treatments and Techniques and Their Relationship to Various Dysarthria Types and Apraxia of Speech (AOS)

Approach	Dysarthria						AOS
	Flaccid	Spastic	Ataxic	Hypo-kinetic	Hyper-kinetic	Unilateral UMN	
Behavioral							
Respiration							
"5 for 5" respiratory tasks	+	+	+	+	+	+	–
Expiratory muscle conditioning	+	+	+	+	+	–	–
Maximum vowel prolongation	++	–	+	+	–	–	–
Postural adjustments	+	+	+	–	–	–	–
Manual push on abdomen	+	+	–	+	+	–	+
Neck breathing	++	–	–	+	–	+	+
Glossopharyngeal breathing	++	–	–	–	–	–	–
Inspiratory checking	++	–	+	–	–	–	–
Inhale more deeply before speech	+	+	+	+	–	–	–
Terminate speech earlier in exhalatory cycle	+	+	+	++	–	–	–
Increase/decrease phrase length	+	+	+	+	–	–	–
Phonation							
Intense, high level phonatory effort	+	+	–	+	+	+	–
Lee Silverman Voice Therapy (LSVT)	++	–	–	++	–	–	–
Effort closure techniques	+	–	–	++	–	–	–
Abrupt glottal attack	++	–	–	+	–	–	–
Lateralize thyroid cartilage	++	–	–	+	–	–	–
Speak at onset of exhalation	+	+	+	–	–	–	–
Breathy onset	–	++	+	+	++	–	–
Continuous voicing of consonants	–	–	–	–	++	–	–
Optimal breath group	+	+	+	+	–	–	–

continues

Table 2-4. *continued*

Approach	Dysarthria						AOS
	Flaccid	Spastic	Ataxic	Hypo-kinetic	Hyper-kinetic	Unilateral UMN	
Resonance							
Continuous positive airway pressure	+	+	−	+	−	−	−
Supine positioning	‡	−	−	−	−	−	−
Occlude nares	‡	−	−	−	−	−	−
Exaggerate jaw movement	+	+	−	−	−	−	−
Increase loudness	+	−	−	+	−	−	−
Reduce pressure consonant duration	‡	+	−	−	−	−	−
Articulation							
Strengthening exercises	+	+	+	+	+	+	+
Stretching	‡	‡	−	−	−	+	−
Integral stimulation	+	+	−	+	−	−	‡
Phonetic placement	+	+	+	+	−	+	+
Phonetic derivation	+	+	+	+	−	+	+
Minimal contrasts	+	+	+	+	−	−	+
Exaggerate consonants	+	+	+	+	−	+	−
Alternative place/manner/voicing strategies	‡	+	−	−	−	−	−
Biofeedback	+	+	+	+	+	+	+
Sensory tricks	−	−	−	−	‡	−	−
Conservation of strength	+	+	−	−	−	−	−
8-Step continuum	−	−	−	−	−	−	‡

Dysarthria

Approach	Flaccid	Spastic	Ataxic	Hypo-kinetic	Hyper-kinetic	Unilateral UMN	AOS
Articulation *continued*							
Sound Production Treatment (SPT)	+	+	+	+	+	+	+
Prompts for Restructuring Oral Muscular Phonetic Targets (PROMPT)	–	–	–	–	–	–	++
Intelligibility drills	+	+	+	+	+	+	+
Referential tasks	+	+	+	+	+	+	+
Rate							
Rate modification	+	+	+	+	+	+	+
Hand/finger tapping	+	+	+	+	+	+	+
Rhythmic or metered cueing	–	–	+	+	–	+	+
Visual/auditory feedback	+	+	+	+	+	+	+
Modify pauses	+	+	+	+	–	+	–
ID first letter on alphabet board	+	+	+	+	+	+	+
Prosody and Naturalness							
Breath group duration	+	+	+	+	+	+	+
Modify syllable duration and pause time	+	+	+	+	+	+	–
Across breath group tasks	+	+	+	+	–	–	–
Chunk by syntactic units	+	+	+	+	–	–	–
Contrastive stress tasks	+	+	+	+	+	+	+
Referential stress tasks	+	+	+	+	+	+	+

continues

Table 2-4. *continued*

Approach	Flaccid	Spastic	Ataxic	Hypo-kinetic	Hyper-kinetic	Unilateral UMN	AOS
Prosthetic							
Abdominal binders/corsets	+	+	+	+	+	–	+
Vocal intensity controller	++	–	–	–	–	–	–
Vocal amplifier	+	+	–	+	+	–	–
Palatal lift	++	+	–	+	–	–	–
Nose clip/nasal obturator	+	+	–	–	–	–	–
Delayed auditory feedback	–	–	–	++	–	–	–
Pacing board	–	–	–	++	–	–	–
Metronome	–	–	–	++	–	–	+
Bite block	+	–	–	–	++	–	+
Neck brace/cervical collar	+	–	+	–	+	–	–
Medical/Surgical							
Medialization laryngoplasty	++	+	–	+	+	–	–
Vocal fold fat/collagen injection	++	–	–	+	–	–	–
Midline lateralization thyroplasty	–	–	–	–	++	–	–
Pharyngeal flap	++	+	–	–	++	–	–
Recurrent laryngeal nerve resection, avulsion, denervation-innervation	–	–	–	–	++	–	–
Botox injection	–	–	–	–	++	–	–

Key: + = may be appropriate; ++ = uniquely appropriate but not necessarily for all patients; – = rarely necessary, of uncertain benefit, or contraindicated

Source: Adapted and abbreviated from Duffy (2005a), with permission.

Examples of these modifications include gaining listener attention before speaking; identifying the topic of conversation; using alphabet board supplementation; reducing the number of listeners, speaker-listener distance, noise, and sources of distraction; maximizing hearing and visual acuity; maintaining eye contact. They can also include training consistent strategies for repair of communication breakdowns when they occur (e.g., repetition, rephrasing, spelling, alphabet supplementation, writing, answering questions).

Principles of Motor Learning

Cognitive and physical "work" is essential for speech-oriented treatments regardless of whether the aim is to reduce impairment or compensate for it; in fact, although often neglected, it is also necessary for communication-oriented treatments. In recent years there has been increased attention to the relevance of general principles of motor learning to the conduct of MSD treatments. Although evidence that principles of motor learning apply to speech motor learning is limited, that which does exist supports their relevance. It seems essential that clinicians who treat MSDs and researchers who design treatment protocols for investigation consider them. Discussion of these principles as they apply to MSDs can be found in several sources (e.g., Caruso & Strand, 1999; Clark, 2003; Duffy, 2005a; Rosenbaum, 1991; Rosenbek & LaPointe, 1985; Schmidt, 1991; Schmidt & Bjork, 1996; Singer, 1980; Wertz, LaPointe, & Rosenbek, 1985; Yorkston, Beukelman, Strand, & Bell, 1999). The following is an illustrative listing of a few principles (some of which may be counterintuitive) that seem essential or at least defensible for the structure of therapy:

1. Drill is essential to motor learning. Multiple opportunities for practice are important.
2. Frequent, brief periods of practice may be more beneficial than less frequent lengthy periods of practice.
3. Although mental practice (thinking about how to speak) can contribute to motor learning, it is less effective than physical practice.
4. Self-learning, or discovery-learning, may lead to better retention and generalization than motor learning that is highly prompted. This suggests that, at the least, instruction should be faded during therapy as soon as possible.
5. Feedback about performance is important, especially in the early stages of motor learning, but infrequent feedback and feedback in summary form may be better for long-term retention and generalization than frequent, immediate feedback.
6. Learning of a motor skill is most effective when it is as specific as possible to the goals of training. This suggests that therapy to improve MSD should generally involve speaking, as opposed to nonspeech exercise.
7. Increasing strength requires that muscles be overloaded in some way and that repetition occurs.
8. Consistent (blocked) practice—an unvarying task performed repetitively—may be better early in motor learning and may increase rate of acquisition and speed of movement. Variable (random) practice may lead to better retention and generalization. Variable practice is more relevant to natural speaking conditions.

Management for Specific MSDs

Communication-oriented approaches to treatment are relatively independent of

MSD type. In contrast, not all speech-oriented treatments are equally appropriate for all MSDs, and some may be contraindicated for some MSD types (Duffy, 2005a). This makes sense because different MSDs reflect different underlying neurophysiologic impairments.

A representative listing of behavioral treatment strategies that are appropriate for different dysarthria types are summarized in Table 2–4. The reader is cautioned that the quality of evidence about their effectiveness is variable. The following points summarize some conclusions about which there is some supportive evidence or at least general consensus. They illustrate how some dysarthria treatments are specific to dysarthria type.

1. Efforts to increase strength or compensate for weakness anywhere in the speech system have the greatest validity for people with flaccid dysarthria. However, efforts to increase strength will be ineffective if lower motor neuron innervation to specific muscles is completely lost. Strengthening exercises are contraindicated for flaccid dysarthria secondary to myasthenia gravis. Speakers with vocal fold paralysis are the best candidates for medialization thyroplasty or vocal fold injections of fat or collagen to assist vocal fold approximation. People with flaccid dysarthria are also the best candidates for palatal lift prostheses and velopharyngeal strengthening exercise, such as continuous positive airway pressure.

2. Efforts to increase vocal fold adduction, whether behavioral or surgical, are generally contraindicated for spastic dysarthria because hyperadduction typically is already present.

3. Surgical and prosthetic interventions that might be helpful for respiratory, phonatory, resonatory, or articulatory problems in flaccid or spastic dysarthria are not appropriate for ataxic dysarthria. Ataxic dysarthria is managed behaviorally with methods directed at motor control and coordination through modification of rate and prosody.

4. Lee Silverman Voice Treatment (LSVT; e.g., Ramig et al., 1995, 2001a, 2001b) is probably the most programmatically investigated behavioral treatment for dysarthria. There is perceptual, acoustic, aerodynamic, and kinematic evidence that it results in improvement, with long-term maintenance, in some patients (Yorkston, Spencer, & Duffy, 2003). It emphasizes intense, high-effort voice and speech exercise designed to increase loudness and vocal fold adduction. It was developed for people with Parkinson's disease (hypokinetic dysarthria). At this time, it is most appropriate for hypokinetic dysarthria, is probably contraindicated for spastic and hyperkinetic dysarthrias, and is of unknown benefit for other dysarthria types. However, "the general principles of motor learning and intensity of treatment upon which LSVT is based may be applicable to the management of MSDs other than hypokinetic dysarthria" (Duffy, 2005a, p. 491).

5. Behavioral strategies for hyperkinetic dysarthrias are primarily compensatory because the underlying abnormal movements appear not to be under voluntary control. Botox injection is effective and the preferred method for treating spasmodic dysphonia, particularly dystonia-based adductor spasmodic dysphonia, and it may also be helpful for hyperkinetic dysarthrias secondary to jaw, face, and lingual dystonias (Duffy & Yorkston, 2003). Botox injection would be contraindicated for most, if not all, other MSDs.

The management of AOS, including CAS, shares many things with dysarthria management, but there are significant differences in specific techniques and their purposes. There are no medical interventions specifically designed to improve AOS for which there is evidence of efficacy (Duffy, 2005a). Mechanical and prosthetic devices are occasionally appropriate but less frequently than for the dysarthrias. AAC systems are certainly appropriate, but may be more challenging to implement than for dysarthrias because of the common co-occurrence of AOS and aphasia.

Treatment of AOS is primarily behavioral (see Table 2–4). Communication-oriented approaches are comparable to those used for dysarthria although they often require modification when aphasia is also present. All speech-oriented approaches place heavy reliance on principles of motor learning. The most frequently used approaches specifically designed for AOS include the 8-Step (integral stimulation) Continuum (e.g., Deal & Florence, 1978; Rosenbek, Lemme, Ahern, Harris, & Wertz, 1973), Sound Production Treatment (SPT; e.g., Wambaugh, 2004; Wambaugh, Kalinyak-Fliszar, West, & Doyle, 1998; Wambaugh, Martinez, McNeil, & Rogers, 1999), Prompts for Restructuring Oral Muscular Phonetic Targets (e.g., Bose, Square, Schlosser, & van Lieshout, 2001; Chumpelik, 1984; Freed, Marshall, & Frazier, 1997), and metronome pacing (Dworkin & Abkarian, 1996; Dworkin, Abkarian, & Johns, 1988; Wambaugh & Martinez, 2000). Data on treatment outcome are limited. However, positive effects for the PROMPT and SPT approaches have been replicated and data on their efficacy seem more adequate than for any other acquired AOS therapy (Duffy, 2005a; Wambaugh, 2002).

AOS and CAS are treated in similar ways. PROMPT treatment was actually originally developed for CAS and it is a prototype for a number of tactile-kinesthetic and gestural cueing approaches used for AOS in children (Square, 1999). Integral stimulation methods, probably the most common treatment for CAS (Strand & Skinder, 1999), are similar in principle and techniques to a number of those associated with the 8-step continuum.

Efficacy, Evidence-Based Practice, and Practice Guidelines

The efficacy and effectiveness of treatment for MSDs have been studied more assertively and systematically in recent years. As is true for medicine in general, convincing data for a substantial number of treatments are still lacking. However, reviews of the available evidence have concluded that, in general, people with dysarthria and AOS do benefit from treatment (e.g., McNeil, Doyle, & Wambaugh, 2000; Yorkston, 1996).

Within the last decade nearly all health care subspecialties have been influenced by the concept and methods of evidence-based practice (EBP) and practice guidelines for the most effective and efficient methods of care. EBP emphasizes the use of published data, combined with clinical experience, as a basis for treatment decision-making. Practice guidelines assist EBP by providing systematic reviews of evidence, with subsequent published guides for clinical conduct when there is some degree of certainty that the value of a treatment is worthwhile and exceeds any associated risks (Frattali & Worrall, 2001; Yorkston, Spencer, Duffy, Beukelman, Golper, Miller, Strand, & Sullivan, 2001b).

The Academy of Neurologic Communication Disorders and Sciences (ANCDS) has taken a leadership role in developing practice guidelines for speech-language pathology; MSDs were the first major area to receive attention. Systematic reviews are now available for respiratory-phonatory dysfunction (Spencer, Yorkston, & Duffy, 2003), velopharyngeal function (Yorkston, Spencer, Duffy, Beukelman, Golper, & Miller, 2001a), spasmodic dysphonia (Duffy & Yorkston, 2003), and speech supplementation techniques (Hanson, Yorkston, & Beukelman, 2004). Additional systematic reviews and guidelines are being developed for other MSD treatments, including AOS. These efforts aim to improve care, but they also identify gaps in knowledge about treatments that require further study.

Future Trends and Goals

The future for MSDs depends in part on demographic realities and the politics and economics of health care. There can be little doubt that the aging of the population and increasing life span will increase the prevalence of neurologic disease and its consequences, including MSDs. This should generate increased demand for improved understanding, diagnosis, and management of MSDs. At the same time, the pending health care crisis and increased competition for research support may combine to reduce access of patients to speech therapy, the ability of clinicians to provide optimal care, and the ability of researchers to advance our understanding of MSDs. Meeting these challenges will be difficult. It will derive from social, political, and societal influences and from efforts within the disciplines of speech-language pathology and speech science. In the context of this chapter, it is most appropriate to focus on the disciplines' efforts. The questions and suggestions that follow should be viewed as examples only. They are divided into areas that address

(1) basic understanding and (2) clinical practice. Answers to nearly all of the questions have implications for both areas, however.

Basic Understanding

1. *To what degree are limb motor control and its disorders similar to speech motor control and MSDs?* In comparison to the limbs, surprisingly little is known about speech motor control, and there are reasons to believe there is not one-to-one correspondence between the workings of the limbs and the bulbar speech muscles. The speech system may have, to some unknown degree, its own neurology, perhaps also influenced by unique characteristics of craniofacial muscles and their developmental patterns and functional properties (Kent & Rosen, 2004). These factors might explain why some neurologic diseases, and medical treatments for them, have different consequences for the bulbar versus limb muscles.

Answers to this question are important because the foundation of the Mayo approach to classifying the dysarthrias is based on assumptions about underlying pathophysiology derived from observations of limb movement disorders. Even if the speech and limb motor system have a high degree of correspondence, the explanations for limb deficits have been refined over the years since the Mayo system emerged. For example, it is now felt that problems with sensory and motor scaling and sensorimotor integration may be involved in some of the movement disorders in Parkinson's disease; to what degree do those problems explain some of the speech characteristics of hyperkinetic dysarthria? Basically, we have a lot to learn about the nature of the sensorimotor impairments that underlie MSDs. The Mayo approach would be strengthened or perhaps considerably modified if its implications for pathophysiology were based more directly on study of the bulbar speech muscles rather than inferences largely based on observations of limb motor system impairment.

2. *What is the nature and strength of the relationship between central nervous system control and movements of speech structures during speech versus nonspeech movements?* The degree of independence between speech and nonspeech movements is largely unknown although it is unlikely that understanding nonspeech control of bulbar muscles will fully explain speech motor control (Duffy & Kent, 2001; Kent & Rosen, 2004; Weismer, 2006). The answer to this question will help determine whether the two areas of study should be separate enterprises or whether examining nonspeech movements of speech structures can inform— more rapidly, simply, validly (e.g., removed from linguistic influences), or thoroughly —our understanding of speech motor control and MSDs. This issue has been a matter of considerable debate (e.g., see Ballard, Robin, & Folkins, 2003; Robin, Solomon, Moon, & Folkins, 1997; Weismer, 2006; Ziegler, 2003a, 2003b). Its clarification will help establish optimal investigative methods and influence the focus and efficiency of future research efforts. Clarification will be of more than theoretical interest; it will likely have implications for how MSDs are evaluated clinically and whether their management can legitimately focus on nonspeech activity.

3. *What needs to be done to make acoustic, physiologic, and neuroimaging studies of MSDs maximally informative?*

The tendency in research has been to compartmentalize effort. This is reflected in the level of the speech system studied (e.g., laryngeal, articulatory), the method of study (acoustic, kinematic, neuroimaging), and the research discipline (e.g., speech science, speech pathology, neurology, genetics, epidemiology). These focused approaches have often been illuminating, but Kent (2000) sees a promising direction in multidisciplinary and multitechnology studies. Weismer (2006) has recommended development of consortiums that can collect data on large numbers of people with MSDs who can be examined using standardized tasks and common equipment and measurement approaches, with questions and methods driven by an integrated theory of speech production. A more complete understanding of MSDs may be derived from simultaneously examining the full operation of the speech system with a variety of methods, and from the perspectives of several disciplines. The degree to which such a comprehensive approach is necessary is certainly highly dependent on the questions being addressed. A case can be made, however, that at the core of any study of MSDs, there should be a characterization of the salient auditory-perceptual characteristics of speech. What we hear is, after all, the goal of all the movements that precede it. To neglect such characterization is to obscure appreciation of what is being studied and our ability to generalize findings. This seems self-evident but even a cursory review of the literature establishes that such descriptive detail is often neglected. Highly sophisticated physiologic and neuroimaging studies of speech disorders will be of limited value without a clear description—if not classification—of the speech abnormalities under study.

Clinical Practice

1. *What deviant speech characteristics and types of MSDs are associated with a broad spectrum of neurologic diseases?* As already discussed, answers to this question can contribute to the localization and diagnosis of neurologic disease, at the very least by permitting statements that certain MSDs are or are not compatible with certain neurologic diagnoses. This work needs to continue, both to refine what we already know about some diseases and to begin to establish the range of possibilities for those not yet studied systematically. Epidemiologic studies may permit the development of probabilities for certain neurologic diagnoses when MSD type and the temporal course (e.g., acute, subacute, progressive) are known; this may be of special value when speech difficulty is the presenting complaint. A related need is to better establish the boundaries between MSDs and normal variants or non-neurologic speech abnormalities. Improved understanding of the effects of normal aging on speech is particularly relevant in this regard. Also relevant is the need, at least in some clinical settings, to distinguish between MSDs and nonorganic/psychogenic speech disturbances. This distinction has implications for medical and neurologic diagnosis, as well as for medical and speech pathology management. This is a challenge for perceptual, acoustic, and physiologic research.

2. *What can acoustic and physiologic techniques contribute to clinical practice?* Quantitative, instrumental acoustic and physiologic methods are increasingly applied to the study of MSDs. Some have expressed the hope that "the speech scientist and clinician of the future will have ready access to tools that meld perceptual judgment and instrumental analysis into a reliable and informative summary" (Duffy & Kent, 2001, p. 284). This is a lofty goal but one worth pursuing. Acoustic analyses are particularly ripe for more widespread clinical use for several reasons, including: availability of normative data for some acoustic parameters; its ability to shed light on the locus and nature of abnormalities, and possible source of reduced intelligibility; its ability to capture the output of the entire system; its representation of the goal of speech motor control; its noninvasiveness, quantifiability, and affordability (Forrest & Weismer, 1997; Weismer, 2006). Establishing the acoustic parameters that are most relevant to quantifying the severity of MSDs would help bring the acoustic laboratory into the clinic. If acoustic analysis reaches a point where it can rapidly predict word or sentence intelligibility from a relatively limited sample of speech, it will almost certainly enjoy immediate clinical applicability. It would reduce the need for time consuming perceptual "testing" of blinded listeners, and would provide a metric against which change can be quantified in a functionally meaningful way.

In general, for acoustic and physiologic analyses to become part of standard clinical practice they will probably have to accomplish one or more of the following:

- Reliably confirm or add something to clinical differential diagnosis of MSD type (not simply description) that cannot be achieved by careful, reliable auditory-perceptual evaluation.
- Provide, in a time-efficient way, quantifiable acoustic or physiologic data that predict intelligibility, efficiency of speech, or other indices of MSD severity.
- Detect acoustic or physiologic changes that reliably predict

changes in intelligibility, efficiency, or other indices of MSD severity.

■ Provide feedback during therapy that can shape subsequent speech attempts in a positive, functionally meaningful direction, and do so with greater effectiveness and cost-effectiveness than that which can be accomplished with noninstrumental feedback.

3. *How can the Mayo and other approaches to classifying the dysarthrias be strengthened or refined?* A number of avenues of research could address this issue; a few examples follow:

■ The assessment, description, classification, and understanding of the dysarthrias and AOS would be enhanced by the development of standard assessment protocols. It is likely that multiple tasks will be needed to capture the multiple purposes for which evaluation may be conducted, but these ideally would be packaged as subtests within a single instrument that has been standardized on the same large sample of speakers.

■ The Mayo system may undergo expansion by identifying sub-types within some of the major dysarthria types. For example, flaccid dysarthria probably should be subdivided according to the cranial or spinal nerves involved, and hyperkinetic dysarthria divided into subcategories based on the type of underlying movement disorder (e.g., tremor, myoclonus, dystonia) and perhaps its locus within the speech system (e.g., laryngeal, jaw, multiple loci). Some recent studies raise the possibility of

subtypes of ataxic and hypokinetic dysarthria (Boutsen, Bakker, & Duffy, 1997;; Kent, Kent, Duffy, & Weismer, 1998). These require further study to establish the validity and bases for such subdivisions.

■ Valid methods to train reliability of auditory-perceptual judgments are needed (Duffy & Kent, 2001). Relatedly, developing some consensus about the core auditory-perceptual features that must be present for a diagnosis of each dysarthria type and AOS would improve clinical and research diagnostic reliability, precision, and communication.

■ The predictive value of the Mayo approach for lesion localization should be formally assessed. The validity of the system for this purpose would be enhanced (or questioned) if this can be formally established.

■ The capacity of visual, tactile, reflex, acoustic, and physiologic measures to improve or refine the predictive localizing (and other) value of the Mayo classification system deserves study.

4. *How should the evaluation, classification, and management of MSDs differ between developmental and acquired forms?* To what degree does what we know about acquired MSDs in adults apply to children with developmental or acquired MSDs? Kent (2000) notes that "disorders that affect speech motor learning in children may be fundamentally different from the disorders that disrupt previously acquired speech motor skills in adults" (p. 412). At the very least, there is a need for developmentally appropriate assessments and treatments, and a theory of childhood MSDs that incorporates developmental information (Caruso & Strand, 1999). At the same time, because acquired MSDs have been studied more thoroughly than developmental MSDs, it may be short-sighted to assume that differences between developmental and acquired MSDs are so great that what we have learned about acquired disorders cannot or should not be applied to developmental MSDs. A basic issue is whether or not the Mayo approach to classification of the dysarthrias is useful for developmental dysarthrias. If it is not, is there an alternative means of classification, one that (hopefully) goes beyond considering developmental dysarthria as a singular disorder, or that simply adopts the broad neurologic diagnosis (e.g., "spastic cerebral palsy")? We also need to ask if principles of motor learning that apply to acquired dysarthria or AOS are equally relevant to developmental dysarthria or CAS.

5. *What approaches to managing MSDs are the most effective and efficient, for whom, and under what circumstances?* With few exceptions, general conclusions that treatment of dysarthrias and AOS is effective are based on relatively limited data; they are sufficient to justify further study, but far from sufficient to conclude that all the important questions have been answered. The variables that require investigation are multiple and complex, ranging from medical, prosthetic, and behavioral speech-oriented and communication-oriented approaches, to the range of MSD types and severity, to the nature and course of the underlying neurologic disease. At this point, it is reasonable to assume that evidence of efficacy, effectiveness, and efficiency for a single approach to treatment for a particular type of MSD, of a given level of severity, due to a particular disease with a given predicted course, is

unlikely to be generalizable to different MSD treatments or populations. Behavioral, speech-oriented treatments aimed at reducing or compensating for physiologic impairments are likely to be the most challenging, but all treatment approaches require considerable study. Resolving the debate about the efficacy of nonspeech oromotor exercises to treat acquired and developmental MSDs seems particularly important because such exercises seem to be fairly pervasively used in clinical practice in spite of meager evidence for their effectiveness or lack thereof.

Acknowledgments. This work was supported in part by research Grant 5 RO1 DC 00319 from the National Institute of Deafness and Other Communication Disorders at the National Institutes of Health.

References

Abbs, J. H., Hunker, C. J., & Barlow, S. M. (1983). Differential speech motor system impairments with suprabulbar lesions: neurophysiological framework and supporting data. In W. R. Berry (Ed.), *Clinical dysarthria* (pp. 21–26). San Diego, CA: College-Hill.

Achilles, R. (1955). Communicative anomalies of individuals with cerebral palsy: I: Analysis of communicative processes in 151 cases of cerebral palsy. *Cerebral Palsy Review, 16,* 15–24.

Agranowitz, A., & McKeown, M. R. (1964). *Aphasia handbook for adults and children.* Springfield, IL: Charles C. Thomas, 1964.

American Speech-Language-Hearing Association. (1995). *Functional communication measure.* Rockville, MD: Author.

Ansel, B. M., & Kent, R. D. (1992). Acoustic-phonetic contrasts and intelligibility in the dysarthria associated with mixed cerebral palsy, *Journal of Speech and Hearing Research, 35,* 296-308.

Aram, D. M., & Nation, J. E. (1982). *Child language disorders.* St Louis, MO: Mosby.

Ballard, K. J., Granier, J. P., & Robin, D. A. (2000). Understanding the nature of apraxia of speech. *Aphasiology, 14,* 969-995.

Ballard, K. J., Robin, D. A., & Folkins, J. W. (2003). An integrative model of speech motor control: a response to Ziegler. *Aphasiology, 17,* 37-48.

Berry, M. F., & Eisenson, J. (1956). *Speech disorders: Principles and practices of therapy.* New York: Appleton-Century-Crofts.

Blakely, R. W. (2001). *Screening test for developmental apraxia of speech* (2nd ed.). Austin, TX: Pro-Ed.

Blumberg, M. (1955). Respiration and speech in the cerebral palsied child. *American Journal of Disorders of Childhood, 89,* 48-53.

Bose, A., Square, P.A., Schlosser, R., & van Lieshout, P. (2001). Effects of PROMPT therapy on speech motor function in a person with aphasia. *Aphasiology, 15*(8), 767-785.

Boutsen, F. R., Bakker, K., & Duffy, J. R. (1997). Subgroups in ataxic dysarthria. *Journal of Medical Speech-Language Pathology, 5,* 27-36.

Cahill, L. M., Murdoch, B. E., & Theodoros, D. G. (2002). Perceptual analysis of speech following traumatic brain injury in childhood. *Brain Injury, 16,* 415-446.

Canter, G. J. (1967). Neuromotor pathologies of speech. *American Journal of Physical Medicine. 46,* 659-666.

Caruso, A. J., & Strand, E. A. (1999). Motor speech disorders in children: Definitions, background, and a theoretical framework. In A. J. Caruso & E. A. Strand (Eds.), *Clinical management of motor speech disorders in children* (pp. 1-27). New York: Thieme.

Catani, M., & ffytche, D. H. (2005). The rises and falls of disconnection syndromes. *Brain, 128,* 2224-2239.

Chapey, R. (2001). *Language intervention strategies in aphasia and related neurogenic communication disorders* (4th ed.). Philadelphia: Lippincott Williams & Wilkins.

Chumpelik (Hayden), D. (1984). The PROMPT system of therapy. In D. Aram (Ed.), *Seminars in Speech and Language, 5,* 139-156.

Clark, H. M. (2003). Neuromuscular treatments for speech and swallowing: A tutorial, *American Journal of Speech-Language Pathology, 12,* 400.

Clement, M., & Twitchell, T. E. (1959). Dysarthria in cerebral palsy. *Journal of Speech and Hearing Disorders, 24,* 118-122.

Crary, M. (1993). *Developmental motor speech disorders.* San Diego, CA: Singular.

Dabul, B. (2000). *Apraxia battery for adults* (2nd ed.). Austin, TX: Pro-Ed.

Darley, F. L. (1967). Lacunae and research approaches to them. In C. Milliken & F. L. Darley (Eds.), *Brain mechanisms underlying speech and language* (pp. 236-240). New York: Grune & Stratton.

Darley, F. L. (1983). Preface. In W. R. Berry (Ed.), *Clinical dysarthria* (pp. xiii-xiv). San Diego, CA: College-Hill Press.

Darley, F. L., Aronson, A. E., & Brown, J. R. (1969a). Differential diagnostic patterns of dysarthria, *Journal of Speech and Hearing Research, 12,* 246-269.

Darley, F. L., Aronson, A. E., & Brown, J. R. (1969b). Clusters of deviant speech dimensions in the dysarthrias, *Journal of Speech and Hearing Research, 12,* 462-496.

Darley, F. L, Aronson, A. E., & Brown, J. R. (1975). *Motor speech disorders.* Philadelphia: W. B. Saunders.

Deal, J. L., & Florance, C. L. (1978). Modification of the eight-step continuum for treatment of apraxia of speech in adults. *Journal of Speech and Hearing Disorders, 43,* 89-95.

Delaney, A. L., & Kent, R. D. (2004, November). *Developmental profiles of children diagnosed with apraxia of speech.* Poster session presented at the Annual Convention of the American Speech-Language-Hearing Association. Philadelphia, PA.

Duffy, J. R. (2003). Apraxia of speech: historical overview and clinical manifestations of the acquired and developmental forms. In L. D. Shriberg & T. F. Campbell (Eds.), *Proceedings of the 2002 Childhood Apraxia of*

Speech Symposium (pp. 3-12). Carlsbad, CA: The Hendrix Foundation.

Duffy, J. R. (2005a). *Motor speech disorders: Substrates, differential diagnosis, and management* (2nd ed.). St. Louis, MO: Elsevier Mosby.

Duffy, J. R. (2005b). Pearls of wisdom—Darley, Aronson, and Brown and the classification of the dysarthrias. *Perspectives on Neurophysiology and Neurogenic Speech and Language Disorders, 15*(3), 22-27.

Duffy, J. R., & Kent, R. D. (2001). Darley's contribution to the understanding, differential diagnosis, and scientific study of the dysarthrias. *Aphasiology, 15*, 275-289.

Duffy, J. R., & Yorkston, K. M. (2003). Medical interventions for spasmodic dysphonia and some related conditions: A systematic review. *Journal of Medical Speech-Language Pathology, 11*, ix.

Dworkin, J. P., & Abkarian, G. G. (1996). Treatment of phonation in a patient with apraxia and dysarthria secondary to severe closed head injury. *Journal of Medical Speech-Language Pathology, 2*, 105-115.

Dworkin, J. P., Abkarian, G. G., & Johns, D. F. (1988). Apraxia of speech: The effectiveness of a treatment regime. *Journal of Speech and Hearing Disorders, 53*, 280-294.

Enderby, P. (1983a). *Frenchay dysarthria assessment*. San Diego, CA: College-Hill Press.

Enderby, P. (1983b). The standardized assessment of dysarthria is possible. In W. R. Berry (Ed.), *Clinical dysarthria* (pp. 109-119). San Diego, CA: College-Hill Press.

Feindel, W. (1999). The beginnings of neurology: Thomas Willis and his circle of friends. In F. C. Rose (Ed.), *A short history of neurology*. Boston: Butterworth Heinemann.

Ferry, P., Hall, S., & Hicks, J. (1975). "Dilapidated" speech: Developmental verbal dyspraxia. *Developmental Medicine and Child Neurology, 17*, 749-756.

Forrest, K., & Weismer, G. (1997). Acoustic analysis of dysarthric speech. In M. R. McNeil (Ed.), *Clinical management of sensorimotor speech disorders* (pp. 63-80). New York: Thieme.

Frattali, C., & Worrall, L. E. (2001). Evidence-based practice: Applying science to the art of clinical care. *Journal of Medical Speech-Language Pathology, 9*, ix.

Freed, D. B., Marshall, R. C., & Frazier, K. E. (1997). Long-term effectiveness of PROMPT treatment in a severely apractic-aphasic speaker. *Aphasiology, 1*, 365-372.

Froeschels, E. A. (1943). A contribution to the pathology and therapy of dysarthria due to certain cerebral lesions. *Journal of Speech Disorders, 8*, 301-321.

Gerratt, B. R., Till, J. A., Rosenbek, J. C., Wertz, R. T., & Boysen, A. E. (1991). Use and perceived value of perceptual and instrumental measures in dysarthria management. In C. A. Moore, K. M. Yorkston, & D. R. Beukelman (Eds.), *Dysarthria and apraxia of speech: Perspectives on management* (pp. 77-93). Baltimore: Paul H. Brookes.

Grewel, F. (1957). Classification of dysarthrias. *Acta Psychiatrica Neurolica Scandinavica, 32*, 325-337.

Guenther, F. H. (1994). A neural network model of speech acquisition and motor equivalent speech production. *Biological Cybernetics, 72*, 43-53.

Guenther F. H., & Perkell, J. S. (2004). A neural model of speech production and its application to studies of the role of auditory feedback in speech. In B. Maassen, R. Kent, H. Peters, P. van Lieshout, & W. Hulstijn (Eds.), *Speech motor control in normal and disordered speech* (pp. 29-49). New York: Oxford University Press.

Guyette, T., & Dietrich, W. (1981). A critical review of developmental apraxia of speech. In N. Lass (Ed.), *Speech and language: Advances in basic research and practice* (Vol. 5, pp. 1-49). New York: Academic Press.

Hadden, W. B. (1891). On certain defects of articulation in children with cases illustrating the results of education of the oral system. *Journal of Mental Science, 37*, 96-105.

Hanson, E. K., Yorkston, K. M., & Beukelman, D. R. (2004). Speech supplementation techniques for dysarthria: A systematic review.

Journal of Medical Speech-Language Pathology, 12, ix.

Hardy, J. C. (1964). Lung function of athetoid and spastic quadriplegic children. *Developmental and Child Neurology, 6,* 378-388.

Hardy, J. (1967). Suggestions for physiologic research in dysarthria. *Cortex, 3,* 128-156.

Head, H. (1926). *Aphasia and kindred disorders of speech.* New York: Macmillan.

Hickman, L. (1997). *Apraxia profile.* San Antonio, TX: Psychological Corporation.

Hiller, H. (1929). A study of speech disorders in Freidreich's ataxia. *Archives of Neurology and Psychiatry, 22,* 75-90.

Hixon, T. J., Hawley, J. L, & Wilson, K. J. (1982). An around-the-house device for the clinical determination of respiratory driving pressure: A note on making the simple even simpler. *Journal of Speech and Hearing Disorders, 47,* 413-415.

Hixon, T. J., & Hoit, J. D. (1998). Physical examination of the diaphragm by the speech-language pathologist. *American Journal of Speech-Language Pathology, 7,* 37-45.

Hixon, T. J., & Hoit, J. D. (1999). Physical examination of the abdominal wall by the speech-language pathologist. *American Journal of Speech-Language Pathology, 8,* 335-346.

Hixon, T. J. & Hoit, J. D. (2000). Physical examination of the rib cage wall by the speech-language pathologist. *American Journal of Speech-Language Pathology, 9,* 179-196.

Hixon, T. J., & Hoit, J. (2005). *Evaluation and management of speech breathing disorders.* Tucson, AZ: Redington Brown.

Hunker, C. J., & Abbs, J. H. (1984). Physiological analysis of parkinsonian tremors in the orofacial system. In M. R. McNeil, J. C. Rosenbek, & A. E. Aronson (Eds), *The dysarthrias: Physiology, acoustics, perception, management* (pp. 69-100). San Diego, CA: College-Hill Press.

Hurst, J. A., Baraister, M., Auger, E., Graham, F., & Norell, S. (1990). An extended family with a dominantly inherited speech disorder. *Developmental Medicine and Child Neurology, 32,* 352-355.

Ingram, T. T. S., & Barn, J. A. (1961). A description and classification of common speech disorders associated with cerebral palsy. *Cerebral Palsy Bulletin, 3,* 57-69.

Irwin, J. (1955). Phonetic equipment of spastic and athetoid children. *Journal of Speech and Hearing Disorders, 20,* 54-57.

Jackson, J. H. (1878). On affectation of speech from disease of the brain. *Brain, 1,* 304-330.

Kaufman, N. (1995). *Kaufman Speech Praxis Test for Children.* Detroit, MI: Wayne State University Press.

Kay Elemetrics. (1993). *Multi-Dimensional Voice Program (MDVP). Computer program.* Pine Brook, NJ: Author.

Kearns, K. P., & Simmons, N. N. (1988). Interobserver reliability and perceptual ratings: more than meets the ear. *Journal of Speech and Hearing Research, 31,* 131.

Kent, R. D. (1996). Hearing and believing: Some limits to the auditory-perceptual assessment of speech and voice disorders. *American Journal of Speech-Language Pathology, 5,* 7-23.

Kent, R. D. (2000). Research on speech motor control and its disorders: A review and prospective. *Journal of Communication Disorders, 33,* 391-428.

Kent, R. D., Kent, J. F., Duffy, J. R., & Weismer, G. (1998). The dysarthrias: Speech-voice profiles, related dysfunctions, and neuropathology. *Journal of Medical Speech-Language Pathology, 6,* 165-211.

Kent, R. D., & Netsell, R. (1978). Articulatory abnormalities in athetoid cerebral palsy. *Journal of Speech and Hearing Disorders, 43,* 353-373.

Kent, R. D., & Rosen, K. (2004). Motor control perspectives on motor speech disorders. In B. Maassen, R. Kent, H. Peters, P. van Lieshout, & W. Hulstijn (Eds.), *Speech motor control in normal and disordered speech* (pp. 285-311). New York: Oxford University Press.

Kent, R. D., Vorperian, H. H., Kent, J.vF., & Duffy, J. R. (2003). Voice dysfunction in dysarthria: Application of the Multi-Dimensional Voice Program™. *Journal of Communication Disorders, 36,* 281-306.

Kent, R. D., Weismer, G., Kent, J. F., & Rosenbek, J. C. (1989). Toward phonetic intelligibility testing in dysarthria, *Journal of Speech and Hearing Disorders, 54,* 482–449.

LaPointe, L. L. (1986). Foreword. In R. Netsell (Ed.), *A neurobiologic view of speech production and the dysarthrias.* San Diego, CA: College-Hill Press.

Liepmann, H. (1913). Motor aphasia, anarthria, and apraxia. *Transaction of the 17th International Congress of Medicine in London,* Section xi, Part 2, 97–106.

Love, R. J. (1992). *Childhood motor speech disability.* New York: Merrill.

Luchsinger, R., & Arnold, G. E. (1965). *Voice-speech-language: Clinical communicology —its physiology and pathology.* Belmon, CA: Wadsworth.

Luria, A. R. (1966). *Higher cortical functions in man.* New York: Basic Books.

Martin, A. D. (1974). Some objections to the term apraxia of speech. *Journal of Speech and Hearing Disorders, 39,* 53–64.

McNeil, M. R. (Ed.). (1997): *Clinical management of sensorimotor speech disorders.* New York: Thieme.

McNeil, M. R., Doyle, P. J., & Wambaugh, J. (2000). Apraxia of speech: a treatable disorder of motor planning and programming. In S. E. Nadeau, L. J. Gonzalez Rothi, & B. Crosson (Eds.), *Aphasia and language: Theory to practice* (pp. 221–266). New York: Guilford Press.

McNeil, M. R., Pratt, S. R., & Fossett, T. R. D. (2004). The differential diagnosis of apraxia of speech. In B. R. Maassen, R. Kent, H. Peters, P. van Lieshout, & W. Hulstijn (Eds.), *Speech motor control in normal and disordered speech* (pp. 389–413). New York: Oxford University Press.

McNeil, M. R., Robin, D. A., & Schmidt, R. A. (1997). Apraxia of speech: definition, differentiation, and treatment. In M. R. McNeil (Ed.), *Clinical management of sensorimotor speech disorders* (pp. 311–344). New York: Thieme.

McNeil, M. R., Rosenbek, J. C., & Aronson, A. E. (1984). *The dysarthrias: Physiology, acoustics, perception, management.* San Diego, CA: College-Hill Press.

Mecham, M. J., Berko, M. J., & Berko, F. G. (1966). *Communication training in childhood brain damage.* Springfield, IL: Charles C. Thomas.

Melo, T. P., Bogousslavsky, J., van Melle, G., & Regli, F. (1992). Pure motor stroke: A reappraisal. *Neurology, 42,* 789–795.

Morley, D. E. (1955). The rehabilitation of adults with dysarthric speech. *Journal of Speech and Hearing Disorders, 20,* 58–64.

Morley, M. E., Court, D., & Miller, H. (1954). Developmental dysarthria. *British Medical Journal, 1,* 8–10.

Morely, M. E., Court, D., Miller, H., & Garside, R. (1955). Delayed speech and developmental aphasia. *British Medical Journal, 2,* 463–467.

Müller, J. Wenning, G. K., Verny, M., McKee, A., Chaudhuri, K. R., Jellinger, K., Poewe, W., & Litvan, I. (2001). Progression of dysarthria and dysphagia in postmortem-confirmed parkinsonian disorders. *Archives of Neurology, 58,* 259–264.

Netsell, R. (1969). Evaluation of velopharyngeal function in dysarthria. *Journal of Speech and Hearing Disorders, 34,* 113–122.

Netsell R. (1984). A neurobiologic view of the dysarthrias. In M. R. McNeil, J. C. Rosenbek, & A. E. Aronson (Eds.), *The dysarthrias: Physiology, acoustics, perception, management* (pp. 1–36). San Diego, CA: College-Hill Press.

Netsell, R. (1986). *A neurobiologic view of speech production and the dysarthrias.* San Diego, CA: College-Hill Press.

Peacher, W. G. (1950). The etiology and differential diagnosis of dysarthria. *Journal of Speech and Hearing Disorders, 15,* 252.

Perkins, W. H. (Ed.). (1983). *Dysarthria and apraxia: Current therapy of communication disorders.* New York: Thieme-Stratton.

Platt, L., Andrews, G., Young, M. & Quinn, P. T. (1980). Dysarthria of adult cerebral palsy: II. Phonemic analysis of articulation errors. *Journal of Speech and Hearing Disorders, 23,* 28–40.

Ramig, L. O., Countryman, S., Thompson, L. L., & Horii, Y. (1995). Comparison of two forms of intensive speech treatment for Parkinson disease. *Journal of Speech and Hearing Research*, *38*, 1232-1251.

Ramig, L. O., Sapir, S., Fox, C., & Countryman, S. (2001a). Changes in vocal loudness following intensive voice treatment (LSVT) in individuals with Parkinson disease: A comparison with untreated patients and normal age-matched controls. *Movement Disorders*, *16*, 79-83.

Ramig, L. O., Countryman, S., Pawlas, A. A., O'Brien, C., Hoehn, M., & Thompson, L. L. (2001b). Intensive voice treatment (LSVT) for individuals with Parkinson's disease: A two year follow up, *Journal of Neurology, Neurosurgery, and Psychiatry*, *71*, 493-498.

Robin, D. A. (1992). Developmental apraxia of speech: Just another motor problem. *American Journal of Speech-Language Pathology*, *1*, 19-22.

Robin, D. A., Solomon, N. P., Moon, J. B., & Folkins, J. W. (1997). Nonspeech assessment of the speech production mechanism. In M. R. McNeil (Ed.), *Clinical management of sensorimotor speech disorders* (pp. 49-52). New York: Thieme.

Rose, F. C. (1999). Three early nineteenth century neurological texts. In F. C. Rose (Ed.), *A short history of neurology*. Boston: Butterworth Heinemann.

Rosenbaum, D. A. (1991). *Human motor control*. San Diego, CA: Academic Press.

Rosenbek, J. C., Kent, R. D., & LaPointe, L. L. (1984). Apraxia of speech: an overview and some perspectives. In J. C. Rosenbek, M. McNeil, & A. E. Aronson (Eds.), *Apraxia of speech: Physiology, acoustics, linguistics, management* (pp. 1-72). San Diego, CA: College-Hill Press.

Rosenbek, J. C., & LaPointe, L. L. (1985). The dysarthrias: Description, diagnosis, and treatment. In D. F. Johns (Ed.), *Clinical management of neurogenic communication disorders* (2nd ed., pp. 97-152). Boston: Little, Brown.

Rosenbek, J. C., Lemme, M. L., Ahern, M. B., Harris, E. H., & Wertz, R. T. (1973). A treatment for apraxia of speech in adults. *Journal of Speech and Hearing Disorders*, *38*, 462-472.

Rosenbek, J. C., McNeil, M. R., & Aronson, A. E. (Eds.). (1984). *Apraxia of speech: Physiology-acoustics-linguistics-management*. San Diego, CA: College-Hill Press.

Rosenbek, J. C., & Wertz, R. T. (1972). A review of 50 cases of developmental apraxia of speech. *Language, Speech, and Hearing Services in Schools*, *16*, 129-131.

Rutherford, B. (1944). A comparative study of loudness, pitch, rate, rhythm, and quality of speech of children handicapped by cerebral palsy. *Journal of Speech and Hearing Disorders*, *9*, 262-271.

Sandyk, R. (1995). Resolution of dysarthria in multiple sclerosis by treatment with weak electromagnetic fields. *International Journal of Neuroscience*, *83*, 81-92.

Schmidt, R. A. (1991). Frequent augmented feedback can degrade learning: Evidence and interpretations. In G. E. Stelmach & J. Requin (Eds.), *Tutorials in motor neuroscience* (pp. 59-75). Dordrecht, The Netherlands: Kluwer.

Schmidt, R. A., & Bjork, R. A. (1996): New conceptualizations of practice: Common principles in three paradigms suggest new concepts for training. In D. A. Robin, K. M. Yorkston, & D. R. Beukelman (Eds.), *Disorders of motor speech: Assessment, treatment, and clinical characterization* (pp. 3-23). Baltimore: Paul H. Brookes.

Sheard, C., Adams, R. D., & Davis, P. J. (1991). Reliability and agreement of ratings of ataxic dysarthric speech samples with varying intelligibility. *Journal of Speech and Hearing Research*, *34*, 285-293.

Shriberg, L. D., Aram, D. M., & Kwiatowski, J. (1997). Developmental apraxia of speech: III. A subtype marked by inappropriate stress. *Journal of Speech, Language, and Hearing Research*, *40*, 313-337.

Shriberg, L. D., Ballard, K. J., Tomblin, J. B., Duffy, J. R., & O'Dell K. H. (2006). Speech, prosody, and voice characteristics of a mother and daughter with a 7;13 translocation affecting FOXP2. *Journal of Speech, Language, and Hearing Research, 49,* 500–525.

Shriberg, L. D., & Campbell, T. F. (Eds.). (2003). *Proceedings of the 2002 Childhood Apraxia of Speech Symposium.* Carlsbad, CA: The Hendrix Foundation.

Singer, R. N. (1980). *Motor learning and human performance: An application to motor skills and movement behaviors.* New York: Macmillan.

Southwood, M. H., & Weismer, G. (1993). Listener judgments of the bizarreness, acceptability, naturalness, and normalcy of the dysarthria associated with amyotrophic lateral sclerosis. *Journal of Medical Speech-Language Pathology, 1,* 151–161.

Spencer, K. A., Yorkston, K. M., & Duffy, J. R (2003). Behavioral management of respiratory/phonatory dysfunction from dysarthria: A flowchart for guidance in clinical decision making. *Journal of Medical Speech-Language Pathology, 11,* xxxix.

Square, P. A. (1999). Treatment of developmental apraxia of speech: tactile-kinesthetic, rhythmic, and gestural approaches. In A. J. Caruso & E. A. Strand (Eds.), *Clinical management of motor speech disorders in children* (pp. 149–185). New York: Thieme.

Strand, E. A. (2001). Darley's contributions to the understanding and diagnosis of developmental apraxia of speech. *Aphasiology, 15,* 291–304.

Strand, E. A., & Skinder, A. (1999). Treatment of developmental apraxia of speech: Integral stimulation methods. In A. J. Caruso & E. A. Strand (Eds.), *Clinical management of motor speech disorders in children* (pp. 109–148). New York: Thieme.

Tikofsky, R. S. (1970). A revised list for the examination of dysarthric single word intelligibility. *Journal of Speech and Hearing Research, 13,* 59–64.

Tikofsky, R. S. (1964). Intelligibility measures of dysarthric speech. *Journal of Speech and Hearing Research, 7,* 325–333.

Traynor, B. J., Codd, M. B., Corr, B., Forde, C., Frost, E., & Hardiman, O. M. (2000). Clinical features of amyotrophic lateral sclerosis according to the El Escorial and Arlie House diagnostic criteria: A population-based study. *Archives of Neurology, 57,* 1171–1176.

van der Merwe, A. (1997). A theoretical framework for the characterization of pathological speech sensorimotor control. In M. R. McNeil (Ed.), *Clinical management of sensorimotor speech disorders* (pp. 1–25). New York: Thieme.

van Mourik, M., Catsman-Berrevoets, C. E., Paquier, P. F., Yousef-Bak, E., & van Dongen, H. R. (1997). Acquired childhood dysarthria: Review of its clinical presentation. *Pediatric Neurology, 17,* 299–307.

Vargha-Khadem, F. (2003). From genes to brain and behavior: The KE family and the FOXP2 gene. In L. D. Shriberg & T. F. Campbell (Eds.), *Proceedings of the 2002 Childhood Apraxia of Speech Symposium* (pp. 27–36). Carlsbad, CA: The Hendrix Foundation.

Vargha-Khadem, F., Watkins, K. E., Price, C. J., Ashburner, J., Alcock, K. J., Connelly, A., et al. (1998). Neural basis of an inherited speech and language disorder. *Proceedings of the National Academy of Sciences USA, 95,* 12695–12700.

Wambaugh, J. L. (2002). A summary of treatments for apraxia of speech and review of replicated approaches. *Seminars in Speech and Language, 23*(4), 293–308.

Wambaugh, J. L. (2004). Stimulus generalization effects of sound production treatment for apraxia of speech. *Journal of Medical Speech Language Pathology, 12,* 77–97.

Wambaugh, J. L., Kalinyak-Fliszar, M. M., West, J. E., & Doyle, P. J. (1998). Effects of treatment for sound errors in apraxia of speech and aphasia, *Journal of Speech, Language, Hearing Research, 41,* 725–743.

Wambaugh, J. L., & Martinez, A. L. (2000). Effects of rate and rhythm control treatment on consonant production accuracy in apraxia of speech. *Aphasiology, 14,* 851–871.

Wambaugh, J. L., Martinez, A. L., McNeil, M. R., & Rogers, M. A. (1999). Sound production treatment for apraxia of speech: Overgeneralization and maintenance effects. *Aphasiology, 13,* 821-837.

Watkins, K. E., Dronkers, N. F., & Vargha-Khadem, F. (2000). Behavioral analysis of an inherited speech and language disorder: Comparison with acquired aphasia. *Brain, 125,* 452-464.

Weismer, G. (2006). Philosophy of research in motor speech disorders. *Clinical Linguistics and Phonetics, 20,* 315-349.

Wepman, J. M., Jones, L., Bock, R. D., & Van Pelt, D. (1960). Studies in aphasia: background and theoretical formulations. *Journal of Speech and Hearing Disorders, 25,* 323-332.

Wepman, J. M., & Van Pelt, D. (1955). A theory of cerebral language disorders based on therapy. *Folia Phoniatrica, 7,* 223-235.

Wertz, R. T., LaPointe, L. L., & Rosenbek, J. C. (1984). *Apraxia of speech in adults: The disorder and its management.* New York: Grune and Stratton.

West, R., Ansberry, M., & Carr, A. (1957). *The rehabilitation of speech.* New York: Harper.

Wolfe, W. G. (1950). A comprehensive evaluation of 50 cases of cerebral palsy. *Journal of Speech and Hearing Disorders, 15,* 234-251.

Workinger, M. S., & Kent, R. D. (1991). Perceptual analysis of the dysarthrias in children with athetoid and spastic cerebral palsy. In C. A. Moore, K. M. Yorkston, & D. R. Beukelman (Eds.), *Dysarthria and apraxia of speech: Perspectives on management* (pp. 109-126). Baltimore: Paul H. Brookes.

York, G. (1999). Hughlings Jackson's evolutionary neurophysiology. In F. C. Rose (Ed.), *A short history of neurology.* Boston: Butterworth Heinemann.

Yorkston, K. M. (1996). Treatment efficacy: Dysarthria. *Journal of Speech and Hearing Research, 39,* S46.

Yorkston, K. M., & Beukelman, D. R. (1981). *Assessment of intelligibility of dysarthric speech.* Tigard, OR: CC Publications.

Yorkston, K. M., & Beukelman, D. R. (1996). *Sentence intelligibility test.* Lincoln, NE: Tice Technology Services.

Yorkston, K. M., Beukelman, D., & Bell, K. (1988). *Clinical management of dysarthric speakers.* San Diego, CA: College-Hill Press.

Yorkston, K. M., Beukelman, D. R., Strand, E. A., & Bell, K. R. (1999). *Management of motor speech disorders in children and adults* (2nd ed.). Austin, TX: Pro-Ed.

Yorkston, K. M., Honsinger, M. J., Mitsuda, P. M., & Hammen, V. (1989). The relationship between speech and swallowing disorders in head-injured patients. *Journal of Head Trauma Rehabilitation, 4,* 1-16.

Yorkston, K. M., Spencer, K. A., & Duffy, J. R. (2003). Behavioral management of respiratory/phonatory dysfunction from dysarthria: A systematic review of the evidence. *Journal of Medical Speech-Language Pathology, 11,* xiii.

Yorkston, K. M., Spencer, K., Duffy, J. R., Beukelman, D., Golper, L. A., & Miller, R. (2001a). Evidence-based practice guidelines for dysarthria: Management of velopharyngeal function. *Journal of Medical Speech-Language Pathology, 9,* 257-274.

Yorkston, K. M., Spencer, K., Duffy, J. R., Beukelman, D., Golper, L. A., Miller, R., Strand, E. A., & Sullivan, M. (2001b). Evidence-based practice guidelines: Application to the field of speech-language pathology, *Journal of Medical Speech-Language Pathology, 9,* 243-256.

Yorkston, K. M., Strand, E. A., & Kennedy, M. R. T. (1996). Comprehensibility of dysarthric speech: Implications for assessment and treatment planning. *American Journal of Speech-Language Pathology, 5,* 55-66.

Yoss, K. A., & Darley, F. L. (1974). Developmental apraxia of speech in children. *Journal of Speech and Hearing Research, 17,* 399-416.

Zentay, P. J. (1937). Motor disorders of the nervous system and their significance for speech. Part I. Cerebral and cerebellar dysarthria. *Laryngoscope, 47,* 147-156.

Zeplin, J., & Kent, R. D. (1996). Reliability of auditory-perceptual scaling of dysarthria. In D. R. Robin, K. M. Yorkston, & D. R. Beukelman (Eds.), *Disorders of motor speech: Recent advances in assessment, treatment, and clinical characterization* (pp. 145–154). Baltimore: Paul H. Brookes.

Ziegler, W. (2003a). Speech motor control is task specific: Evidence from dysarthria and apraxia of speech. *Aphasiology, 17,* 3–36.

Ziegler, W. (2003b). To speak or not to speak: Distinctions between speech and nonspeech motor control. *Aphasiology, 17,* 99–105.

Zyski, B. J., & Weisiger, B. E. (1987). Identification of dysarthria types based on perceptual analysis. *Journal of Communication Disorders, 20,* 367–378.

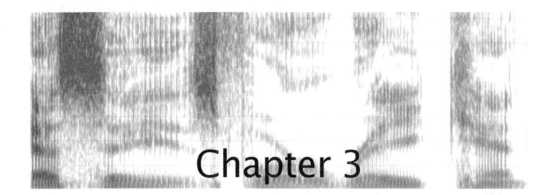

Chapter 3

NEURAL PERSPECTIVES ON MOTOR SPEECH DISORDERS
Current Understanding

Gary Weismer

This chapter presents a neuroanatomic and *functional neurologic* framework for the student of motor speech disorders, but does not present detailed information typically covered in a chapter on the neurologic underpinnings of speech production. For example, material on the anatomy and physiology of neurons, the structure and variation of motor units, and the detailed structure of fiber tracts and nuclei is assumed to be generally familiar or easily accessible to readers. Rather, the focus of this chapter is on a model of sensorimotor structures, pathways, and functions of the brain that can be referenced to the Mayo classification system described in Chapter 2 and summarized below under *Preliminaries*. Students interested in alternative presentations of material on brain mechanisms for speech should consult Duffy (2005, Chapter 2), Kent and Tjaden (1997), and an older text by Kuehn, Lemme, and Baumgartner (1989).

The organization of this chapter is as follows. First, a model of brain structures relevant to sensorimotor control is presented, accompanied by a general discussion of what the term "speech motor control" means in this text. Parts of the model are then taken one at a time and discussed in further detail not only in terms of general structure and function but also with respect to possible pathophysiology and its effect on speech production. Throughout the chapter, components of the traditional speech motor examination are described and discussed.

The Model: A Brief Description

Figure 3–1 is a box-and-arrows diagram of the parts of the brain thought to be involved in sensorimotor control in general,

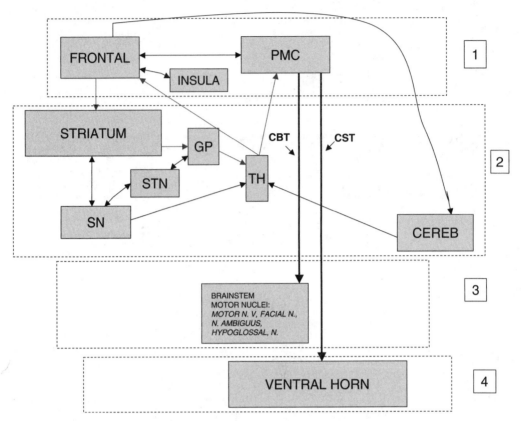

Figure 3–1. Box-and-arrows schematic diagram of central nervous system (CNS) structures involved in sensorimotor control. Section 1 contains cortical structures (PMC = primary motor cortex); Section 2, the basal nuclei and cerebellum (GP = globus pallidus; SN = substantia nigra; STN = subthalamic nucleus; TH = Thalamus; CEREB = cerebellum); Section 3, the brainstem motor nuclei; Section 4, the ventral horn of spinal cord. CBT = corticobulbar tract; CST = corticospinal tract. Single-headed arrows indicate fiber tracts going to the structure where the arrowhead points; double-headed arrows indicate pairs of structures with fiber tracts going in both directions. See text for additional details.

and speech motor control in particular. Two general points about this diagram and its interpretation should be made at the outset of this discussion. First, we use the term *sensori*motor control to designate the likely role of different forms of sensory information in shaping and maintaining "good" motor behavior. The most obvious case for speech is auditory and tactile/proprioceptive information (e.g., in the latter case, tongue-palate contact in the accurate production of certain high vowels and many consonants), but there are other more subtle forms of sensory information that enter into the production of smooth, accurate movements. Second, much of our current information on sensorimotor control is based on studies of limb and hand (paw) movements produced by humans and animals. Knowledge of the precise mechanisms of *speech* motor control lags that of limb motor control—and even orofacial control in animals—precisely because there is no animal model of speech production. Much of what is currently thought to be known about speech motor control, therefore, is inferential, based on "natural" experiments in which humans suffer localized brain damage and have speech production deficits specific to the affected structures. In fact, as reviewed in Chapter 2 and discussed below, this is the conceptual basis of the Mayo Clinic classification system of dysarthria. Knowledge of speech motor control mechanisms is increasing with brain imaging techniques. One of the claims from this work, in its infancy, is that speech motor control mechanisms in the brain are widely distributed across many structures. The possibility of speech production requiring diverse and sometimes unexpected brain mechanisms is reflected by the several cortical mechanisms shown in Figure 3–1. To add to the complication but to make a clinically relevant point, the precise mechanisms involved in speech production may depend on the kind of speech being produced (Blank, Scott, Murphy, Warburton, & Wise, 2002).

It is useful to separate the model into four general sections, as shown by the dashed-line rectangles in Figure 3–1. Sections 1 and 2 include cortical and subcortical structures known to be important to motor control. The cortical "boxes" in the model represent several areas, including the primary motor cortex, the premotor cortex, the supplementary motor area and Broca's area, the latter three gathered in the box labeled "Frontal," and parts of the insular cortex. Not shown among the cortical areas are the primary sensory cortex and Wernicke's area, both of which have

been implicated in some studies as active during speech production. Cells in the primary motor cortex and the premotor cortex receive either direct or indirect connections from the other cortical areas. Primary and premotor cortex send axons to make direct connections to the motor cells in the brainstem and spinal cord. The corticobulbar tract (CBT in Figure 3–1) makes these connections between cortex and brainstem, the corticospinal tract (CST in Figure 3–1) between cortex and spinal cord. These direct connections carry the processed and integrated output of many sources of cortical and subcortical activity. Note also the lack of specification for the hemisphere affiliation of the cortical areas shown in Figure 3–1. It is, of course, well accepted that for most individuals the left hemisphere is dominant for speech and language production and reception, but both hemispheres show activity during speech production as would be expected because many of the muscles of the head and neck receive bilateral innervation (see below) from the cortical primary and premotor areas.

Section 2 of the brain model in Figure 3–1 shows the basal nuclei, the thalamus, the cerebellum, and connections between these structures. The doubled-headed arrows between certain structures indicate information flowing in both directions; these connections are described more fully below. The basal nuclei (often called the basal ganglia) include the caudate and putamen which together constitute the striatum, the substantial nigra, the subthalamic nucleus, and the globus pallidus (other structures not mentioned here are sometimes included as part of the basal nuclei). The thalamus is made up of many nuclei that relay information from several different locations throughout the brain and spinal cord to the cortex; sometimes it is called the main sensory relay for neural signals in transit to the cortex. The thalamus also contains several "motor nuclei" which are described later in this chapter. The cerebellum, a massive, phylogenetically older part of the brain located beneath the cerebral hemispheres and posterior to the brainstem, contains nuclei connected by large fiber tracts to many different parts of the brain.

Section 3 of the model includes nuclei in the brainstem associated with the cranial nerves that innervate head and neck muscles, as well as nuclei for audition. The motor neurons (neuron cell bodies connected to muscle fibers by means of an axon) associated with cranial nerves V (trigeminal), VII (facial), IX (glossopharyngeal), X (vagus), XI (accessory), and XII (hypoglossal), can be considered the final common pathways for motor control. In other words, signals originating in these brainstem motor neurons and conducted via the cranial nerves to muscles represent the combined influences of all cortical, subcortical, and cerebellar processing reflected in the descending input signal delivered to a motor nucleus in the brainstem. Auditory nuclei in the brainstem receive information from the auditory nerve, one of the two divisions of cranial nerve VIII (the other is the vestibular portion, important for balance and orientation in space). Auditory mechanisms are included in our model because they have a prominent role in our definition of speech motor control. In the simplified diagram of Figure 3-1, connections between the brainstem and other structures of the brain, including the cerebellum, subcortical nuclei, and spinal cord, have been omitted.

Finally, section 4 represents spinal motor neurons and their innervation of the muscles of respiration. The cell bodies of these motor neurons are located in the ventral horn of the spinal cord. As in the brainstem, they and the spinal nerves that issue from them can be considered the final common pathway to the muscles of the thorax, diaphragm, and abdomen.

The Model and Speech Motor Control

The model in Figure 3-1 is a schematic representation of the mechanisms involved in motor control in general, and speech motor control in particular. The following question can (and should) be asked, "Is a model of general motor control, based largely on studies of limb and hand behavior sufficient for and appropriate to an understanding of *speech* motor control?" For the purposes of this text, we believe the answer to this question is "no," even though principles of general motor control most certainly apply to aspects of speech motor control. Speech motor control is different from limb motor control because the goals of speech production appear to be the acoustic results of particular vocal tract shapes and changes in those shapes over time. In this conception of speech motor control, consistent with recent research and emerging theories of speech production behavior (e.g., Guenther, Hampson, & Johnson, 1998), the acoustic signal produced by the speech mechanism is part of the motor control process, not separate from it; this is why parts of our model shown in Figure 3-1 contain auditory processing components. As children are learning and refining the acoustic consequences of the changing configurations of the vocal tract they store these associations as a set of expectations, namely, that certain movements will produce certain acoustic consequences. The mature speaker uses this set of expectations as a form of quality control over her speech movements. If there is a mismatch between a movement and the acoustic consequence, some updating of this particular expectation would be required to re-establish the correct relationship. This perspective on the nature of speech motor control also explains why evaluation of the speech mechanism by oromotor, nonverbal tests (e.g., such as generating maximum strength efforts with the lips, jaw, or tongue, or wagging the tongue laterally at maximum speed) has limited application to the understanding of a *speech* motor control deficit: a task with no acoustic output, even if performed by parts of the speech mechanism, is not speech and therefore is subject to different control strategies and potential deficits. The acoustic output of the vocal tract is not the result of speech motor control, it is an integral part of it.

In the remainder of this chapter we consider each section of the model in Figure 3–1 in somewhat more detail, with emphasis on how damage to its components may assist in diagnosis of specific neurologic disease and how it may affect speech motor control. To "build up" the system, we begin with section 4, and work our way "up" the nervous system to the cortex. Because signs and symptoms of different types of neurologic damage are discussed within the framework of the model, some preliminary material is discussed to allow detailed consideration of the model. These preliminaries are standard concepts of neurologic description as available in any basic text on neurologic disease and diagnosis.

Preliminaries

This section presents some general concepts useful to understanding the link between neuroanatomy and neuropathology. These include the notion of *signs and symptoms* of neurologic disease, and the specific differences between upper and lower motor neuron disease. These specific differences, in fact, are mostly defined in terms of unique signs and symptoms. Finally, a brief review of the Mayo Clinic classification system of motor speech disorders is presented, stressing the presumed, underlying neuroanatomic damage associated with each of the categories in the system.

Signs and Symptoms

There is a technical difference between a sign and a symptom of a neurologic disease (or any disease). *Signs* are observable, by visual examination and in some cases through more formal testing. *Symptoms* are complaints made by patients when telling health care professionals about their problem. Signs and symptoms taken together typically constitute the basis for diagnosis of disease. A good example of a neurologic sign that is relevant to the current discussion is the patient who enters an SLP's office with feet widely spaced and a slightly staggering gait. As described below, this is a sign of cerebellar disease. A symptom of cerebellar disease might be the patient's complaint of frequently losing his or her balance without warning.

For the remainder of this chapter the terms signs and symptoms are used interchangeably or jointly, as in, "The signs and symptoms of Parkinson disease are tremor, rigidity, and bradykinesia." This recognizes that certain symptoms may technically become signs when they are observed (e.g., the observation of a sudden loss of balance by a patient with cerebellar disease is technically both a sign and, by the patient's report, a symptom).

Classical Signs of Neurologic Disease

The concept of "classical signs of neurological disease" is central to an understanding of motor speech disorders as categorized within the Mayo classification system. Different neurological diseases are often associated with unique signs and symptoms, the latter most typically based on limb characteristics. For example, when a patient has damage to the fiber tracts connecting cortical cells with motor neurons in either the brainstem or spinal cord, the lesion is said to be in the upper motor neuron (explained in detail immediately below). Patients with this kind of damage often have a group of limb signs/ symptoms that include an excess of tone, overactive reflexes, and weakness. These classical symptoms of upper motor neuron disease, although based on limb characteristics, are used in the Mayo classification system to "explain" the speech characteristics of spastic dysarthria, the kind of dysarthria typically seen in persons with upper motor neuron damage. This is a case, then, where limb motor characteristics are taken as directly applicable to speech motor control. As stated earlier, this is a controversial and unproven aspect of the discipline of motor speech disorders. The concept of "classic" signs/ symptoms of neurologic diseases as based

primarily on limb characteristics should be kept in mind for the remainder of this chapter.

Upper Versus Lower Motor Neuron

The terms *upper* and *lower motor neuron* are used to describe locations of structures within the nervous system, as well as disease types, as in *upper motor neuron disease* or *lower motor neuron disease*. The terms can be explained with reference to the simple schematic diagram in Figure 3–2. This drawing shows boxes with connecting lines, the boxes representing cell groups and the lines representing fiber tracts running between the cell groups. The top two boxes represent motor cells of the cortex in the right and left hemispheres; for the sake of simplicity, we assume these cells to be located in primary motor cortex. The middle two boxes represent motor nuclei in the brainstem, which contain the motor neurons that innervate muscles of the head and neck. The two boxes represent the two sides of the brainstem; all motor nuclei (and sensory nuclei) in the brainstem are paired, with one on the left and the other on the right side. These nuclei, as listed in Figure 3–1 and described below, include the motor nucleus of V, the facial motor nucleus, the nucleus ambiguus, and the hypoglossal nucleus. Finally, the lower two boxes represent the motor neurons in the ventral horn of the spinal cord. These cells send axons to muscles of the limbs and respiratory system, as well as other muscles of the trunk.

The tracts in Figure 3–2 include those that connect cortical motor cells with motor neurons in the spinal cord. This is

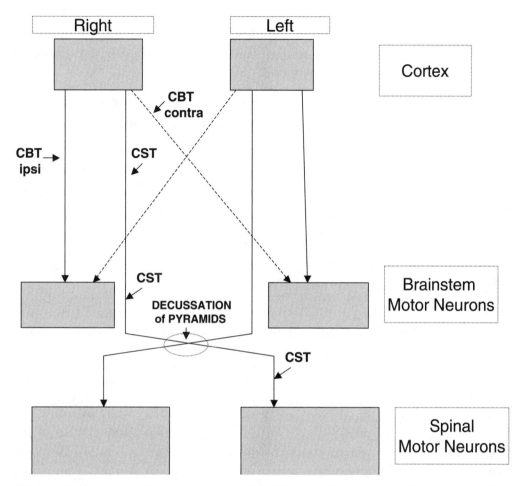

Figure 3–2. Box-and-arrows schematic diagram showing simple way to understand the difference between upper and lower motor neuron. Top two boxes represent cortical cells in primary motor cortex, middle two boxes the brainstem motor neurons, and the bottom two boxes the motor neurons in the ventral horn of the spinal cord. CST is the corticospinal tract, the fibers of which cross from the cortical side in which they begin to the opposite side to make synapses with the motor neurons in the ventral horn; the crossover point is in the lower medulla. A lesion in the cortex where the CST begins or anywhere in the tract before the synapse with the ventral horn motor neurons is an upper motor neuron lesion; a lesion in the ventral horn motor neurons or of the nerves issuing from them to the muscles they innervate is a lower motor neuron lesion. CBT ipsi is part of the corticobulbar tract that runs from one side of the cortex to the same side of the brainstem motor neurons; CBT contra is part of the corticobulbar tract that runs from one side of the cortex to the opposite side of the brainstem motor neurons. A lesion in the cortex or these tracts before the synapse with the brainstem motor neurons is an upper motor neuron lesion; a lesion in the brainstem motor neurons or the nerves issuing from them to the muscles they innervate is a lower motor neuron lesion.

shown in Figure 3–2 by the line labeled CST, which stands for *corticospinal tract*; the line is labeled only on a single side, but it can be seen that the tract runs on both sides of the brain. This tract, which descends from each hemisphere first as the *corona radiata*, is then gathered into a tighter bundle called the *internal capsule*, which enters and passes through the brainstem as the *cerebral peduncles* and eventually forms the columnlike *pyramids* on the ventral surface of the medulla. At the base of the medulla the great majority of fibers from one hemisphere cross over to the other side and continue running down this side of the spinal cord, giving off fibers along the entire length of the cord to the motor neurons in the ventral horn of the central gray matter. The crossover of the corticospinal tracts is indicated in the schematic drawing by the small, dotted line oval placed at the bottom of the brainstem level; the crossover point is called the *decussation of the pyramids*. This contralateral innervation of spinal motor neurons explains why a stroke that damages the left cerebral hemisphere will result in weakness or paralysis of limb muscles on the right side of the body, and vice versa.

With an understanding of how the corticospinal tract connects motor cells in the cortex with those of the spinal cord, the difference between upper and lower motor neuron disease can be explained. When a lesion occurs above a motor neuron in the spinal cord—that is, in the cortex, or anywhere along the corticospinal tract prior to a synapse with a motor neuron—it is called an upper motor neuron lesion. Damage within the motor neuron (in the ventral horn of the spinal cord) or along the peripheral nerve connecting the motor neuron with a muscle is called a lower motor neuron lesion. The diseases produced by such lesions—upper motor neuron versus lower motor neuron disease—produce different sets of symptoms.

Symptoms of Upper Motor Neuron Disease

Upper motor neuron disease is likely to produce any or all of the following signs in muscles of the limbs: spasticity (a form of hypertonia), weakness, and hyperreflexia. In addition, some patients may show emotional lability.

Spasticity

Spasticity describes the characteristics of muscle tone when an examiner asks the patient to relax and then assesses the effects of passive displacement of a limb. For example, if the patient places her arm in front of her, slightly bent with the hand roughly at mid-torso level, the examiner can displace the arm away and toward the body and evaluate how much resistance it offers to the passive motion. A limb with normal tone will offer a small amount of resistance to passive displacement, but a limb with spasticity will offer a great deal of resistance when displaced away from the body, but not toward the body. The resistance to displacement may also be sensitive to the speed of passive displacement, with greater resistance as speed increases. Spasticity is a form of hypertonicity, or abnormally high muscle tone.

Weakness

Weakness needs little description; patients with upper motor neuron disease typically cannot produce strength efforts like those of neurologically healthy persons of comparable age, gender, and general health.

Hyperreflexia

Hyperreflexia implies a heightened sensitivity of certain reflexes. A classic example of hyperreflexia relevant to orofacial mechanisms is the jaw-jerk reflex, elicited by tapping down on the chin while the mandible is slightly open and relaxed. A neurologically healthy individual will either have no obvious response or a very small, upward movement of the mandible in response to the tap. The patient with upper motor neuron disease may have an exaggerated jaw-jerk reflex, seen as a large upward movement of the mandible in response to the tap. Hyperreflexia of the jaw-jerk, together with certain other symptoms (see below) is sometimes used as one of the diagnostic signs for amyotrophic lateral sclerosis (ALS).

Emotional Lability

Emotional lability has been observed in some patients with upper motor neuron disease, especially following strokes that damage the internal capsule. In severe cases, patients may laugh and cry for no apparent reason, and when asked if they are sad (e.g., when crying) deny the feelings. In less severe cases the emotional reaction may be tied to a meaningful situation but may be exaggerated. The reasons for this symptom of upper motor neuron disease, seen in perhaps one quarter of patients who survive stroke and more often in the earlier phases of recovery, are not well understood.

Symptoms of Lower Motor Neuron Disease

Lower motor neuron disease is likely to produce any or all of the following effects in the muscles of the limbs: reduced mus-cle tone (hypotonia), atrophy (wasting), hyporeflexia, weakness, and fasciculations.

Reduced Muscle Tone, or Hypotonicity

This is a symptom revealed when an examiner passively displaces a limb, as described above. In this case, the limb offers an unusually low amount of resistance to passive displacement. In extreme cases a hypotonic limb may appear to offer no resistance to displacement, giving an impression of "floppiness."

Atrophy

Atrophy, sometimes referred to as *wasting*, is the loss of muscle tissue over time. Atrophy is typically not seen in upper motor neuron disease and so can become a distinguishing characteristic between upper and lower motor neuron disease. Atrophy occurs in lower motor neuron disease because the damage to the motor neuron or peripheral nerve interferes with or eliminates the production and transport of nutrients from the nerve cell to the muscle.

Hyporeflexia

This is the condition wherein reflexes observed in neurologically healthy individuals are either reduced in magnitude or completely absent.

Weakness

Weakness is a pervasive feature of lower motor neuron disease.

Fasciculations

Observed on the surface of a muscular structure at rest, fasciculations are small, local muscle twitches. These involuntary contractions of small bundles of muscle fibers create an appearance on a structure's surface of rising and falling bumps. Some fasciculations are normal (as in the common experience of eyelid twitches), but when paired with atrophy and weakness are indicative of lower motor neuron disease. In the speech mechanism, fasciculations are most often observed on the tongue surface of patients with lower motor neuron disease.

The tracts shown in Figure 3–2 also include the pair that connects cortical motor cells with motor nuclei in the brainstem. This is called the *corticobulbar tract* (labeled CBT in Figure 3–2), which first descends from the cortex within the *corona radiata*, is then gathered into a tighter bundle called the *internal capsule*, and enters the brainstem as the *cerebral peduncles,* which give off fibers to motor nuclei. Some of these fibers connect one side of the cortex with the motor nuclei in the brainstem on the opposite side; this *contralateral connection* (CBT-contra in Figure 3–2) is like that of the corticospinal tract, described above. Other fibers connect a side of the cortex with the brainstem motor nuclei on the same side; this is referred to as an *ipsilateral* connection (CBT-ipsi in Figure 3–2). There are many cases in which cells from both sides of the cortex connect to a motor nucleus in the brainstem via both an ipsilateral and contralateral fiber tract. A motor nucleus in the brainstem that receives such connections is said to be *bilaterally innervated* from the cortex. In a few cases, a motor nucleus in the brainstem, or a subset of the cells within a motor nucleus, will receive only contralateral connections via the corticobulbar tract. There are no reports in the literature of a corticobulbar tract having only ipsilat-

eral connections with a paired motor nucleus in the brainstem (but see below, description of Accessory Nucleus and cranial nerve XI). A reasonable summary statement is that the motor nuclei in the brainstem receive either bilateral or contralateral innervation from the cortex, via the corticobulbar tract.

The definition of upper and lower motor neuron lesions for the corticobulbar tract and its target brainstem nuclei can be understood in exactly the same way as described above for the corticospinal tract. An upper motor neuron lesion will be in the corticobulbar tract, prior to the synapse in a motor nucleus of the brainstem; a lower motor neuron lesion will be in the brainstem motor nucleus or the nerve (cranial nerve) issuing from the nucleus to the muscle(s). To a first approximation, the signs and symptoms of upper versus lower motor neuron lesions are as described above, but with the proviso that the evaluation of certain aspects of muscle or structural function in the speech mechanism may be more difficult or complicated than in the limbs.

For example, determination of spasticity requires passive displacement of a structure, an easy task with the limbs but somewhat more challenging even with the more accessible structures of the speech mechanism such as the jaw. Passive displacement of the tongue, vocal folds, and soft palate, at least for the clinical evaluation of spasticity, is clearly not realistic. This is more than an intellectual exercise in the limits of neurologic evaluation because spasticity is often invoked as an explanation of, for example, the strain-strangled voice quality and slow speaking rate of persons with bilateral upper motor neuron lesions—those patients often diagnosed with spastic dysarthria. Very often, the speech-language pathologist will infer a particular neurologic sign from the speech symptoms and knowledge of lesion location. Once again, the student should note the correspondence of this aspect of diagnosis to the conceptual foundations of the Mayo Clinic classification system.

Finally, weakness is a feature of both upper and lower motor neuron disease. The degree of weakness will vary according to the severity of the disease and may not be uniform across the different structures of the speech mechanism. As described below, clinical tests of strength of speech mechanism structures are largely confined to the lips, jaw, and tongue. Many of these tests are evaluated subjectively, as when the patient is asked to push his or her tongue against the inside of the cheek with maximal effort while the examiner offers resistance by pressing against the tongue, on the outside of the cheek. Some strength tests can be implemented with instruments that measure either maximal force or pressure applied by a speech mechanism structure. Whether the tests are subjective or objective, there are two specific cautions about their use in understanding a speech production deficit in a suspected or known motor speech disorder. First, the clinician must be aware that normal speech production requires far less muscular strength than the maximal capabilities of speech mechanism structures. According to several theoretical and experimental estimates, speech requires somewhere between 5 to 20% of the maximal strength capabilities of structures such as the jaw, lips, and tongue (see Bunton & Weismer, 1994). The interpretation of weakness with respect to speech production skills, therefore, must currently be regarded as indeterminate, especially in cases where the weakness is detectable but not profound. Second, the types of orofacial muscular contractions typically used to assess weakness are quite different from the muscular contractions used in speech. Pressing the tongue into the cheek or compressing the lips or closing the jaw with maximal effort are not like the gestures used to create speech. This further complicates the use of this information for understanding the speech production deficit in motor speech disorders.

Mayo Clinic Classification of Motor Speech Disorders

The history and many other aspects of the Mayo classification system were covered in Chapter 2. Students are encouraged to read the original research papers that form the experimental basis of the Mayo classification system (Darley, Aronson, & Brown, 1969a, 1969b). The summary here is meant as a general framework for the student to return to and reflect on as the remainder of the chapter is read. The summary includes some more recent additions and modifications of the original Mayo Clinic classification system.

Flaccid Dysarthria

Associated with lower motor neuron damage, the lesions may be in the motor neurons of the brainstem or spinal cord, in the peripheral nerves leading from those motor neurons to the muscles of the head and neck and respiratory system, or at the neuromuscular junction where the peripheral nerve makes contact with the muscle. Breathiness, hypernasality, and imprecise consonants are among the frequent voice and speech problems noted with this form of dysarthria.

Spastic Dysarthria

Associated with bilateral upper motor neuron damage, the lesions may be anywhere within the corticobulbar or corticospinal tracts, provided they are above the motor neurons. Strained-strangled (stenotic) voice, slow speaking rate, and imprecise consonants are among the "signature" speech and voice abnormalities in this dysarthria.

Ataxic Dysarthria

Associated with damage to the cerebellum or the fiber tracts connecting it to other parts of the brain (in this case, the spinal cord, brainstem, and cerebral hemispheres), ataxic dysarthria is often characterized by harsh voice, prosodic abnormalities including equal and excess stress on multisyllabic words which may contribute to a perceptual impression of scanning speech, and an overall impression of slurred, drunk-sounding speech.

Hypokinetic Dysarthria

Hypokinetic dysarthria is most often associated with Parkinson's disease, in which the neurotransmitter dopamine is depleted in the basal nuclei as a result of cell death in the substantia nigra; hypokinetic dysarthria may also occur in diseases that produce Parkinsonism. Weak voice, possible faster-than-normal speaking rate of an episodic nature (termed "short rushes of speech"), and imprecise consonants are typical speech characteristics of hypokinetic dysarthria.

Hyperkinetic Dysarthria

Associated with damage to one of several structures of the basal nuclei, the nature of hyperkinetic dysarthria may vary according to which basal nuclei structure sustains the lesion. For this reason, it is difficult to list a central group of speech characteristics associated with hyperkinetic dysarthria because they will depend, to some degree, on the nature of the disease process.

Mixed Dysarthria

"Mixed" is a designation for dysarthrias that result from damage to two or more of the areas described above. For example, both upper and lower motor neuron lesions are typical of ALS in fully developed form. The dysarthria in these cases is referred to as a mixed flaccid-spastic type. Another example is multiple sclerosis (MS) in which lesions are typically found in the cerebellum and upper motor neuron. When a dysarthria exists in these cases, it is said to be a mixed spastic-ataxic type. In theory, any of the Mayo categories could be heard as coexisting in the same patient, hence a variety of combination (mixed) dysarthrias can occur.

Unilateral, Upper Motor Neuron Dysarthria

This is a recently documented form of dysarthria involving damage on a single side of the brain, presumably in the corticobulbar tract. At one time it was thought that dysarthria associated with upper motor neuron disease had to involve bilateral lesions. Stated otherwise, unilateral lesions of the corticobulbar tract were not expected to produce dysarthria because of the extensive bilateral innervation of speech mechanism musculature. Based on reviews of a fair number of cases, however, it now seems clear that unilateral upper motor neuron damage can produce dysarthria, albeit of a mild and often temporary kind. Interestingly, as described by Duffy (2005), when this dysarthria is diagnosed, it does not necessarily sound like spastic dysarthria.

Apraxia of Speech

Not regarded as a dysarthria because the disorder is supposed to exist in the absence of muscular weakness or paralysis, apraxia of speech is often thought to be a result of cortical lesions, but the precise location is highly controversial; in some instances apraxia of speech has been claimed to occur with subcortical lesions. The speech characteristics include difficulty initiating speech which may be evident by the patient groping for the correct articulatory posture, slow, effortful articulatory behavior, and exaggerated articulatory difficulty with phonetically complex material. These problems are thought to be a reflection of programming difficulties, wherein the patient cannot plan the articulatory sequence efficiently or correctly even though the execution part of speech production—control over the muscles—appears to be normal.

The major speech characteristics of different types of motor speech disorders are offered as typical characteristics, but these are by no means definitive. Within a given dysarthria type there will be substantial variation in the specific speech characteristics regarded as abnormal, but the *type* may still be recognizable. This is an important distinction for the aspiring and working clinician: it may be possible to group patients as having the same type of dysarthria even when their specific speech characteristics are not the same. This point is made in Chapter 2, that the identification of type of dysarthria is a complex, pattern recognition task that is not very well understood. Moreover, iden-

tification of type of motor speech disorder is not necessarily reliable, even among trained clinicians.

The Model: A Closer Look

Section 4: Spinal Mechanisms

Muscles of respiration are controlled by motor neurons spanning almost the entire length of the spinal cord; these motor neurons are located in the ventral horn of the central gray matter. As shown in Figure 3-3, motor nerves exit the ventral horn and travel as part of the peripheral nervous system to the muscles they innervate. In general, the level of motor neurons within the spinal cord correspond to the level within the torso of the muscle they innervate. For example, many of the accessory muscles of inspiration—those having origins outside the rib cage but insertions on the higher ribs, such as the scalenus group, the sternocleidomastoids, and the pectoralis major and minor muscles—have motor neurons in the cervical (C1–C8) part of the spinal cord. Similarly, the intercostal muscles (external and internal) are innervated from the thoracic parts of the spinal cord (T1–T11), at roughly the same level along the long axis of the torso as the ribs. Muscles of the abdominal wall are mostly innervated from low thoracic and high lumbar portions of the spinal cord (roughly T7–L2). The one remarkable, clinically relevant exception to this is the motor neuron pool that innervates the diaphragm, the massive muscle of inspiration that separates the thorax from the abdomen. The highest point of the domed diaphragm is roughly at the level of the 6th thoracic

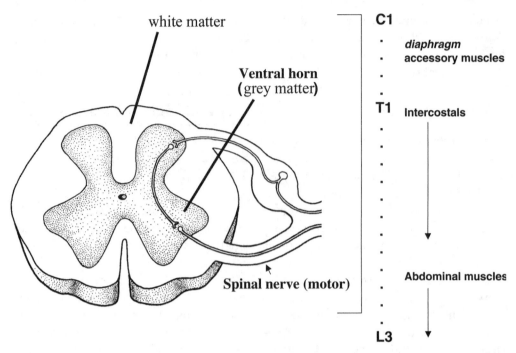

white matter

Ventral horn
(grey matter)

Spinal nerve (motor)

C1
· diaphragm
· accessory muscles
·
·
T1 Intercostals
·
·
·
·
·
·
·
·
·
· **Abdominal muscles**
·
·
L3

Figure 3–3. Drawing of a transverse slice of the spinal cord from a thoracic level, showing white matter (fiber tracts) and central gray matter (cell bodies), the ventral horn of which contains the motor neurons for respiratory muscles. The right side of the figure provides a sketch of the range of spinal segments that innervate respiratory muscles, most notably the innervation of the diaphragm from cervical segments of the cord. See text for additional detail.

vertebra (T6), but its motor neurons are located in the cervical region of the spinal cord, between C3 to C5. Thus, a transection of the spinal cord below C5 will paralyze all the "main" thoracic and abdominal muscles, but will leave the diaphragm intact. Because the diaphragm is a powerful muscle of inspiration, a patient with a spinal transection below C5 will be able to breathe for life without assistance, and will also be able to inflate the lungs for speech production, albeit of a type where voice loudness cannot be maintained throughout an utterance. A spinal transection between C3 and C5 will result in some paresis (weakness) of the diaphragm and such a patient may need some assis-

tance in breathing for life. Obviously, a transection higher than C3 will paralyze the diaphragm and a ventilator will be required to sustain life.

Spinal cord damage involving motor neurons at any level of the spinal cord will result in paresis or paralysis of the affected muscles. Over time, the muscle tissue innervated by the damaged or destroyed motor neurons may atrophy as well. Weakness or paralysis of major inspiratory and expiratory muscles may affect speech breathing. When it does, the patient will have a flaccid dysarthria. The specific effects on speech production of the kind of flaccid dysarthria associated with damage restricted to the spinal cord may include problems with voice loudness and phrasing, and may create difficulty in the production of certain kinds of stress contrast that depend on rapid changes in lung pressure. An excellent presentation of speech breathing problems in cases of spinal cord injury is available in Hixon and Hoit (2005). What follows here is a brief summary of speech breathing manifestations of dysarthria.

Voice Loudness

When a patient has thoracic and abdominal muscle weakness and/or paralysis as a result of damage to spinal motor neurons, voice loudness will generally be insufficient. This is because the loss of muscular ability undermines the patient's ability to make and *sustain throughout an utterance* the muscular contribution required for normal voice intensity. The physiology of normal voice loudness for speech is described in Chapter 4.

Phrasing

Weakness or paralysis of respiratory muscles may result in a reduced number of syllables per utterance. Speech breathing is characterized by quick inspirations to prepare the respiratory system for an utterance. The utterance is produced on expiratory airflow and therefore a decreasing volume of air within the lungs, until the next preparatory inspiration is made. "Phrasing" is a term applied to speech breathing that can have several meanings, one of which is the number of syllables produced during an utterance, that is, during one of the expiratory events whose beginning and ending boundaries are the inspiratory "refills" just described. A reduced number of syllables per utterance may be a result of respiratory muscle weakness because the loss of muscular control makes it difficult to control the pressure developed in the lungs, resulting in utterances that are terminated after an unusually brief duration. The patient's ability to produce only a few syllables per utterance may also result in the termination of utterances at unusual locations—such as within, rather than at the end of a grammatic phrase—that adds to the communication difficulty experienced by both listener and speaker.

Stress Contrasts

Multisyllabic words in English typically have one syllable that is more prominent than the other(s). The prominence of one syllable relative to another is heard by listeners as a stress contrast. Syllable prominence or stress within a word is related to complex speech production events, including changes in fundamental frequency (F_0), vowel duration, vowel quality, and voice loudness. Similarly, speakers often choose to make a word within an utterance more prominent than the other words, to emphasize a point or indicate a contrast with something already spoken or assumed as part of the conversation. This is called sentence stress or prominence, and it is implemented by roughly the same production mechanisms as word stress. The increased loudness associated with prominent/stressed syllables is accomplished by small but rapid increments in lung pressure relative to the overall lung pressure used to produce an utterance. These pressure increments require rapid and precise contraction of expiratory muscles, which may be compromised in cases of respiratory muscle weakness or paralysis resulting from spinal motor neuron damage.

Section 3: Brainstem Mechanisms

Section 3 of the model includes the brainstem nuclei containing the motor neurons and sensory cells associated with muscles of the larynx, pharynx, tongue, velum, jaw, lips, and other facial muscles. These nuclei are located in the pons and medulla and contribute to five cranial nerves that have a motor component. Figure 3–4 shows a schematic diagram of the brainstem, in coronal view. The positions of the paired nuclei are shown, as are the fiber tracts running within the brainstem (shown as dotted-lines) before they exit as cranial nerves. The rough location of the cranial nerve exits from the brainstem are labeled. Also shown is the accessory nucleus, which is located in the upper cervical spinal cord and is the origin of cranial nerve XI. As in the spinal cord, damage to these nuclei or the nerves issuing from them will generally result in paresis or paralysis, and atrophy, of the relevant muscle tissue. Sensory nuclei within the brainstem receive information about touch, proprioception (position of a structure in space), pain, temperature, and of course taste. Here the nuclei are described briefly, followed

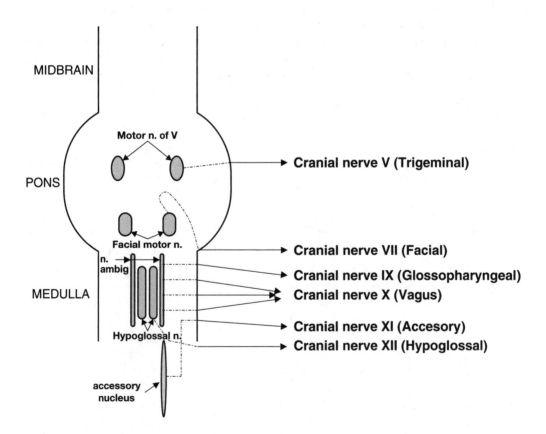

Figure 3–4. Schematic diagram of the location of brainstem and spinal motor nuclei for head and neck musculature, as well as the cranial nerves associated with those nuclei. The view is coronal.

by a brief description and discussion of the cranial nerves typically tested in the speech mechanism examination.

Motor Nucleus of V

The motor nucleus of V is paired (like all the nuclei to be discussed), with one nucleus on each side of the brainstem midline. As depicted in Figure 3-4, the nucleus is an oval-shaped, compact group of cells located approximately midway between the superior and inferior borders of the pons. The input to the motor nucleus of V—the information delivered to it from cortical levels via the corticobulbar tract—is bilateral, meaning that both cerebral hemispheres send fibers to the nucleus on its same and opposite side. Axons from the motor nucleus travel laterally and ventrally (forward) and exit the brainstem approximately at mid-pons level as part of cranial nerve V (trigeminal). Soon after it exits the pons the trigeminal nerve separates into three major divisions—ophthalmic, maxillary, and mandibular—but motor fibers are found only in the mandibular division. The motor fibers innervate the muscles that close and open the mandible, the mylohyoid muscle (floor of the mouth), the tensor veli palatini (a muscle of the velopharynx important for opening the auditory tube), and the tensor tympani (a muscle of the middle ear whose action can damp vibration of the ossicular chain).

Jaw motions during speech have been studied more than other structures of the speech mechanism. This is probably because the jaw is easily accessible for monitoring of motions (unlike, say, the tongue and velum) that are fairly simple for speech (unlike, say, the motions of the tongue). It is widely assumed, and probably for good reason, that unilateral, upper motor neuron damage will not have much or any effect on jaw motions because the motor nuclei of V are innervated bilaterally. It is not known how unilateral, lower motor neuron damage might affect jaw motions for speech.

Evaluation of Motor Integrity of Motor Nucleus of V. Evaluation of the integrity of the motor nucleus of V can be performed using the masseter bulge test. The patient is asked to relax with her mouth closed, and the tester places the index and middle fingers of both hands roughly at the ear lobes of a patient and slowly moves them forward along the side of the face, toward the mouth. As the fingers are moving forward the examiner will reach a point where her fingers move inward, as if a ridge has been reached where the fingers "drop off" toward the midline of the mouth. This ridge is the anterior edge of the masseter muscle, one of the important jaw closers for both mastication and speech. If the fingers are positioned against this ridge and a patient is asked to bite (clench), the masseter muscles will bulge as they shorten, pushing the fingers toward the examiner. It is quite easy to feel this movement in a healthy masseter muscle.

A unilateral, lower motor neuron lesion will result in an asymmetric masseter bulge when the teeth are clenched, with a weak or absent bulge on the affected side and a normal bulge on the healthy side. If both sides have a weak or absent bulge, there is some ambiguity in interpretation because either bilateral lower motor neuron or bilateral upper motor neuron damage could produce this result. One way to resolve the ambiguity of lesion location is to test the jaw-jerk reflex, mentioned above. The normal response is very subtle, and perhaps absent to the naked eye, but in cases of upper motor neuron lesions a strong, upward movement of the mandible will follow the downward tap. This is consistent with the general symptom of hyperexcitable reflexes in upper motor neuron disease. The combination of a hyperexcitable jaw-jerk reflex with observation of fasciculations of the tongue can be diagnostic of ALS, which often has both upper and lower motor neuron damage.

The presence of a unilateral, lower motor neuron lesion can also be evaluated by asking the patient to slowly open her mandible while the clinician offers some resistance to the motion. During the opening motion the jaw will deviate toward the affected side if there is a unilateral lesion of the motor nucleus of V.

Facial Motor Nucleus

The facial motor nucleus is located in the lower pons, slightly more medial than the more superior motor nucleus of V (see Figure 3–4). The nucleus sits approximately halfway between the fourth ventricle (at the posterior border of the pons) and the ventral surface of the pons. Axons emerging from the facial motor nucleus run within the brainstem posteriorly toward the floor of the fourth ventricle (shown for the sake of illustration as an upward course in the schematic of Figure 3–4), loop around the abducens nucleus (associated with cranial nerve VI which supplies motor innervation to muscles of the eye), and then course ventrolaterally to emerge at the junction of the pons and medulla as cranial nerve VII. Cranial nerve VII innervates all muscles of facial expression as well as several other muscles (including the stapedius muscle in the middle ear, the contraction of which is the end product of the acoustic reflex).

The facial motor nucleus receives a fairly complex input from cortical and subcortical parts of the brain. The motor neurons that control muscle fibers from approximately mid-face and up receive bilateral innervation from cortical cells, but motor neurons serving the lower facial muscles receive only contralateral innervation from the cortex. As explained more fully below, this innervation pattern means that a unilateral cortical lesion in the face area is likely to have little effect on upper facial muscles (such as those of the forehead), but will result in weakness and possibly paralysis of the lips and other central/lower facial muscles on the side of the face opposite to the lesion location. The facial motor nucleus also receives complex innervation from parts of the limbic system, which plays a major role in emotional expression. The separation of input to the facial motor nucleus from cortex and limbic system most certainly explains the clinical observation in certain stroke patients whose capacity for facial expressions elicited in emotional situations is at odds with their relative inability to produce volitional manipulation of facial muscles.

The integrity of cranial nerve VII is important in speech production because of the role it plays in control of lip motions and the resulting configurations of the labial orifice. Lip motions are not only important for English consonants such as bilabial stops and labiodental fricatives, but the shaping of the lip orifice—what is often called the rounding-spreading dimension, but is better understood as the area and length of the space between the lips—is crucial to vowel production. This is especially the case in languages where there are vowel contrasts critically dependent on the shape of the lip orifice, such as the /i/-/y/contrast in Swedish (/y/ is very much like an /i/ produced with rounded lips). Here the tongue configuration for the two vowels is essentially identical and the goodness of the articulatory contrast depends on the ability to create a difference in the area of the labial orifice (English does not have these kinds of vowel contrast). To date, there are no studies of labial configuration characteristics for speech in persons with upper or lower motor neuron damage affecting facial muscle control.

Evaluation of Motor Integrity of Facial Motor Nucleus and Cortical Facial Area. There are simple rules for evaluating the integrity of the motor pathways associated with facial muscle control. A unilateral, lower motor neuron lesion will cause *all* ipsilateral muscles of the face to be weak or paralyzed. A lesion in the facial motor nucleus or on cranial nerve VII near its exit from the brainstem will therefore affect all facial muscles from forehead to chin. This will be apparent by viewing the patient's face at rest, where the smoothing of the furrows of the forehead and of the nasolabial fold on the affected side, as well as drooping of the corner of the mouth on the same side, will indicate loss of facial muscle control. This scenario can be contrasted with the case of a unilateral, upper motor neuron lesion, where the primary deficit will only be seen in the central/lower face on the side opposite the lesion. Thus, even though the forehead on the side contralateral to the lesion will be normally furrowed, the nasolabial fold will be smoothed and the corner of the mouth will droop. The apparently normal forehead appearance coupled with a weak or paralyzed lower face is indicative of an upper motor neuron lesion of the side opposite the facial evidence.

There are additional tests for the integrity of facial motor pathways. It is often said, for example, that individuals with unilateral, upper motor neuron lesions will show some asynchrony of the two corners of the mouth when asked to smile voluntarily (with the affected side, opposite the lesion, lagging the lateral movement of the healthy side). These same patients, however, may show symmetric movements when smiling spontaneously. In contrast, patients with unilateral, lower motor neuron damage will present with a deficit on the affected side that will be the same in voluntary and spontaneous smiles. Also, facial muscle weakness can be demonstrated by asking the patient to lift her eyebrows, where marked asymmetry of the gesture indicates weakness on the side with the lower eyebrow; or to have the examiner attempt to open the patient's eyes when the latter forcefully closes them—intact musculature for closing the eyes should prevent the examiner from lifting the eyelid and exposing the eye. Because these are tests of upper-face control, weakness confined to one side would only be expected with an ipsilateral, lower motor neuron lesion. Weakness on both sides of the upper face could indicate either a bilateral lower or upper motor neuron lesion.

A test of central/lower facial control is to ask the patient to forcefully close the lips while the examiner attempts to open them. Any weakness of the relevant muscles should allow the examiner to separate the lips, but a healthy facial motor pathway should allow the patient to maintain lip closure against this effort. A unilateral, upper motor lesion would affect the control of lip muscles on the side opposite the lesion and could reduce the patient's ability to maintain lip closure for this test; the same situation would apply to a unilateral lower motor neuron lesion. Bilateral lesions, either of the lower or upper motor neuron, should clearly weaken the muscles of the central/lower face and prevent the patient from resisting the examiner's attempt to separate the lips.

Nucleus Ambiguus

The nucleus ambiguus is a column of cells running almost the entire length of the medulla (see Figure 3–4). This column of cells is located about midway between the ventral and dorsal surfaces of the brainstem, and somewhat lateral to the midline. Motor neurons in the nucleus ambiguus innervate the constrictor muscles of the pharynx, muscles of the velopharynx (such as the levator veli palatini), intrinsic muscles of the larynx, and a single muscle of the tongue (the palatoglossus, or anterior faucial arch). These motor neurons receive bilateral input from the cortical areas in which the muscles are represented. Motor axons exit the nucleus ambiguus and run more or less laterally and somewhat ventrally within the brainstem until they emerge as a series of rootlets from the lateral aspect of the medulla as parts of cranial nerves IX (glossopharyngeal) and X (vagus). Fibers in cranial nerve IX innervate only one muscle, the stylopharyngeus; the remaining muscles are innervated by cranial nerve X.

Evaluation of the Motor Integrity of the Nucleus Ambiguus and Cranial Nerves IX and X. The motor function of cranial nerves IX and X cannot be evaluated separately because there is no unique test for the stylopharyngeus muscle. Thus, evaluation of the motor function of the two nerves and their common brainstem nucleus is combined. Tests of the integrity of the relevant muscle groups, and by inference cranial nerves IX and X and the nucleus ambiguus, typically focus on the velopharynx and larynx. The weakness or paralysis associated with a unilateral lesion in the nucleus or cranial nerve X would likely produce a breathy voice quality and some hypernasality, depending on the extent of the damage. A suspected, unilateral lower motor neuron lesion involving the nucleus ambiguus/cranial nerve X can also be evaluated by asking the patient to open her mouth and breathe quietly so the position of the relaxed soft palate can be observed. At rest the velum should have a symmetric appearance. When the patient is asked to phonate a vowel, the observable movement of the soft palate and posterior wall of the pharynx—raising of the soft palate and tensing of the pharyngeal muscles—should be symmetrical if there is no damage to the nucleus or nerve. In the case of a unilateral, lower motor neuron lesion, when the patient phonates the soft palate will raise asymmetrically, with higher elevation on the healthy side and the uvula pulled off the midline in the same direction (the same patient may show a similar, but more subtle asymmetry with the velum at rest). Normally the primary muscles of velopharyngeal closure, the levator veli palatini and the superior pharyngeal constrictor, apply equal force on the two sides of the velopharynx and therefore produce symmetric movements around the orifice. A unilateral, lower motor neuron lesion will produce weakness or paralysis of the muscles on the same side, allowing the healthy muscles on the opposite side to "overpower" the affected muscles and pull the structures in the unaffected direction.

The interpretation of a breathy voice quality as a sign of a unilateral, lower motor neuron lesion is more complicated, as are some of the other laryngeal tests for the motor integrity of cranial nerves X and the nucleus ambiguus. Vocal fold vibration is produced by a combination of aerodynamic, mechanical, and muscular forces, the latter being required for overall settings of the larynx but not strictly for the vibration, even if they are desirable for "good" phonation and the full range of phonatory ability (see Chapter 5). In other words, the vocal folds can vibrate in response to aerodynamic and mechanical forces even when the laryngeal muscles are weak or paralyzed, and especially when the muscles on only one side are affected by a unilateral, lower motor neuron lesion. Moreover, the range of "normal" voice qualities is enormous, with some people having breathy qualities in the absence of any known neural pathology. Breathy voice quality as a sign of lower motor neuron disease is probably most reasonable when co-occurring signs (such as hypernasality) are present.

A more direct evaluation of laryngeal muscular integrity is to have the patient cough forcefully or produce a series of staccatolike /i/ sounds, the latter sometimes called laryngeal diadochokinesis. Both tasks require forceful adductory efforts, produced by some combination of the lateral cricoarytenoid, interarytenoid, and vocalis muscles. An inability to produce a sharp cough and "hard" onsets of successive /i/ sounds could indicate a lower motor neuron lesion although there is no way to identify which side the lesion is on (including the possibility of bilateral lesions) unless the vocal folds are imaged with indirect or direct laryngoscopy studies (e.g., stroboscopy, high-speed digital imaging).

Unilateral, upper motor neuron lesions in cell bodies or fiber tracts associated with velopharyngeal and laryngeal musculature will likely produce little effect on resonance or phonation because of the bilateral innervation of the lower motor neurons, described above. As reviewed by Duffy (2005), however, a unilateral upper motor neuron lesion *can* result in phonatory and resonatory effects despite the bilateral innervation. The interested reader is encouraged to read the careful coverage of unilateral, upper motor neuron dysarthria in Duffy (2005) and Chapter 2 of the present text.

Accessory Nucleus

The accessory nucleus is a column of cells in the ventral horn of the upper five or six cervical segments of the spinal cord. These cells give the appearance of a spinal continuation of the nucleus ambiguus (see Figure 3–4), the two nuclei being more or less in line with each other. The accessory nucleus supplies innervation to the sternocleidomastoid and the trapezius muscles. Cortical input to the accessory nucleus is ipsilateral for the motor neurons supplying the sternocleidomastoid muscle, and contralateral for the trapezius muscle.

The accessory nucleus is included here because it is the origin of cranial nerve XI, the accessory nerve. Fibers from the motor neurons of the accessory nucleus exit the spinal cord and ascend along its surface until reaching the level of the medulla where the most caudal fibers of cranial X exit the brainstem (see the dotted-line from the accessory nucleus). There the accessory fibers join with vagus fibers and together (also with cranial nerve IX) they exit the skull and then separate to their respective muscle targets. The main functions of the two muscles innervated by the accessory nucleus and cranial nerve XI are to rotate the head to the side opposite the contracting muscle (sternocleidomastoid) and to elevate the shoulder on the same side of the contracting muscle (trapezius). These muscles are potentially of interest to evaluation of the speech mechanism because both have points of attachment on the clavicle, upper ribs, and sternum and so can function as secondary (accessory) muscles of inspiration. Such muscles do not typically come into use in normal respiration or speech breathing, but may be recruited for deep inspiration during exercise or in cases of spinal cord injury that weaken diaphragmatic mechanisms of inspiration. The standard neurologic tests for the integrity of these muscles are described in many textbooks (see Wilson-Pauwels, Akesson, Stewart, & Spacey, 2002).

Hypoglossal Nucleus

The hypoglossal nucleus is a column of cells running on either side of the midline of the medulla (Figure 3-4). The nucleus is in the posterior part of the medulla with its rostral end in the floor of the fourth ventricle. The motor neurons of the hypoglossal nucleus innervate all intrinsic muscles of the tongue and three extrinsic muscles of the tongue (genioglossus, styloglossus, hyoglossus; recall that palatoglossus is innervated from the nucleus ambiguus via cranial nerve X). Axons from the hypoglossal nucleus first run forward (ventrally) in the medulla; midway between the dorsal and ventral surfaces the fibers bend obliquely to exit the brainstem in a series of rootlets as cranial nerve XII (hypoglossal nerve). The cortical input to the hypoglossal nucleus is primarily bilateral, with the exception of the genioglossus muscle which is innervated contralaterally (left side of cortex innervates

hypoglossal motor neurons on the right side of the medulla, right side of cortex innervates hypoglossal motor neurons on the left side of the medulla).

Evaluation of the Integrity of the Hypoglossal Nucleus and Cranial Nerve XII. The distinction between intrinsic and extrinsic tongue muscles is a long-debated aspect of speech motor control. Some scientists believe the intrinsic muscles play more of a role in shaping the tongue (as in the case of grooving for lingual fricatives) and the extrinsic muscles in positioning the tongue within the vocal tract (as in the position difference between front and back vowels). There is probably more cooperation than strict difference between the two sets of muscles in creating tongue shapes and positions, and this may be reflected in the fact that there are no neurologic evaluations permitting isolated evaluation of intrinsic and extrinsic tongue muscles. Like evaluations of the motor integrity of other cranial nerves, the focus for the tongue is on differentiating upper from lower motor neuron lesions.

If a healthy patient is asked to protrude her tongue it will emerge from the mouth along the midline, without remarkable deviation to either the right or left side. The genioglossus muscle—the paired muscle that inserts along the entire length of the tongue, and is often said to compose its bulk—produces the protrusion motion by applying equal force on its two sides. If one side of the genioglossus muscle is weak because of an upper or lower motor neuron lesion the protruding tongue will deviate markedly to the weak side, pushed that way by the healthy, stronger muscle. Upon seeing such a deviation, the examiner can be reasonably certain there is a neurologic problem but cannot, in the absence of other evidence, pinpoint the location of the lesion. This is because unilateral weakness of the genioglossus could result from two different lesion locations: (1) an ipsilateral, lower motor neuron lesion that affects the hypoglossal nucleus and/or cranial nerve XII, or (2) a contralateral, upper motor neuron lesion affecting the cortical tongue cells or the corticobulbar fibers that run from the cortical tongue area of one hemisphere and cross in the brainstem before terminating in the hypoglossal nucleus on the other side.

For example, a unilateral, lower motor neuron lesion of the left hypoglossal nucleus and a unilateral, upper motor neuron lesion of the cortical tongue area in the right cerebral hemisphere will both result in weakness of the left genioglossus. Both lesion locations, therefore, produce the same sign, a deviation of the protruded tongue to the weak (left) side. What, then, distinguishes a unilateral upper from lower motor neuron lesion of motor neurons and fibers serving the tongue? SLPs and neurologists typically rely on the appearance of the tongue at rest, inside the mouth, where fasciculations and atrophy of one side of the tongue will indicate an ipsilateral lower motor neuron lesion. As described above, upper motor neuron lesions are not typically associated with either of these symptoms. Therefore, a protruded tongue that deviates to the left and shows no atrophy or fasciculations is suggestive of a cortical or cortibulbar tract lesion (upper motor neuron), on the side opposite the deviation.

Lower Motor Neuron Disease and Speech Production

As reviewed above, flaccid dysarthria is typically associated with lower motor neuron disease. Presumably, the weakness and/or paralysis following damage to motor neurons or the peripheral nerves to muscles results in the symptoms of flaccid dysarthria: breathiness because weak adductory forces makes the closing phase of vocal fold vibration relatively less effective; hypernasality as a result of the weak musculature (levator veli palatini, superior constrictor, musculus uvuli) typically involved in closure of the velopharyngeal orifice; and imprecise consonants as a result of weakness of the lingual muscles. Flaccid dysarthria associated with either isolated brainstem damage or specific lesions of peripheral nerves has not been studied as much as some of the other types of dysarthria, so the precise speech production characteristics are not well understood. Moreover, lesions whose effects are restricted to specific parts of the speech mechanism are unusual because the motor nuclei of the brainstem are contained within a very small volume of tissue. Thus, structural damage or deterioration within the brainstem is unlikely to involve a single motor nucleus. One interesting feature of flaccid dysarthria to emerge from the Mayo studies was the absence of speaking rate abnormalities among this group of patients. Certainly some patients with damage to brainstem structures or peripheral nerves will produce abnormally slow speaking rates, but available data do not implicate rate as a major feature of flaccid dysarthria. This would suggest that the slow speaking rates characteristic of some of the other types of dysarthria and in some cases of apraxia of speech cannot be attributed to weakness of speech mechanism structures.

Upper Motor Neuron Disease and Speech Production

Spastic dysarthria has traditionally been associated with bilateral, upper motor neuron lesions. The hypertonicity—specifically the spasticity—of upper motor neuron disease has been thought to contribute to the strain-strangled voice quality (too much adductory force) and perhaps the slow speaking rate observed so often in spastic dysarthria. The role, if any, of hyperexcitable reflexes in the specific speech characteristics of spastic dysarthria is unknown.

Auditory Nuclei

A series of nuclei from the medulla to the thalamus serve as processing and relay points for the delivery of auditory information to the primary auditory cortex, located in the superior and lateral parts of the superior gyrus of the temporal lobe.

Information is delivered to the first of the brainstem nuclei, the cochlear nucleus in the medulla (see Figure 3–5), from the auditory part of cranial nerve VIII. The auditory nerve codes in neural form the frequency and intensity analysis performed by the cochlea. As the coded information travels up the auditory pathway to the cortex a variety of analyses produce the perceptual experiences we know as pitch, loudness, sound localization, sound quality, and sound sequence (that is, the relative simultaneity or sequential nature of multiple auditory stimuli). The relationship between the physical attributes of a signal, such as frequency, intensity, and phase relations, and the just mentioned perceptual characteristics is fairly well understood thanks to the long-established

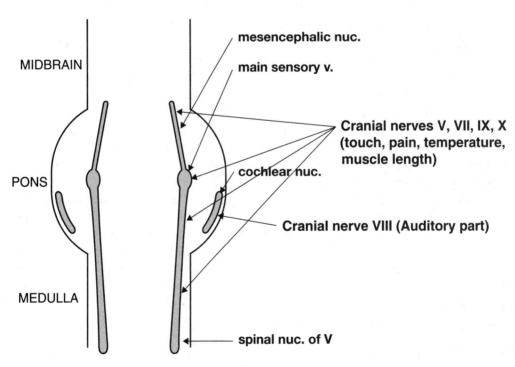

Figure 3–5. Schematic diagram of the location of the cochlear nucleus—the first brainstem structure in the central auditory pathways—and the sensory nucleus of V. See text for additional details.

and productive discipline of psychoacoustics. Moreover, the science of psychoacoustics has been translated into clinical practice; many of its findings form the basis for tests used in diagnostic audiology.

Missing from the above list of auditory analyses is speech. Clearly, analyses along the auditory pathway and in the cortex that yield percepts of pitch, loudness, and quality, are related to the perception of speech. But the discipline of speech perception, which has a history almost as long as that of auditory psychophysics, has not produced definitive explanations concerning the perception of speech and how it might be related to speech production. Standard audiologic evaluations of the speech reception threshold (SRT) or speech discrimination ability may provide some very coarse-grained information on auditory abilities, but these tests are far removed from the phenomena linking speech perception with speech production abilities. For the time being, then, we have to rely on the very gross connection between a patient's general hearing ability and their speech production capabilities. In patients with hearing impairment and no other known neurologic disease, a general expectation is that the more severe the hearing loss the greater the impact on speech production ability. Thus, the speech intelligibility deficits of persons with neuromotor disease and substantial hearing loss, as for example sometimes observed in persons with the athetoid form of cerebral palsy, most likely reflect the combined influence of hearing loss and neuromotor deficits on speech production.

Sensory and Other Brainstem Nuclei

Section 3 of the model as shown in Figure 3–4 does not include sensory nuclei associated with head and neck structures because the focus in clinical evaluation is typically on motor functions. This does not mean that sensory function is unimportant for speech production. Tactile integrity, proprioceptive function, even sensation of air pressures and flows are likely to be important to speech production skill and probably especially so during speech development. Unfortunately, clinical tests for the evaluation of orosensory integrity are controversial, partly because there is no agreement on proper tests or their interpretation. The clinician should know, however, that tactile, pain, temperature, and proprioceptive sensation is processed by the sensory nucleus of the trigeminal nerve, a long, paired nucleus that runs virtually the entire length of the brainstem. This nucleus has three subnuclei, including a top part in the midbrain called the mesencephalic nucleus of V, a middle part in the pons called the main (or primary) sensory nucleus of V, and the bottom part (in the medulla) called the spinal nucleus of V. The nucleus is named for the trigeminal nerve because so much sensory information from the head and neck is carried through the three nerve branches of cranial nerve V. For example, touch sensation from the face and the anterior two-thirds of the tongue is delivered to the brainstem through cranial nerve V. Most of this information projects to the main sensory nucleus of V, in the pons. Other cranial nerves, however, also deliver information on touch, pain, and temperature to the sensory nucleus of V. This includes cranial nerve VII (facial nerve) which carries sensory information from parts of the pinna and the ear-canal side of the tympanic membrane; cranial nerve IX (glossopharyngeal nerve), from the pharynx, the posterior one-third of the tongue, the middle ear side of the tympanic membrane, and some skin around the ear; and cranial nerve X (vagus), from the larynx and external ear.

The sensory nerves and nuclei for audition (just the cochlear nucleus), touch, pain, and temperature are summarized schematically in Figure 3-5. Note how several cranial nerves deliver sensory information to the sensory nucleus of V. An interesting chapter on possible functions and evaluations of the sensory components of the speech mechanism is available in Kent, Martin, and Sufit (1990).

The brainstem also contains nuclei serving other functions in the head and neck region. These nuclei include those that receive taste information and control salivatory and other glandular secretions. The interested student is referred to Wilson-Pauwels et al. (2002) for a more detailed but accessible presentation.

Section 2: Basal Nuclei and Cerebellum

Section 2 of the model includes the several groups of cells in the basal nuclei, the thalamus, and the cerebellum. The schematic diagram in Figure 3-6 shows the interconnections between these structures. These structures are grouped together because of what is presumed to be their joint role in movement planning, initiation, and coordination.

Basal Nuclei

The basal nuclei include the *putamen* and *caudate*, which together are called the *striatum*; the *substantia nigra*, the *globus pallidus*, and the *subthalamic nucleus*. These structures are interconnected in complex ways as shown by connecting

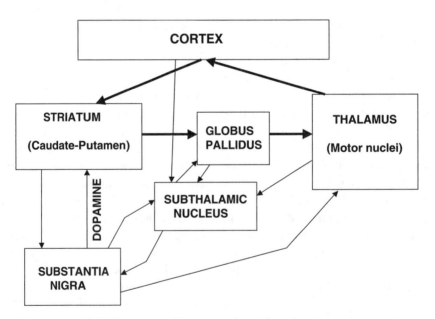

Figure 3–6. Schematic diagram showing the interconnections between basal nuclei structures, and the motor loop between the basal nuclei and cortical structures (the latter shown by the heavy arrows). Note the dopaminergic pathway between the substantia nigra and the striatum.

arrows in Figure 3-6. Many of the structures are connected reciprocally (for example, see the arrows in both directions between the substantia nigra and the striatum). Most importantly, for our purposes, most of the outputs from the basal nuclei converge on the globus pallidus which sends its output to the thalamus. The thalamus then relays this information to motor parts of the cortex (different areas of the cortex are lumped together for this schematic), which as shown in the figure sends the information back to the basal nuclei. Thus, the basal nuclei receive their own, processed output via the globus pallidus→thalamic→cortical→basal nuclei loop. This is shown in Figure 3-6 by the thick lines connecting these structures.

The putamen is thought to be primarily involved with learning and execution of complex movements. The caudate nucleus is believed to have a similar function, but is often implicated in more cognitive aspects of planning and execution of complex movement sequences. Lesions in either the putamen or caudate nucleus will result in movement disorders, which may be accompanied by personality and/or mood disorders. The substantia nigra is found in the midbrain and contains cells that manufacture the neurotransmitter dopamine. Dopamine is transported to the striatum (see the labeled pathway in Figure 3-6) where it plays a critical role in the regulation of movements. To a first approximation, Parkinson's disease has its onset and progression as a result of cell death in the substantia nigra and the ensuing loss of sufficient amounts of dopamine in the striatum.[1] The classic symptoms

of Parkinson's disease are tremor, rigidity (a type of hypertonus, differing from spasticity because the excessive tone is not dependent on the direction of limb movement), and bradykinesia (slowed preparation, initiation, and production of movements). The subthalamic nucleus receives input from the cortex and thalamus, as well as other parts of the basal nuclei, and sends its output primarily to the globus pallidus. The output of the subthalamic nucleus is thought to modulate the activity of the globus pallidus. Because the globus pallidus is the terminal nucleus in the basal nuclei-thalamic-cortical-basal nuclei loop, the subthalamic nucleus may play an important role in shaping the output of the basal nuclei and, therefore, the form of motor behavior. Lesions in the subthalamic nucleus cause choreiform movements (brief, tic- or jerklike movements of the distal extremities [like the fingers] and the face, sometimes resembling fragments of movements but not having a real purpose) and ballism (involuntary, large-scale jerks involving the proximal limbs, sometimes in the form of "throwing" movements). Interestingly, lesions or deep-brain stimulation of the subthalamic nucleus may be used therapeutically to relieve symptoms of Parkinson's disease. Finally, the globus pallidus is, as mentioned above, the main output of the basal nuclei; this output is delivered to the thalamus, which in turn sends the information to motor areas of the cortex. Isolated lesions of the globus pallidus are very rare (Kuoppamäki et al., 2005), but when they have been reported they seem to produce some symptoms like those seen

---

[1]This is an oversimplification of the neurotransmitters that play an important role in the basal nuclei. There are other neurotransmitters of importance, but the scope of this chapter does not permit full coverage of their role in normal and disordered movement. See Kandel, Schwartz, and Jessell (2000) for excellent treatment of neurotransmitters and movement.

in Parkinson's disease. Deep-brain stimulation of the globus pallidus (particularly of the more medial, internal segment) has also been used to relieve symptoms of Parkinson's disease.

Three or four nuclei in the thalamus receive the output of the globus pallidus and send that information to various motor areas of the cortex, such as the supplementary motor cortex, the premotor cortex, and the primary motor cortex. In this way, the basal nuclei are thought to influence motor commands in the descending corticospinal and corticobulbar tracts. Isolated lesions of these thalamic regions—typically referred to in the contemporary literature as the motor thalamus—are rare, but consequences for complex motor behavior can be assumed. Parts of the motor thalamus have also been targets for neurosurgery to relieve the tremor symptoms of Parkinson's disease and other neuromotor disorders.

Symptoms of Basal Nuclei Disease

The concepts of upper versus lower motor neuron disease are not typically applied to signs and symptoms associated with diseases of the basal nuclei. In the older neurologic literature and even in some contemporary writings diseases of the basal nuclei are said to produce *extrapyramidal signs and symptoms*. *Extrapyramidal* refers to structures and lesion effects outside of the *pyramidal tract*, the term used to describe the corticospinal and corticobulbar tracts which form the "direct" pathways from cortex to motor neurons in the spinal cord and brainstem. The basal nuclei have only indirect connection to these "direct" tracts, via the loop described above (Figure 3–6), hence the term extrapyramidal.

There are many symptoms of basal nuclei disease. There are also some predictable effects of basal ganglia disease on speech production. These are summarized here.

Tone. Parkinson's disease is the result of dopamine deficiency in the basal nuclei. One of the classic symptoms of Parkinson's disease is *rigidity*, a form of hypertonus. A rigid limb, when passively displaced, will feel stiff and offer a great deal of resistance to the motion. This high degree of resistance will be felt when the limb is displaced either away from, or into, the body, and is not likely to be sensitive to speed or range of displacement (contrast this with spasticity, another form of hypertonus discussed earlier).

Certain diseases of the basal nuclei may be associated with tone that fluctuates from hyper- to hypotonia. Diseases such as athetosis (one of the categories of cerebral palsy, thought to involve primary damage to the putamen) and Huntington's disease (a genetic disease affecting cells in the striatum—most notable the caudate nucleus) may produce this kind of fluctuating tone.

Dyskinesias. Dyskinesias are impairments of voluntary movement and may be seen in a variety of neurologic diseases and sometimes as a result of treatment of those diseases. Some of the more common dyskinesias include *tics, jerks,* and *dystonias.* The impaired movements may be spasmodic, as in a slow buildup of muscular contraction that is maintained for an unusual amount of time. When this happens, the disorder is called a dystonia. In other cases the impaired movements may be sudden and brief, as in the facial tics of Tourette's syndrome, or jerky and repetitive as in *myoclonus*.

Basal Nuclei Disease and Speech Production. The many diseases of the basal nuclei and their connections may result in a variety of speech symptoms. This discussion is limited to a selected few. In the Mayo classification system, basal nuclei disease may be associated with hypokinetic and hyperkinetic dysarthria, and in cases where there is basal nuclei disease plus damage to other parts of the brain as well, mixed dysarthria. Hypokinetic dysarthria is typically associated with Parkinson's disease, and is often characterized by reduced voice loudness with breathy quality, imprecise consonants which may be a function of a faster-than-normal speaking rate (episodic or chronic), and a general reduction of articulatory gestures. The extent to which these speech symptoms are directly related to, or can be explained by, the triad of classic neurologic signs of the disease—tremor, rigidity, and bradykinesia—is unknown. There seem to be logical links between rigidity and bradykinesia and the speech symptoms of reduced articulatory gestures and voice loudness; after all, it makes sense that stiff muscles would result in smaller-than-normal movements and difficulty initiating and moving speech structures. But the logic of the link shows some weakness when the effects of therapeutic drugs on nonspeech (e.g., limb) and speech symptoms are observed. Drugs meant to supplement dopamine often relieve the classic symptoms of Parkinson's disease, but have little effect on the severity of the hypokinetic dysarthria (for a good review of drug effects on hypokinetic dysarthria, see Schulz, 2002; and Pinto et al., 2004). This suggests a more complex relationship, or perhaps an indeterminate relationship, between the signs and symptoms of Parkinson's disease and the nature of hypokinetic dysarthria.

Hyperkinetic dysarthria is a cover term for dysarthrias associated with a number of basal nuclei structures and may encompass several, unique forms of the speech disorder. A good illustration of the difficulty of relating the classic motor signs of neurologic disease to speech motor symptoms is found in the dysarthria of athetosis, a subtype of cerebral palsy usually associated with damage to the striatum. Athetosis is characterized by slow, writhing movements, often but not exclusively of the hands and feet, and may be accompanied by a related movement disorder called chorea in which rapid, jerky, and often large movements seem to travel across the body with no apparent purpose. When chorea and athetosis occur together the movements are called choreoathetotis. In the case of speech, the random movements of athetosis or choreoathetosis have been thought of as a form of "motor noise" that contribute in an important way to the dysarthria seen in this form of cerebral palsy. Such a view would predict that speakers with the athetoid form of cerebral palsy and dysarthria would, if asked to produce multiple repetitions of a single utterance, have much more variable articulatory behavior than neurologically normal controls. In this view, the random motions of athetosis or choreoathetosis—the motor noise—would create abnormal movement variability on each repetition. Many years ago Neilsen and O'Dwyer (1984) tested this notion by recording electrical activity from speech muscles in a group of adults with the athetoid form of cerebral palsy and in neurologically healthy (control) speakers. Neilsen and O'Dwyer's findings were surprising and provocative: Athough the speakers with athetosis had clearly abnormal muscle activity for repeated utterances, the variability of the muscle activity across repetitions was no greater than observed for the control speakers. Neilsen and O'Dwyer's conclusion was that the random movements and fluctuating tone typically said to be classic signs of athetosis did not explain the speech disorder, or at least not the observed muscle activity of articulators producing speech.

One final observation can be made concerning hyperkinetic dysarthria and its tenuous relationship to underlying pathophysiology. The two most common forms of cerebral palsy—spastic and athetotic—are supposed to have very different underlying pathophysiologies (the characteristics of spasticity have been described above). Yet repeated attempts to demonstrate clear distinctions—that is, different types of dysarthria—between speakers with the two forms of this disease have not proved successful (see Jeng, Weismer, & Kent, 2006). If the link between neurologic signs and symptoms and characteristics of the speech production deficit were clear, the two types of cerebral palsy

should be associated with fairly different types of dysarthria.[2]

Cerebellum

The cerebellum, like the basal nuclei, is part of what we can call a "motor loop." The cerebellar loop is depicted in Figure 3–7. The cortex of the cerebellum sends fibers to a nucleus deep in the cerebellum (dentate nucleus), which then sends a fiber tract via the pons to the motor thalamus, which in turn projects to the motor cortex. The loop is closed by fibers from the motor cortex that are sent back to the cerebellum, via the pons. This loop is thought to be critical in the sequencing of complex movements and in adjusting the forces applied by different muscles and, hence, the scale of motion of structures moved by those muscles. The cerebellar loop also seems to be involved in motor learning, the trial-by-trial adjustments in muscle force and movement sequencing that transform unskilled to skilled behavior.

---

[2]The quest to show differences between the hyperkinetic dysarthria of athetoid cerebral palsy and spastic dysarthria of spastic cerebral palsy is more complicated than space allows us to explore in this chapter. Patients with so-called "pure" forms of the disease are difficult to identify, for one thing, meaning that some studies that have failed to find different dysarthria types between the two forms may simply be reporting data on groups that are not that different neurologically. Because several different studies have failed to find the dysarthria difference between the two types, however, it is safe to conclude that an easy link between neurologic signs and symptoms and specific speech production deficits cannot be made at this time.

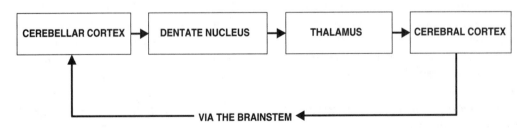

Figure 3–7. Schematic diagram showing the motor loop between the cerebellum and cortex.

Symptoms of Cerebellar Disease

As might be expected, damage to the cerebellum or parts of the cerebellar motor loop result in a disorganization of smooth movement. Muscles are not contracted at the correct times and contractile forces are not scaled appropriately to the needs of the task. Specific neurologic tests of cerebellar disease, which may be associated with strokes, tumors, head injuries, and degenerative conditions, are summarized here.

Tone. When cerebellar disease results in a tone disorder it will typically be in the form of hypotonia. Passive displacement of a limb will create the impression of little resistance, and muscles may feel flabby to the touch.

Weakness. As in most neurologic diseases with a significant motor component, patients with cerebellar disease will not be able to generate much strength and may fatigue easily.

Dysmetria. Patients with cerebellar disease will have problems in the scaling and timing of movements. If asked to point to an object the patient will likely overshoot it and may produce an oscillatory motion around the target. Dysmetria can be shown clearly when the patient is asked to produce a repetitive movement, such as making a repetitive and rhythmic motion with the wrist (typically, a pronating-supinating sequence) or closing and opening the forefinger and thumb with a highly regular pattern. The pattern produced by the patient is likely to appear irregular both in time and space; the motions will appear to lack the smoothly repetitive structure (time) of the neurologically normal person and may vary in amplitude (space) as well, with smaller and larger movements produced across the sequence.

Decomposition of Movement. In cerebellar disease, complex gestures are often broken down into their simple components, giving movements a piece-at-a-time appearance very much at odds with normal movements. The great World War I neurologist Gordon Holmes provided a detailed description of decomposition of movement by observing soldiers with penetrating head injuries to the cerebellum getting out of their field-hospital beds. Neurologically normal individuals typically swing their trunk upright from the bed as they lower their legs to stand, the whole action seeming to be one integrated gesture. In contrast to this, Holmes watched as the injured soldiers moved one leg, then the next, and only rotated their trunks when other required movements for rising from bed were completed. Decomposition of movement gives the appearance of a compensatory strategy, one allowing the patient to accomplish a goal such as getting out of bed without too much jerky movement and incoordination.

Ataxia. The term "ataxia" is often used as a general cover description for the production of clumsy, incoordinated, but purposeful movements; it is also used to designate the staggering, wide-base posture that characterizes walking movements of many persons with cerebellar disease. Reading this, the student may notice that the term "ataxia" seems to encompass the characteristics, summarized above, of dysmetria and decomposition of movement. In fact, Holmes viewed "ataxia" as a cover term for several of the commonly observed motor problems of cerebellar disease, and it is probably best to understand the term in this way.

Cerebellar Disease and Speech Production. Ataxic dysarthria has several prominent characteristics that seem to be consistent with the classic neurologic symptoms of cerebellar disease. For example, patients with ataxic dysarthria are often perceived to have "scanning speech," in which each syllable and possibly each sound seems to be metered out as an independent event, almost as if the smooth flow of speech has been broken apart. In the Mayo studies (Darley, Aronson, & Brown, 1969a, 1969b), excess and equal stress was identified as a common abnormality in patients with cerebellar disease, and it is easy to see how this would contribute to the scanning speech impression. Scanning speech seems to be a speech manifestation of decomposition of movement, wherein the apparently separate sound or syllable events is a simplification of a complex set of movements, perhaps to avoid loss of coordination among the articulators. The drunken-sounding speech and tendency for sudden bursts of voice loudness among persons with ataxic dysarthria seem to reflect the problems in cerebellar disease with control of the scale of motor behavior. Excessive changes in intonation (most notably in the fundamental frequency contour) and sudden increases in voice loudness seem to fit the idea of a motor system that is subject to sudden changes in control.

Section Summary

Section 2 of the model includes two important motor loops, one between the basal nuclei and the cortex, and the other between the cerebellum and the cortex.

Both loops are clearly involved with the selection, planning, and execution of complex movements; both loops almost certainly play a role in the learning of such movements. The involvement of these loops in speech motor control is best exemplified by the effects on speech of lesions to the relevant structures and connections between them.

Section 1: Cortical Mechanisms

Section 1 of the model includes several different areas thought to be involved in either the planning or execution of speech production skills. Traditionally, cortical mechanisms have not been considered relevant to a strict definition of dysarthria.[3] Rather, these mechanisms, and their breakdown as a result of neurologic disease, have more often been associated with aphasia and apraxia of speech. Apaxia of speech, originally (and still, by many: see Hillis et al., 2004) thought to involve lesions in Broca's area, was conceived of as a disorder in which the problem was not in the execution stage of speech production, but in the planning stage. The kinds of neuromuscular control problems seen in dysarthria—paralysis, weakness, incoordination—were thought to be absent in patients with apraxia of speech, or at least not responsible for the disordered speech characteristics. Cortical damage was thought to disrupt a patient's ability to plan articulatory sequences, resulting in hesitations, articulatory gropings, impaired prosody, and disproportionate impairment with increased complexity of an articula-

---

[3]Cortical lesions that result in dysarthria are thought to be rare, but have been reported to occur when small strokes create highly localized lesions in the motor cortex serving face and tongue areas (Kim, Kwon, & Lee, 2003).

tory sequence (such as with the addition of syllables to an utterance or increased articulatory complexity within syllables, such as complicated consonant clusters).

Damage to the face, tongue, and/or laryngeal areas of the primary motor cortex is an upper motor neuron lesion and, therefore, would be expected to result in spastic dysarthria. This expectation is consistent with preliminary evidence that unilateral, upper motor neuron lesions at *any* location along the corticobulbar tract—in the cortex, internal capsule, or cerebral peduncles (the portion of the corticobulbar tract running in the brainstem but above the level of the brainstem motor nuclei)—produces a uniform kind of dysarthria (Urban et al., 2006).[4] Whether or not this same conclusion applies to *bilateral* lesions along the corticobulbar tract is unknown. For now, the notion that bilateral cortical lesions in face/tongue/larynx areas would produce the same kind of dysarthria as bilateral lesions in the internal capsule must be considered a hypothesis, albeit a reasonable one.

In recent years the role of cortical mechanisms in speech production has been re-examined, largely due to a small number of brain imaging studies of both neurologically normal speakers and persons with speech disorders. Many different areas of the cortex, including the SMA, the insula, the postcentral gyrus (primary sensory cortex), and parts of the premotor cortex, have been implicated in speech production skills. In particular, the anterior insular cortex of the left hemisphere has been claimed to be a sort of clearing house for the coordination of the many muscles involved in normal speech production (Ackermann & Riecker, 2004).

If this is so, we would expect lesions of the anterior insula to result in articulatory coordination problems, which would certainly fit with the often assumed presence of coordination difficulties in certain dysarthrias. Interestingly, the insula has also been implicated in apraxia of speech (Dronkers, 1996; but see Hillis et al., 2004, for a different view), which, like certain dysarthrias, has been claimed to have articulatory incoordination as a prominent characteristic (see the review in McNeil, Robin, & Schmidt, 1997). The student should understand that a particular characteristic of speech production, such as incoordination, cannot necessarily be used to differentiate types of dysarthria from one another, or dysarthria from apraxia of speech. The different speech disorders share many characteristics, and there is also some degree of disagreement over the proper diagnosis for some patients. For now, we can say that cortical areas are clearly involved in the production of speech, most likely from the planning to execution stages. Small cortical lesions that produce dysarthrias are likely to resolve quickly, perhaps leaving a mild, residual speech disorder.

Cortical Damage and Speech Production

Presumably, as reviewed above, cortical damage of speech mechanism cells in the primary motor cortex (that is, for the face, tongue, larynx, and so forth) causes a mild dysarthria that often resolves shortly after the onset of the lesion. It is not known how or if these dysarthrias fit into the Mayo system. Damage either in Broca's area, or to the anterior tip of the insular

---

[4]Urban et al. (2006) do not report a *type* of dysarthria among their patients, but simply that the nature of the dysarthria was the same regardless of the lesion location along the corticobulbar tract.

cortex has been claimed to result in apraxia of speech. Patients with apraxia of speech are said to have increasing speech production difficulty with increasing phonetic complexity; this particular observation, in the absence of easily detectable weakness or other classic neurologic signs (such as hypertonicity) has led clinicians to regard apraxia of speech as a programming disorder. The increased speech production difficulty with increasing phonetic complexity occurs, according to this view, because greater phonetic complexity requires greater programming resources. It is not known, however, if speakers with dysarthria might also produce more errors and have more difficulty initiating speech with increasing phonetic complexity.

Summary

This chapter presented information on brain structures and functions, in the context of motor speech disorders and the Mayo classification system. Emphasis was placed on relationships between what certain regions of the brain are thought to do in the control of movement, and how these functions may affect speech. There is a good deal of uncertainty about the precise relations between lesions of specific areas of the brain and their effects on speech, but a working knowledge of the material presented here is critical to an SLP's skill set, especially as a member of a healthcare team treating persons with neurogenic speech disorders. The student should also keep in mind that much of the information on structures and connections in the nervous system has been presented in schematic form. Fortunately, there are excellent, general resources on neuroanatomy, neurophysiology, and neuropathology, some of which are included in the reference list for this chapter.

References

Ackermann, H., & Riecker, A. (2004). The contribution of the insula to motor aspects of speech production: A review and hypothesis. *Brain and Language*, *89*, 320–328.

Blank, S. C., Scott, S. K., Murphy, K., Warburton, E., & Wise, R. J. S. (2002). Speech production: Wernicke, Broca, and beyond. *Brain*, *125*, 1829–1838.

Bunton, K., & Weismer, G. (1994). Evaluation of a reiterant force-impulse task in the tongue. *Journal of Speech and Hearing Research*, *37*, 1020–1031.

Darley, F. L., Aronson, A. E., & Brown, J. R. (1969a). Differential diagnostic patterns of dysarthria. *Journal of Speech and Hearing Research*, *12*, 246–269.

Darley, F. L., Aronson, A. E., & Brown, J. R. (1969b). Clusters of deviant speech dimensions in the dysarthrias. *Journal of Speech and Hearing Research*, *12*, 462–496.

Dronkers, N. F. (1996). A new brain region for coordinating speech articulation. *Nature*, *384*, 159–161.

Duffy, J. R. (2005). *Motor speech disorders* (2nd ed.). St. Louis, MO: Mosby.

Guenther, F. H., Hampson, M., & Johnson, D. (1998). A theoretical investigation of reference frames for the planning of speech movements. *Psychological Review*, *105*, 611–633.

Hillis, A. E., Work, M., Barker, P. B., Jacobs, M. A., Breese, E. L., & Maurer, K. (2004). Re-examining the brain regions crucial for orchestrating speech articulation. *Brain*, *127*, 1479–1487.

Hixon, T. J., & Hoit, J. D. (2005). *Evaluation and management of speech breathing disorders: Principle and methods*. Tucson, AZ: Redington Brown LLC.

Jeng, J-Y., Weismer, G., & Kent, R. D. (2006). Production and perception of Mandarin tone in adults with cerebral palsy. *Clinical Linguistics and Phonetics, 20*, 67-87.

Kandel, E., Schwartz, J. H., & Jessell, T. M. (2000). *Principles of neural science* (4th ed.). New York: Elsevier.

Kent, R. D., Martin, R. E., & Sufit, R. L. (1990). Oral sensation: A review and clinical prospective. In H. Winitz (Ed.), *Human communication and its disorders* (pp. 135-191). Norwood, NJ: Ablex Press.

Kent, R. D., & Tjaden, K. (1997). Brain functions underlying speech. In W. J. Hardcastle & J. Laver (Eds.), *The handbook of phonetic sciences* (pp. 220-255). Oxford, UK: Blackwell Publishers.

Kim, J. S., Kwon, S. U., & Lee, T. G. (2003). Pure dysarthria due to small cortical stroke. *Neurology, 60*, 1178-1180.

Kuehn, D. P., Lemme, M. L., & Baumgartner, J. M. (Eds.) (1989). *Neural bases of speech, hearing, and language.* Boston: College-Hill Press.

Kuoppamäki, M., Rothwell, J. C., Brown, R. G., Quinn, N., Bhatia, K. P., & Jahanshahi, M. (2005). Parkinsonism following bilateral lesions of the globus pallidus: Performance on a variety of motor tasks shows similarities with Parkinson's disease. *Journal of Neurology Neurosurgery and Psychiatry, 76*, 482-490.

McNeil, M. R., Robin, D. A., & Schmidt, R. A. (1997). Apraxia of speech: Definition, differentiation, and treatment. In M. R. McNeil (Ed.), *Clinical management of sensorimotor speech disorders* (pp. 311-344). New York: Thieme.

Neilson, P. D., & O'Dwyer, N. J. (1984). Reproducibility and variability of speech muscle activity in normal and cerebral palsied subjects: EMG findings. *Journal of Speech and Hearing Research, 27*, 502-517.

Pinto, S., Ozsancak, C., Tripoliti, E., Thobois, S., Limousin-Dousey, P., & Auzou, P. (2004). Treatments for dysarthria in Parkinson's disease. *The Lancet: Neurology, 3*, 547-546.

Schulz, G. M. (2002). The effects of speech therapy and pharmacological treatments on voice and speech in Parkinson's disease: A review of the literature. *Journal of Current Medicinal Chemistry, 9*, 1241-1253.

Urban, P. P., Rolke, R., Wicht, S., Keilmann, A., Stoeter, P., Hopf, H. C., & Dieterich, M. (2006). Left-hemispheric dominance for articulation: A prospective study on acute ischaemic dysarthria at different localizations. *Brain, 129*, 767-777.

Wilson-Pauwels, L., Akesson, E. J., Stewart, P. A., & Spacey, S. D. (2002). *Cranial nerves in health and disease* (2nd ed.). Hamilton, Ontario: B. C. Decker.

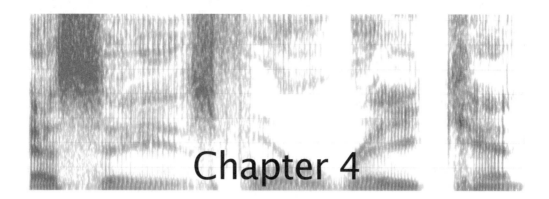

Chapter 4

SPEECH BREATHING IN MOTOR SPEECH DISORDERS

Gary Weismer

*T*his chapter presents information on speech breathing, how it may be disrupted in motor speech disorders, and the potential effects of those disruptions on speech intelligibility and other aspects of communication. An overall goal of this chapter is to show how a relatively simple, noninstrumental assessment of speech breathing in persons with motor speech disorders may suggest behavioral goals with potentially large-scale effects on communication effectiveness.

The speech-language pathologist should have a working knowledge of the physiology of speech breathing and how that knowledge can be exploited to improve a patient's speech production abilities. Therefore, the first part of this chapter presents a brief review of the anatomy and physiology of speech breathing. A brief review of the research literature on speech breathing in speakers with dysarthria follows. This is meant to survey known speech breathing patterns in dysarthria and to place them within a context of problems that can be addressed in a clinical

setting. The third part of the chapter is concerned with the assessment of speech breathing and stresses a noninstrumental approach, one that can be used by any knowledgeable clinician. Finally, some management guidelines are proposed.

Speech Breathing Anatomy and Physiology

Detailed reviews of respiratory structures can be found in Hixon (1973), Hixon and Hoit (2005), and Seikel, King, and Drumright (2000). This section focuses on anatomic knowledge that is directly related to the function of the respiratory system in general and the process of speech breathing in particular. That knowledge includes (1) the elastic nature of respiratory structures and (2) the muscular parts of the respiratory system that can compress or expand air within the lungs, and thus change alveolar (lung) pressures.

Elastic Nature of Respiratory Structures

All structures of the respiratory system, including muscular tissues, bones, and cartilages of the rib cage and pectoral girdle, large membranes (such as the pleural membranes), and other connective tissues, are elastic. This means that, when these structures are not subjected to any external forces, they will assume a rest configuration, depending on their natural properties. When they are subjected to forces that alter the rest configuration—such as stretches or compressions—they will exert a restoring force directed toward that rest configuration. The magnitude of the restoring force will be proportional to the degree to which the structure has been displaced from the rest position.

The properties of elasticity can be appreciated by considering properties of an ordinary mattress spring. If the spring is placed on a surface, as shown in Figure 4–1A, the spring's length can be used as a representation of its rest configuration;

here the spring is not affected by compressing or expanding forces and therefore generates zero force. In Figure 4–1B and 4–1C the spring has been lengthened by two expanding forces, one that stretches it a little away from its rest length (Figure 4–1B) and one that stretches it a lot away from rest (Figure 4–1C). For the purpose of comparison, the spring's rest length is shown immediately above these two stretched conditions. At these new, stretched lengths, the springs generate compressing forces in the direction of the rest length. These are the restoring, or recoil, forces described above. Imagine for a moment that the springs in Figures 4–1B and 4–1C have been stretched by pulling at each end and are being held at the lengths shown in the figure. In this case, the restoring or recoil forces will not produce motion toward the rest length because opposing forces, of equal but opposite magnitude to the recoil forces, are being applied at either end of the stretched spring to hold it at the new length. In Figures 4–1B and 4–1C, the stretching forces

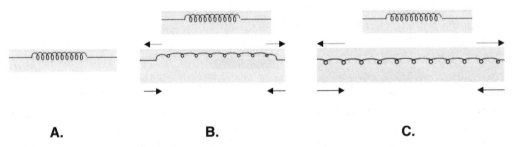

A.   **B.**   **C.**

Figure 4–1. Ordinary mattress springs at rest and at two different degrees (lengths) of stretch. **A.** Spring at rest, no forces applied to it, therefore the spring generates no force. **B.** Spring stretched somewhat relative to rest length (spring at rest length shown above the stretched spring). The dotted arrows above the spring and facing away from the rest length show the direction of force required to hold the spring at the stretched length, the solid arrows below the spring and facing toward the rest length indicate the direction of the recoil force. **C.** Spring stretched from rest length to a greater degree than in (B), arrows interpreted as in (B).

(the forces exerted to hold the spring at the stretched lengths) are shown above the stretched springs as dashed lines ending in outward arrowheads, whereas the recoil forces are shown below the stretched springs by solid lines ending in inward arrowheads.

What happens if the opposing forces are released? The spring will recoil back toward the rest position, and, neglecting any inertial forces for the purposes of this discussion, will stop at the rest position because at this length the spring generates zero force (and hence no motion). If we draw graphs of the compressive recoil force exerted by the spring over time as it changes length from the stretched position to the rest length, the results would look like those shown in Figure 4-2. The graphs on the left and right show how the recoil force of a single spring would change with decreasing length after being released from a relatively smaller stretch (12 cm) and a relatively larger stretch (18 cm), respectively. After a 12-cm stretch (left graph), the force generated by the spring decreases rapidly and becomes increasingly small as the rest length (0 cm on the *x*-axis) is approached. The same pattern is followed when the spring is stretched to 18 cm (right graph), but note the much higher value of force at the beginning of recoil from the 18-cm, as compared to 12-cm, stretch. This is consistent with the statement made above concerning elastic objects: The magnitude of the recoil force

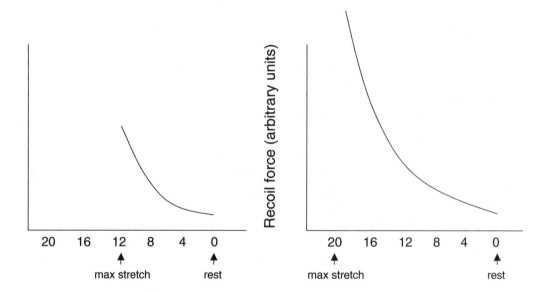

Figure 4–2. Recoil force in arbitrary units (*y*-axis) as a function of spring length (*x*-axis). "0" on the *x*-axis is the rest length, all positive numbers on the *x*-axis are increasing stretches of the spring. Graphs show that the greater the stretch, the greater the recoil force. The left graph corresponds to the lesser degree of stretch as depicted in Figure 4–1B, the right graph to the greater degree of stretch as shown in Figure 4–1C.

will be proportional to the degree to which the structure has been displaced from its rest position.

Exactly the same description of events would apply if the spring was initially compressed from its rest position—that is, made shorter than the rest length. The compression would result in a recoil force exerted in an expanding direction, toward the rest position. Just as in the case of the different magnitudes of stretch shown in Figure 4–2, the greater the initial compression, the greater the recoil force.

These considerations on the nature of elasticity have direct application to the structures of the respiratory system and its use in the production of speech. The elastic nature of the various structures of the respiratory system means that each has a rest configuration, and each will generate a recoil force when that configuration is changed. For example, imagine the lungs removed from the chest cavity and separated from the other structures to which they are normally attached. The spongy, saclike lungs will, if placed on a flat surface, collapse almost completely, to a very small size. Why does this happen? Because this small size is the elastic rest position of the lungs. If we stretch the lung tissue by pumping air into the sacs, the tissue will generate a recoil force proportional to the volume of air pumped in; this recoil force will be directed toward the collapsed rest position.

Now imagine that the pump has inflated the lungs somewhat and there is a passageway between the lungs and atmosphere, via a tube such as the trachea. The end of the trachea can either be shut completely, or opened to allow the free passage of air between the lungs and atmosphere, in either direction. This arrangement is shown in Figure 4–3, where the inward-pointing arrows symbolize the recoil force

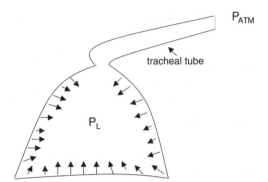

Figure 4–3. Schematic drawing of inflated lungs, generating a recoil force (depicted by the inward directed arrows from the lung walls) to return to the lung rest position. A tube leading to the atmosphere, the trachea, is shown here as closed (dotted line covering the outlet of the tube). See text for additional details.

generated by the stretched lungs and the trachea is shown closed at its outlet by a dotted line. Under these conditions, the air within the lungs (and the tracheal tube) can be considered a closed volume within which air molecules are subjected to the recoil force generated by the stretched lung tissue. The recoil force applied to the closed volume of air effectively decreases the volume by forcing the molecules to be closer together than they were before the force was applied. One of the basic gas laws, *Boyle's law*, states that in a closed volume of air the product of volume and pressure ($P \times V$) is constant (when air temperature is held constant). Thus, if the recoil force results in an effectively smaller volume of air, the air pressure inside the lungs (P_L in Figure 4–3) must be raised above atmospheric pressure (P_{atm} in Figure 4–3) in accordance with Boyle's law. As long as the tracheal outlet remains closed and there are no other forces acting on the air molecules within the lungs,

P_L will remain at the value produced by the recoil force. In this case P_L is said to be a positive pressure, because it is greater than the reference pressure, which is P_{atm}; if P_l was less than P_{atm}, it would be referred to as a negative pressure. The situation is directly analogous to the stretched springs shown in Figure 4–1 which exert a recoil force but are not producing motion because of an equal force exerted in the opposite direction. In Figure 4–3 the opposing force is generated by the closed end and walls of the trachea.

If the tracheal outlet is opened to the atmosphere under the recoil conditions shown in Figure 4–3, air will flow from the lungs to atmosphere as long as the pressure inside the lungs (P_L) exceeds that outside the lungs (P_{atm}). In accordance with our spring model, this will be the case until the lungs recoil back to their rest position; at rest, there will be no pressure difference between P_L and P_{atm} because there is no recoil force to compress the air molecules within the lungs. Air will flow between two locations only when there is a difference in pressure between the locations.

This simple example of how recoil force affects air pressure within the lungs can now be generalized to a more realistic anatomic and physiologic set of conditions. The lungs do not exist as an independent structure within the thoracic cavity, but are tightly connected to the inside of the ribs and the cranial surface of the diaphragm by means of *pleural linkage*. In addition, muscles, ligaments, and other membranes are also directly or indirectly connected to the lung and ribs, so the elasticity of the respiratory system must be considered as reflecting the combined (linked) elastic characteristics of all these structures. It is reasonable to ask, then, what is the elastic rest position of the entire, linked system?

The answer to this question, and its implication for speech breathing, can be discussed with reference to Figure 4–4. The chart in panel 4–4A is a respirometric record of lung volume (*y*-axis) as a function of time (*x*-axis); the record shows three tidal breaths followed by a vital capacity maneuver. The *y*-axis is scaled in percent vital capacity (VC), with 100% reflecting the volume of air that can be exhaled from the lungs following a maximal inhalation and 0% the volume in the lungs after a maximal exhalation. When someone asks, "What lung volume did the patient use to initiate her utterance?" or "What lung volume did the patient reach at the end of rest (tidal) exhalation?" they are asking for the percentage of vital capacity at which an utterance was begun or at which the patient finished their rest breathing cycle. We use this terminology to refer to lung volume events for the remainder of the chapter. In the respirometric record of Figure 4–4, 35% VC has special significance because it is the lung volume corresponding to the end of the rest (tidal) breathing cycle. This is shown clearly in Figure 4–4A by the three tidal breaths each "finishing" at 35% VC. The lung volume at which the tidal breaths "finish"—the end of tidal expiration—is referred to as the *resting expiratory level* (REL) because for most people it is the mechanical rest position of the linked respiratory structures. The choice of an REL of 35% VC for the present example is not at all unusual for young adult persons in the upright posture, but the elastic rest volume may vary somewhat within and across individuals depending on factors such as age, body type, and health status. The important issue here is that the end of rest expiration can be taken as a good estimate of the elastic rest position of the linked respiratory structures.

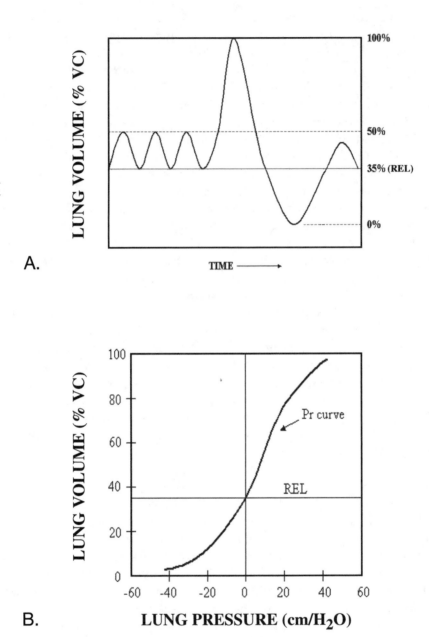

Figure 4–4. A. Spirometric record showing lung volume (percent vital capacity) on the *y*-axis and time on the *x*-axis. Three tidal breaths are shown, followed by a vital capacity maneuver. **B.** Relaxation pressure curve with lung volume shown on the *y*-axis and alveolar pressure on the *x*-axis. "0" pressure on *x*-axis = atmospheric pressure. The curve shows the pressures developed in the lungs solely on the basis of elastic forces generated by respiratory structures. REL = resting expiratory level, or the lung volume at which the elastic properties of the respiratory system are at rest.

If we apply our analogy of the mattress spring to lung volume, REL corresponds to the spring's rest length; lung volumes in excess of REL (>35% VC in Figure 4-4) are like stretches applied to the spring, whereas lung volumes below REL (<35% VC) are like compressions. Following the example presented in Figure 4-1, at lung volumes above REL, the recoil forces exerted by the stretched, linked respiratory structures will be in the compressive direction because the stretched "spring" will attempt to recoil to its smaller, rest position size. In the absence of any other forces applied to the air in the lungs, these compressive recoil forces will raise P_L above P_{atm}. Similarly, at lung volumes below REL, recoil forces exerted by the compressed, linked respiratory structures will be in the expanding direction because the compressed "spring" will attempt to recoil to its larger-sized rest position. When the recoil forces are directed in this expanding direction, the air volume within the lungs is effectively increased and P_L decreased, consistent with Boyle's law. In the absence of other forces and with the tracheal tube open to atmosphere, the negative P_L will result in a flow of air from the atmosphere to the lungs until the increase in lung volume reaches REL.

In 1946, Rahn, Otis, Chadwick, and Fenn performed a famous experiment in which they demonstrated how P_L, resulting *solely* from recoil forces of the respiratory system, varied as a function of lung volume. Participants sat in a chair with a cork in each nostril. Threaded through the middle of one of the corks was a small, hollow tube, the nasal end of which protruded slightly past the cork and into the nasal cavity. The other end of the tube was attached outside the body to a pressure transducer, a device that terminates in a closed chamber and is used to measure air

pressure. A first step in this experiment was the determination by respirometry (Figure 4-4A) of each participant's vital capacity, and based on this value the calculation of percentage increments of VC from 0 to 100% in 5% steps. Each participant breathed into the spirometer to one of these VC increments, took his mouth off the spirometer tube, closed his lips, opened his glottis, and relaxed completely. Under these conditions, the volume of air contained within the lungs, mouth, and nasal cavities could be considered a *closed volume* because no air was moving between the lungs and atmosphere or vice versa. In other words, all pathways between the lungs and atmosphere were blocked (at the lips, nostrils, and in the closed-chamber of the pressure transducer). Moreover, under these conditions any compression or expansion of the air within the closed volume could be assumed to be uniform throughout the entire volume. This is important because the pressure sensed by the tube in the nostril and converted to an electrical signal by the pressure transducer could be regarded as representative of the pressure within the lungs, P_L.

The success of this experiment depended completely on the ability of the participants to relax completely after inhaling or exhaling to a particular increment of lung volume and then closing their lips to prevent air from escaping to the atmosphere. By asking the participants to relax completely, the experimenters were hoping to eliminate any contractile activity among the respiratory muscles—muscles of the neck, thorax, and abdomen—capable of compressing or expanding lung tissue and, hence, air within the lungs. When they made their air pressure measurements, the investigators wanted to be quite certain that the only forces applied to the volume of air within the lungs were those resulting from elastic recoil of respiratory structures. This is a good assumption if a participant is able to "turn off" all respiratory muscles, but how does an experimenter know if this is what a participant has done—if they are truly relaxed? Rahn et al. (1946) reasoned that if a participant produced the same pressure measurement multiple times at a specific increment of lung volume (say, 55% VC), muscular contraction at that volume was highly unlikely. The inference that there was no muscle contraction seemed reasonable because the same pressure reading obtained multiple times at the same lung volume would require exactly the same muscular effort on each of the repeated trials. Because the elastic characteristics of a biological system are not "voluntary," meaning they are not controlled but rather are inherent characteristics of the tissue, it makes sense that in the absence of muscular contraction the same recoil force (and hence the same air pressure within the lungs) would be produced every time the system was stretched or compressed to the same degree. Rahn et al. therefore only used "good relaxers" in their experiment, these being participants who produced reproducible pressures on multiple trials at the same lung volumes. Relaxation pressures were recorded at 5% increments throughout the entire vital capacity range.

Rahn et al. obtained the results shown in Figure 4–4B. This chart is often referred to as a *relaxation pressure curve*, with the plotted pressure symbolized as P_r. P_r is the pressure inside the lung (P_L) due solely to the recoil forces produced by the stretched or compressed respiratory structures. It is called relaxation pressure to signify the absence of muscular forces contributing to the pressure inside the

lungs and to recognize how the data are collected experimentally. In the terminology of respiration, elastic forces and the lung pressures resulting from them are often referred to as *passive* forces and pressures, respectively. Thus, the curve in Figure 4–4B can also be referred to as a *passive lung pressure curve*.

The chart in Figure 4–4B shows %VC on the y-axis and lung pressure (also called alveolar pressure) on the x-axis. Pressure is scaled on the x-axis in two ways, one using the units "centimeters of water" (cm/H_2O) which is typical of much of the classic literature on speech aerodynamics, and the other using the units "kilopascal" (kPa), which is more common in contemporary publications. "Zero" on both scales is equivalent to atmospheric pressure, our reference point for all positive (greater than P_{atm}) and negative (less than P_{atm}) air pressures. P_r data in Figure 4–4B can be summarized in a way that follows directly from the basic concepts of elasticity discussed above. At the elastic rest position (35%VC), the P_r is zero; at lung volumes greater than REL (>35% VC on the chart) P_r is positive with increasing magnitude as lung volume increases. This makes sense because the recoil force developed by a stretched spring is proportional to the degree to which the spring is displaced from the rest length. 80% VC is therefore a greater "stretch" than 60% VC, relative to the rest "length" of 35% VC. Thus, the recoil force (and the lung pressure it causes) should be higher at 80% VC than at 60% VC. Casual examination of the chart suggests this to be the case; the P_r at 80% VC and 60% VC is about 24 cm/H_2O (or 2.353 kPa) and 11 cm/H_2O (or 1.078 kPa), respectively.

The spring-lung volume analogy applies in the same way for lung volumes below REL, where P_r is always negative and becomes more negative as lung volume decreases to lower values. Here the decreasing lung volumes are like greater compressions of a spring relative to its rest length; the greater the compression, the greater the recoil force in the *expanding* direction. Therefore, 10% VC is a greater compression than 30%, a claim that can easily be verified in Figure 4–4B by visual estimation of the more negative P_r values at 10% VC as compared to 30% VC (the actual values are roughly −21 cm/H_2O [or −2.059 kPa] at 10% VC and −3 cm/H_2O [or −0.294 kPa] at 30% VC).

The significance of the relaxation pressure curve to speech breathing can now be made clear by first summarizing the nature of the P_r-lung volume relationship and then introducing two new facts.

Summary of P_r-Lung Volume Relationship

P_r, an air pressure within the lungs resulting solely from elastic (nonmuscular) forces generated by stretched or compressed respiratory structures, varies as a function of lung volume. P_r is zero (atmospheric pressure) at the rest position of the respiratory structures, which typically is located at the lung volume reached at the termination of the expiratory phase of tidal breathing. For most individuals in the upright posture this volume is around 35 to 40% VC and is called REL. For all lung volumes above REL, P_r is positive because the recoil forces are exerted in the compressive direction; increasing lung volume above REL results in increasingly greater P_r values because the recoil forces increase. For all lung volumes below REL, P_r is negative because the recoil forces are in the expanding direction; decreasing lung volume below REL results in increas-

ingly negative P_r values because the recoil forces increase.

Because these pressures are the result of forces generated by the structural characteristics of respiratory anatomy, they can be considered constants of the system. In other words, if an individual participated in an experiment such as the one conducted by Rahn et al. (Figure 4–4B) and was shown to have a P_r value of 10 cm/H_2O (0.981 kPa) at 60% VC, each and every time that individual breathed to 60% VC the pressure generated by the recoil forces would be exactly 10 cm/H_2O. Extending this logic to the entire P_r curve, if P_r was collected for the same individual 10 separate times at 10% increments of lung volume (10, 20, 30 . . . 100% VC) and these points were connected to show a curve such as the one in Figure 4–4B, the curves would be identical—the experimental results would be replicated *exactly*. This follows because these are not controlled, active pressures, but passive pressures resulting from the inherent elasticity of the respiratory structures. The dependency of P_r on lung volume is a key point in the application of respiratory physiology to speech breathing in motor speech disorders, as explained below.

New Fact #1: P_r Can Be Combined with Voluntary (Muscular) Lung Pressures in an Additive Way

The distinction made above between passive and active forces is very important. The fact that individuals do not have control over relaxation pressures means that at a particular lung volume there will always be an elastic force resulting in some value of lung pressure. The elastic forces of respiratory structures, however, are not the only forces available to compress or expand the air volume within the lungs. Muscular forces, generated by inspiratory and expiratory muscles of the thorax, the diaphragm, which is exclusively an inspiratory muscle, and muscles of the abdomen, which are exclusively expiratory, will produce compressions and expansions of the lung tissues, which in turn will affect the volume of air and hence the pressure within the lungs. Just as lung pressures produced by elastic (passive) forces are called relaxation pressures, lung pressures produced by muscular (active) forces are called muscular pressures and are symbolized as P_m. For example, when $P_m = 10$ cm/H_2O (0.981 kPa) at a given lung volume, the muscular mechanisms of the respiratory system are producing compression of the lungs that would result in a P_L of 10 cm/H_2O *independently of whatever P_r exists at that lung volume.* The overall, or net, pressure within the lungs will simply be the sum of the pressure due to elastic forces and the pressure due to muscular forces. More generally, at any point in time (stated otherwise, at any given lung volume) P_L will be the arithmetic sum of pressures due to recoil forces and pressures due to muscular forces. In the Rahn et al. experiment, the investigators "set" the P_m value to zero at every lung volume by requiring their subjects to relax completely. In normal, everyday use of the respiratory system, however, and especially in the case of speech breathing, the pressure generated inside the lung is always the sum of recoil and muscular pressures.

Two worked examples will make the concept of "net lung pressure" clear. Assume a participant exerts an expiratory muscular effort at 60% VC that would cause an increase in P_1 of +5 cm/H_2O.

At 60% VC, the P_r is approximately 10 cm/H_2O (see above, and Figure 4–4B), so the net P_L at this volume is $P_m + P_r = 5$ cm/H_2O + 10 cm/H_2O = 15 cm/H_2O. Now, assume exactly the same muscular effort at 30% VC, where the P_r is -3 cm/H_2O —what is the P_L? The answer is again given by $P_m + P_r = P_L$, or 5 cm/H_2O + (-3 cm/H_2O) = 2 cm/H_2O.

The actual pressure measured in the lungs is always a sum of the relaxation pressures available at a given lung volume and the muscular forces exerted at that volume. Relaxation pressures, of course, are a "fixed" characteristic of the respiratory system, with positive values above REL and negative values below, as explained above. Muscular pressures are more complex, because they may—and in speech production, often do—reflect simultaneous combinations of inspiratory and expiratory muscular effort. For example, if the external intercostals, an important muscle of inspiration that expands the lungs by raising and rotating the ribs outward, exert a muscular pressure of -5 cm/H_2O and the abdominal muscles (all expiratory) exert a muscular pressure of 10 cm/H_2O at a given lung volume, the *net* P_m at that volume will be $(-5) + 10 = 5$ cm/H_2O.

Figure 4–5 summarizes the forces that contribute to the pressure inside the lung. The passive forces are due to the elastic characteristics of respiratory structures, and are lung volume dependent (Figure 4–4B). These combine with whatever forces are exerted by voluntary muscular effort, produced by muscles of the respiratory system. This combination is shown in Figure 4–5, inside the center oval, by the summation of P_r and (P_m). The parentheses around P_m indicate that its value is potentially a net result of simultaneous inspiratory and expiratory muscular effort

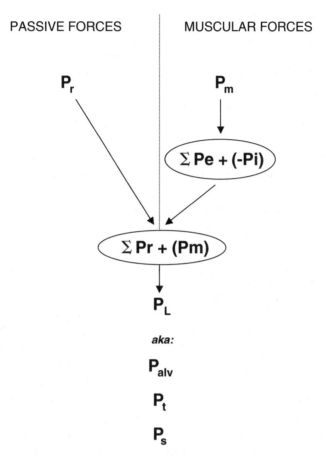

PASSIVE FORCES | MUSCULAR FORCES

P_r

P_m

$\Sigma\, Pe + (\text{-}Pi)$

$\Sigma\, Pr + (Pm)$

P_L

aka:

P_{alv}

P_t

P_s

Figure 4–5. Schematic diagram showing the forces generated by respiratory structures and how they are combined. P_r = relaxation pressure, P_m = muscular pressure. P_r is a nonvoluntary pressure that is lung-volume dependent, as explained in text, and P_m is due to voluntary muscular effort and can reflect the sum of simultaneous expiratory and inspiratory muscular force. At any one point in time (stated otherwise, any point in lung volume), the alveolar pressure is the result of the sum of relaxation and muscular pressures, indicated by the expression in the center oval. For the purposes of this chapter, P_{alv}, P_t, P_L, and P_s are regarded as the same, namely, the pressure measured in the trachea immediately below the vocal folds.

at a given lung volume. This is shown by the summation operator in Figure 4-5 where $P_m = \Sigma\, P_e + (-P_i)$. Moreover, the net outcome of simultaneous inspiratory and expiratory muscular effort may be positive (that is, an overall expiratory muscular pressure) or negative (an overall inspiratory muscular pressure) or, in theory, zero when the magnitudes of P_m and $-P_m$ are the same. This latter point bears emphasis, that at a given lung volume there can be simultaneous expiratory (P_m) and inspiratory ($-P_m$) muscular pressures of the same magnitude which therefore cancel, leaving a net P_m of zero. In this case, only the passive forces at that lung volume contribute to the value of P_L. This concept is important because under these specific conditions P_L is equal to the value of relaxation pressure but the respiratory system is clearly under active muscular control. In fact, this specific set of conditions does occur during certain forms of speech production, such as the sustained vowel tests (e.g., maximum phonation time) so common in speech diagnostic procedures (see below).

The net combination of passive and active pressures, $\sum P_r + (P_m)$, produces the pressure within the lung, to this point called P_L. In Figure 4–5 P_L is given several aliases, including alveolar pressure (P_{alv}), tracheal pressure (P_t), and subglottal pressure (P_s). For our purposes, these terms all mean the same thing, namely, the pressure below the vocal folds. The air spaces including those contained within the lungs and bronchial and tracheal tubes are treated here as a single volume that can be compressed or expanded by the forces described above. For the remainder of this chapter we will adopt the term tracheal pressure (P_t) to denote the lung pressure generated by respiratory forces.

New Fact #2: The Typical P_t Used for Speech Production Is Between 5 and 10 cm/H_2O (0.490-0.980 kPa)

The importance of P_t, of course, is that it is the "power supply" for speech production and furnishes the aerodynamic energy for the creation of different speech sound sources. Among these sound sources, phonation, produced by the vibrating vocal folds, is the most prominent and provides an excellent model of how the pressures developed by the respiratory system are converted to sound energy for speech production. When the appropriate, prephonatory muscular adjustments are made by laryngeal muscles and there is a pressure difference across the larynx, the vocal folds are set into vibratory motion. In the case of vowels, the pressure difference across the larynx is P_t, or the difference between the pressure in the trachea and the pressure immediately above the vocal folds, which is P_{atm} when the vocal tract is open (as it is for vowels). The vibratory motion of the vocal folds will be sustained by aerodynamic and mechanical forces as long as P_t is greater than some minimum value. This minimum P_t value is called the *phonation threshold pressure*, and is typically around 2 cm/H_2O (0.196 kPa) but may be substantially higher at very high fundamental frequencies or when the vocal folds are relatively dry (see Titze, 1994, pp. 102–105). When the vocal folds are set into motion the quasi-periodic vibrations create sound waves that have a spectrum characterized by a fundamental frequency and a consecutive-integer series of harmonics; this acoustic energy serves as the sound source for vowels, semivowels, and voiced consonants.

When people produce conversational speech, they typically generate P_t values of 5 to 10 cm/H_2O. The actual value of P_t for a given utterance will depend on a number of factors, but for our purposes there are two general observations relevant to speech breathing. First, the average value of P_t for an utterance will depend on how loud the speaker wishes to be because there is a relationship between P_t and the sound pressure level (SPL) of voice: the greater the P_t, the greater the voice SPL and, hence, the greater the perceived loudness of the voice. Second, when a speaker produces a multisyllabic phrase the P_t will be more or less constant across the utterance, with rapid rises and falls at the beginning and end of the utterance and perhaps some intrautterance, brief increases in P_t associated with heavily stressed syllables. A typical P_t trace for the first utterance of a well-known reading passage—The Grandfather Passage—is shown schematically in Figure 4-6. The utterance is bounded at its start and end by inhalations, which is why the P_t values are slightly negative before and after the phrase. For this utterance we are assuming emphasis on the word "all." Note the essentially constant P_t value of approximately 7 to 8 cm/H_2O throughout the utterance, with a brief increase for the emphasized word. This figure is meant to emphasize an important axiom of speech breathing: *the task of the respiratory system for speech production is to develop and maintain an essentially constant P_t throughout an utterance.*

The implications of this axiom for speech breathing can now be made clear by studying Figure 4-7. As in Figure 4–4B, this graph shows the relaxation pressure (P_r) curve but now with the pressure labeled P_t (*x*-axis); lung volume (% VC) is on the *y*-axis. An important addition to Figure 4-7 is the vertical dashed line extending along the *y*-axis from approximately 80% VC to 20% VC. This vertical line intersects the P_t axis at only a single point, corresponding roughly to a value of 7 cm/H_2O. Thus, Figure 4-7 shows a constant value of P_t realized over a relatively large range of lung volumes. How is this accomplished by muscular and nonmuscular forces of the respiratory system?

The answer to this question is found in a comparison of the P_r at a given lung volume with what we call the "target" P_t, or the pressure desired for speech production. In the present case the target P_t is 7 cm/H_2O, indicated by the dashed vertical line. Figure 4-7 shows a P_r at approximately 80% VC that is clearly greater than the P_t "target" of 7 cm/H_2O. The P_r at 80% VC (roughly 23 cm/H_2O) is the result of elastic, nonvoluntary forces which must be offset to produce the lower target pressure of 7 cm/H_2O. The solution is to generate a net inspiratory muscular force of approximately −16 cm/H_2O. The overall

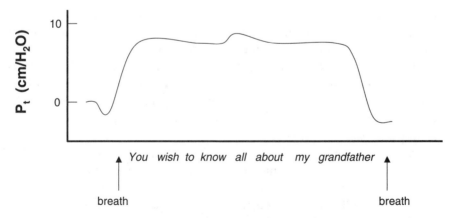

Figure 4–6. Tracheal pressure depicted for the first sentence of "The Grandfather Passage." Note that the pressure is essentially constant across the entire utterance, except for a brief, slight increase on the word "all." See text for additional details.

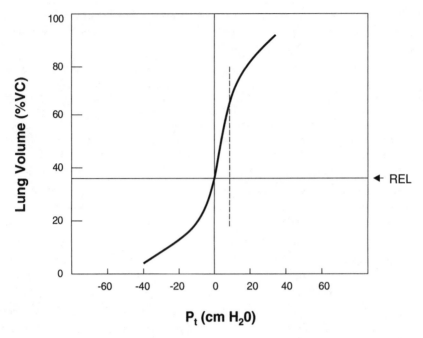

Figure 4–7. Relaxation pressure (P_r) curve but with x-axis labeled as P_t; lung volume (% VC) is on the y-axis. A vertical dashed line extends along the y-axis from approximately 80% VC to 20% VC, intersecting the P_t axis at 7 cm/H_2O. The vertical line is meant to indicate a tracheal pressure that is maintained at 7 cm/H_2O for an utterance produced across the 80 to 20% VC range.

pressure at 80% VC will then be $P_r + (-P_m)$ = P_t, or $23 + (-16) = 7$ cm/H_2O, or the desired target P_t.

This seems simple enough, but the generalization of this logic to other lung volumes shows the complexity of the task of maintaining a constant P_t as lung volume decreases. The pressure available from the elastic characteristics of the respiratory system—the P_r—changes as a function of lung volume, as described above and shown in Figure 4-7. Thus the precise balance between nonmuscular forces and muscular forces required for a constant P_t changes as a function of lung volume. Clearly, the act of speaking involves a constantly decreasing lung volume because air moves from the lungs to

the atmosphere as an utterance is produced. A speaker must constantly adjust the balance of non-muscular and muscular forces as lung volume decreases to achieve a relatively constant P_t for the utterance.

The precise quantitative balance between the two kinds of forces is not of interest here, rather our concern is with more general rules:

1. To achieve a target P_t at a given lung volume, the *amount* of muscular force that must be added to the available P_r is dependent on the difference between the target P_t and the P_r. For example, when the target P_t and the available P_r are fairly similar, as at 60% VC in Figure 4-7, very little net

muscular force will be required to generate the target P_t. Conversely, at 20% VC the difference between target P_t and P_r is quite large, and will require a relatively substantial muscular effort to generate the P_t.

2. The *sign* of the net muscular effort required to achieve a target P_t at a given lung volume depends only on the magnitude of P_r relative to the magnitude of the target P_t. When P_r is greater than the target P_t at a given lung volume, a net inspiratory, or negative muscular effort $(-P_m)$ will be required. For lung volumes where P_r is less than the target P_t, a net expiratory, or positive muscular effort (P_m) will be needed. In those cases where P_r = target P_t—as in Figure 4–7 where the P_r curve crosses the P_t target value, just below 70% VC—the net muscular effort in the respiratory system will be zero, either because there is no muscular effort (i.e., all muscles are relaxed) or because there is inspiratory and expiratory muscular effort of the same magnitude which therefore cancels and results in $P_m = 0$.

These general rules require a few explanatory notes. First, the relationship between P_r and the P_t target is always stated with the qualifier, "at a given lung volume," because the solution to combining forces to achieve a P_t target is dependent on lung volume. The combination of nonmuscular and muscular forces required to achieve a constant P_t changes as lung volume decreases during an utterance, reflecting the changing P_r curve. For example, imagine an utterance such as a sustained vowel starting at 80% VC and continuing to 20% VC, with the P_t shown (i.e., 7 cm/H_2O) in Figure 4–7. Because the P_r is greater than the P_t target at 80% VC,

the utterance would begin with a net inspiratory muscular effort that would decrease smoothly in magnitude until the lung volume is just below 70%, where the P_r curve crosses the target P_t. As the sustained vowel continues below this point, P_r values decrease with lung volume, meaning that increasing amounts of net expiratory muscular effort are required to meet the P_t target. Thus, the task of maintaining a constant P_t as lung volume decreases during speech appears to be one of balancing nonmuscular and muscular forces, the solution depending on a particular lung volume because the available P_r depends on a particular lung volume.

If one thinks about the overall solution of combining nonmuscular and muscular forces to achieve a constant P_t as a series of lung volume-dependent balances, speech breathing seems to be a task of fine motor control, with constant "grading" of muscular effort relative to the volume-dependent P_r. When viewed this way, it is not surprising that persons with dysarthria often have speech breathing problems. From the inability to generate sufficient muscular effort, as sometimes seen in hypokinetic dysarthria, to an inability to control the graded muscular effort required across decreasing lung volume, as may be the case in ataxic dysarthria, the motor control demands of speech breathing present numerous challenges to the speaker with dysarthria.

The final explanatory note is really a reminder of an important fact mentioned in conjunction with Figure 4–5. When describing respiratory muscular effort for speech breathing, the terms "net inspiratory effort" and "net expiratory effort" are used to acknowledge the possibility of simultaneous positive and negative muscular activity. Although this seems counterintuitive, there is experimental evidence of expiratory and inspiratory muscles being active at the same time during vocalization. This seems to be the case especially for tasks where a speaker begins vocalizing at a very high lung volume, where P_r is likely to be greater than the P_t target, and continues vocalizing to lower lung volumes where P_r values are less than the P_t target. Exactly this set of circumstances will occur when a patient is asked to perform the maximum phonation time (MPT) task. The patient is asked to take a maximal inhalation and to phonate until she or he runs out of air. For many patients, the P_t generated for this task is likely to be less than the P_r at very high lung volumes and more than the P_r at very low lung volumes, as described above. When the lung volume is reached where $P_r = P_t$, the respiratory system is still controlled by positive and negative muscular forces which have been gradually changing their magnitudes from the beginning of the task. At the outset of the task there is much greater inspiratory, as compared to expiratory, muscular effort. The balance between the opposing muscular forces is gradually changed as the lung volume where $P_r = P_t$ is approached, but the muscles are never "turned off." During speech breathing, therefore, the respiratory system is never controlled exclusively by nonmuscular forces even though muscular forces may cancel each other out; the presence of these muscular forces is still evidence of active control of the respiratory system for speech.

Why Clinicians Should Know About Efficient Lung Volume Usage for Speech

The preceding discussion leads to the clinically important claim of an *efficient lung volume range for speech production*, and

by implication ranges of lung volume that are not very efficient. This idea has a simple, intuitive appeal: to the extent possible, when generating a target P_t, take advantage of nonmuscular forces and minimize the necessity of muscular forces. With typical P_ts for speech between 5 and 10 cm/H_2O, the most efficient lung volume range would be the one where the P_rs are best matched to these typical P_t values. If a target P_t of 7 cm/H_2O is assumed, a starting lung volume of approximately 60% VC would match the P_r very well to the pressure needs at the onset of the utterance. As the utterance proceeds and lung volume decreases, P_r will decrease and a steadily increasing magnitude of net expiratory muscular effort will be required to achieve a constant P_t. The magnitude of the net expiratory muscular effort will not be too great, however, if a relatively restricted lung volume range is used for utterances. This is illustrated in Figure 4-8, which replots Figure 4-7 but now includes a shaded area extending from about 60% VC to REL. The shaded area indicates the magnitude of muscular effort required to produce the P_t of 7 cm/H_2O. Within this lung volume range, the magnitude of net muscular effort required to achieve a P_t of 7 cm/H_2O never exceeds +7 cm/H_2O; thus, if a speaker begins at 60% VC, talks down to about 35 to 40% VC and then refills the lungs to the same starting lung volume for the next utterance, she will never have to expend much muscular effort to generate an adequate P_t for conversational speech loudness.

Why are other lung volume ranges less efficient than the one shown in Figure 4-8? Could it not be argued that beginning speech at very high lung volumes and continuing to speak well past REL, into low lung volumes, would maximize a speaker's ability to transmit information in a timely manner? From the speaker's perspective,

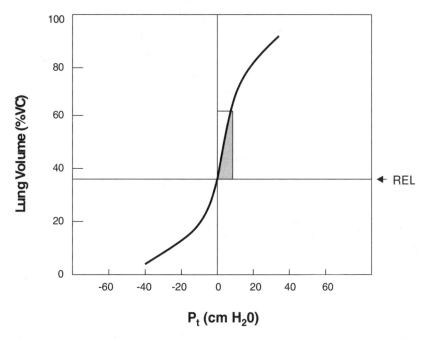

Figure 4–8. A replot of Figure 4–7 but now including a shaded area extending from about 60% VC to REL. The shaded area indicates the magnitude of muscular effort required to produce the P_t of 7 cm/H_2O. See text for additional detail.

initiating an utterance at a very high lung volume and with a conversational loudness (meaning, a value of P_t somewhere between 5-10 cm/H_2O) would require a substantial, net inspiratory muscular effort to offset the very high P_r. Similarly, continuing an utterance well below REL would require a large, net expiratory muscular effort to supplement the negative P_r values and produce the positive pressure for speech. In short, speech produced at very high or very low lung volumes requires a substantial muscular effort to produce the typical P_t values associated with conversational utterances; in contrast, conversational speech produced within the midrange of lung volumes requires only a modest muscular effort.

Patients with dysarthria will often make inefficient use of their lung volume range for speech, and most often will begin utterances at volumes close to REL (see Bunton, 2005). In such cases patients will quickly reach low lung volumes where P_rs are negative and must be supplemented by relatively large expiratory muscular efforts. Less likely are cases where patients begin speaking at very high lung volumes, but if such a patient is encountered they will have to employ large muscular efforts to avoid shouting.

Later in the chapter a simple technique for assessing a patient's starting lung volume for speech is presented, and some recommendations are made for management of inefficient lung volume usage in speech production. Here, it is worthwhile to note the potential linkage between lung volume range for speech and problems of loudness in patients with dysarthria. Many patients with dysarthria, and those with hyopkinetic dysarthria in particular, are known to have inadequate loudness for speech. There are several hypotheses for this symptom, including inadequate closure of the vocal folds during vibration, and a starting lung volume that is too low (or, a combination of the two). The impact of poor closure of the vocal folds on vocal loudness is discussed in detail in Chapter 5, but here we note that vocal fold vibration with weak or absent closure produces an acoustic spectrum with weak or absent energy in higher frequency harmonics. The result of this reduction of energy in the upper spectrum is an overall reduction of voice SPL, which is a major factor in the perception of a weak voice. A low starting lung volume for speech might produce the same overall effect, but for a different reason. If a patient must produce relatively substantial expiratory muscular efforts to supplement negative P_r at low lung volumes but does not have the ability to do so, the P_ts produced for conversational speech will likely be lower than normal. The result will be a relatively low voice SPL—because of the more or less direct relationship between P_t for speech and voice SPL—and the perception of a weak voice. This is one reason why it is so important to assess a patient's lung volume usage for speech, because a simple adjustment, if effective, may reduce the effort required by the patient to produce voice with reasonable energy.

How Does the Respiratory System Achieve the Graded Balance Between Muscular and Nonmuscular Forces?

The clinician should know how the respiratory system deploys muscular mechanisms to produce the constant P_t of conversational utterances. The following discussion considers the parts of the respiratory system that, by applying muscular force to the lungs, can contribute to P_t. A "part" of the respiratory system is a functional anatomic unit that by its net muscular actions can affect the volume (and therefore P_t) of the lung by compressing or expanding it. The behaviors of these parts for a typical utterance are also considered. The parts include (1) the rib cage, (2) the diaphragm, and (3) the abdomen.

The rib cage contains both inspiratory and expiratory musculature and so is capable of generating positive and negative muscular pressures. The abdomen is composed only of expiratory muscles and, therefore, contributes only to positive muscular pressures. The diaphragm, which can be considered a massive muscular barrier between the rib cage and abdomen, is an inspiratory muscle and can only produce negative muscular pressures. These three parts—rib cage, diaphragm, abdomen—are referred to collectively as the *chest wall*.

The chest wall creates volume changes within the lungs by creating air pressure changes that cause air to flow from lungs to atmosphere (expiration) or from atmosphere to lungs (inspiration). Compression of the lungs, caused by muscular mechanisms of the rib cage and abdomen, will cause air to flow from the lungs to the atmosphere and, hence, reduce lung volume. Expansion of the lungs, caused by muscular mechanisms of the rib cage and diaphragm, will cause air to flow into the lungs from the atmosphere. The direction of the flow is of course related to the magnitude of P_t relative to the pressure in the atmosphere (P_{atm}). Air flows from regions of higher to lower pressure, so compressive forces that raise P_t will cause air to flow from them and, hence, reduce their volume. This is the way phonation is produced, which is to say that speech is produced on expiratory flow and, therefore, a decreasing lung volume. Expansive forces that lower P_t will cause air to flow in from the atmosphere, thus increasing lung volume. Negative muscular pressures are used to refill the lungs after volume is lost as a result of expiratory flow. Obviously, when people speak, they will have to refill their lungs for successive utterances, and relatively frequently if they want to remain in the efficient lung volume range described above. An utterance that is produced on one continuous interval of expiratory flow and is bounded at its beginning and end by an inspiratory refill is called a *breath group* (see Figure 4-6, *You wish to know . . .*).

The general muscular mechanisms described here, as discussed above, are superimposed on the pressures created by the elastic recoil characteristics of the respiratory system. Importantly, the three parts of the chest wall can create the necessary pressures and resulting flows and volume changes by means of different combinations of the forces exerted by each of the parts. What follows is a "typical" profile of chest wall control of speech production, but it is by no means the only profile; there are certain aspects of this typical profile, however, that are essential to efficient speech breathing.

The simplest way to describe chest wall control of speech breathing is to provide an account of the sequence of muscular activities for a single utterance. Consistent with information provided above on typical speech pressures and lung volumes, this account will assume a P_t of 7 cm/H_2O with speech initiated at a lung volume of 60% VC and continuing to REL, where an inhalation will refill the lungs for the next utterance.

1. The lungs must be filled to the starting lung volume of 60% VC, accomplished primarily if not in some cases exclusively by contraction of the diaphragm. For the great majority of interutterance, inspiratory refills that prepare the respiratory system for a subsequent utterance, diaphragmatic contraction is the muscular mechanism of choice.

2. As the utterance is initiated, expiratory muscular activity in both the abdomen and rib cage provides whatever additional compression is needed to supplement the P_r and achieve the desired P_t. At the beginning of the utterance the magnitude of this net expiratory muscular effort will be small; it will increase steadily throughout the utterance to maintain the constant P_t. These graded increases are achieved by expiratory muscular efforts of both the rib cage and abdomen. Note the absence of any *inspiratory* muscular activity during conversational speech production. In conversational speech, there is typically no need for inspiratory muscular activity during the utterance because the starting lung volumes are typically associated with values of P_r roughly equal to or slightly less than the P_t target.

The muscular activity of the abdomen in speech breathing deserves special comment. Abdominal muscles are *always* active during speech; the effect can be seen as a rapid, inward movement of the abdominal surface immediately preceding the onset of an utterance. Abdominal muscle activity during speech can be thought of, partly, as a "posture" of the chest wall that allows the expiratory muscles of the rib cage to compress the lungs very efficiently. When the expiratory muscles of the rib cage apply force to the lungs, together with whatever positive P_r is available, the positive pressure generated in the lungs will be applied to their bottom surface, which is the cranial surface of the diaphragm. The diaphragm creates volume changes of the lungs by flattening its dome and, hence, expanding the lungs. Because the diaphragm cannot contract in a way that compresses the lungs, it cannot decrease lung volume directly but may do so indirectly. This occurs when it is pushed upward by contraction of the abdominal muscles, thus compressing the lungs. If the abdominal muscles were not contracted during speech, the positive air pressure developed within the lungs and applied to the cranial surface of the diaphragm would push it downward, compromising the compressive effort of the expiratory rib cage muscles. The compromise would occur because an effort to compress the lungs, made by the rib cage muscles, would actually result in some expansion of the lungs as the diaphragm is pushed downward by the positive air pressure. Constant activity of the abdominal muscles during speech holds the diaphragm in place even as the positive pressure is applied to it, preventing counterproductive expansion of the lungs by footward displacement of the diaphragm. Under these conditions the compressive efforts of the rib cage muscles are more efficient as they operate against the "high resistance" offered by the diaphragm via the contraction of the abdominal muscles. This is another example of efficiency during speech breathing, and it is a very important piece of clinical knowledge. The patient who has weak or paralyzed abdominal muscles will have the challenge of losing some of her compressive, rib cage efforts to produce a positive P_t for speech to the downward displacement of the diaphragm. Clinical approaches to this problem are discussed below.

Evaluating Speech Breathing in Patients With Dysarthria

Based on our description of efficient, speech breathing physiology, lung volume usage and vocal level are clearly two important components of the clinical evaluation of speech breathing. In fact, these components may be strongly interrelated, as a patient's ability to produce an acceptable voice level may depend on the lung volume range in which she is producing speech. It is also important to evaluate the patient's use of the chest wall to produce speech, as well as the patient's "packaging" of linguistic content within an utterance.

It is reasonable to ask, do speakers with dysarthria typically have problems with speech breathing? Several studies (Bunton, 2005; Murdoch et al., 1989; Putnam & Hixon, 1984; Solomon & Hixon, 1993) have described some speakers with dysarthria who use an inefficient lung volume range. Moreover, there is some evidence of abnormal chest wall behavior in some speakers with dysarthria (Murdoch, Chenery, Bowler, & Ingram, 1989; Lethlean, Chenery, & Murdoch, 1990; Murdoch, Chenery, Stokes, & Hardcastle, 1991; Murdoch, Theodoros, Stokes, & Chenery, 1993). These abnormal behaviors range from a tendency to "overuse" the abdomen for lung volume change, perhaps because the rib cage is stiff and not effective in contributing to lung volume change (e.g., Solomon & Hixon, 1993), to clear examples of paradoxic breathing where the rib cage and abdomen move in opposite directions during speech (see below for more information on paradoxic breathing; Murdoch, Chernery, Stokes, & Hardcastle, 1991; Murdoch & Hudson-Tennent, 1993). Many speakers with dysarthria will show problems with phrasing and speaking rate (see any of the articles cited here), both of which could be direct consequences of inefficient lung volume usage and abnormal coordination of chest wall parts. In some cases, abnormal chest wall behaviors among speakers with dysarthria are seen in maximum performance tasks (e.g., sustained vowels) but not in conversational speech (Thompson & Murdoch, 1995).

Each patient has to be evaluated as an individual, and one cannot assume the presence or absence of a speech breathing problem as part of a dysarthria. In many of the studies cited in the preceding paragraph, there were some speakers with Parkinson's disease, cerebellar, motor neuron, and upper motor neuron disease who showed *no* problems with speech breathing. Moreover, when a speaker with neurologic disease has difficulty with speech characteristics such as phrasing (phrases too short or long, or terminated at inappropriate boundaries), it is difficult to know if the problem can be attributed to speech breathing problems alone, laryngeal problems alone, or perhaps a combination of the former and latter. Finally, it is not always the case that an apparent speech breathing anomaly results in a problem requiring clinical attention. For example, a person with dysarthria may have what appears to be an unusual use of the chest wall during speech but be quite intelligible and report little or no problem with effort in producing speech. Thus the evaluation of speech breathing must always be done within the context of the patient's communication effectiveness; the physiologic data, in and of themselves, are not

always easy to interpret. With these cautionary notes in mind, evaluation of speech breathing is now described.

Lung Volume Usage

The most efficient lung volume range for the production of speech is the one requiring the least muscular effort. As described above, for the kinds of P_t used in conversational speech, the desired lung volume range is approximately between 60% VC and REL (around 35–40% VC in the upright posture). Not every patient, however, will be able to produce a "normal" voice level (see below, Vocal Level), and not every patient will be consistently able to confine her utterances to the relatively narrow range of lung volumes between 60% VC and REL. A more general goal is to have the patient begin her utterances at a lung volume somewhat above REL and finish utterances around REL; lung volumes below REL should be avoided for speech production. A therapy plan to meet this goal requires a determination of where in lung volume the patient is typically speaking, and a technique for teaching both utterance initiation above REL and utterance termination around REL.

A general determination of lung volume usage for speech can be made without instruments, by applying knowledge of respiratory physiology. REL, the mechanical rest position of the respiratory system, is defined as the lung volume at end-expiratory tidal (rest) breathing. During tidal breathing the inspiratory phase, which begins at REL and involves a volume increase of approximately half a liter of air (~500 milliliters), is produced primarily by contraction of the diaphragm. When the diaphragm contracts the volume of the lung is increased which results in a momentary drop in P_l and, hence, inspiratory airflow. The contractile flattening of the diaphragm pushes on the incompressible abdominal contents—they can be likened to a bag of water—and forces the ventral abdominal wall outward. When the diaphragm relaxes after contracting it moves upward into the thorax and pulls the abdominal contents with it, an action resulting from the elastic recoil of respiratory structures. Thus, during tidal breathing the ventral abdominal surface will move outward during the inspiratory phase and inward during the expiratory phase.

The clinician can therefore estimate REL by monitoring the motion of the abdominal surface as the patient breathes quietly, preferably in a seated position. The simplest way to do this is to place the palm of the hand on the abdomen (with the patient's permission, of course) and feel the cyclic outward-inward motions associated with inspiratory-expiratory phases of tidal breathing. The point during this cycle when the inward motion is complete and the outward motion is just about to begin is a good estimate of REL.

While continuing to monitor abdominal motion the patient can now be engaged in conversation. If the patient is refilling her lungs before each utterance, the clinician should be able to feel the outward motion of the abdominal surface prior to the utterance. If the patient is initiating utterances too close to REL or even below REL, the clinician will monitor an abdominal position close to the position estimated at end-expiratory tidal breathing as the patient begins speaking. An excellent way to get a sense of this simple procedure is to practice it with friends and fellow students.

If the patient is beginning utterances around REL and, thus, using a lung volume range in which she is not taking advantage

of positive relaxation pressures to contribute to P_t, she will have to generate a larger than desired muscular effort to compress the lungs; she may even be unable to generate an adequate phonatory level because of the muscular effort required. In this case, the clinician has three diagnostic questions to address: (1) is the patient stimulable for modifying the lung volume at which she initiates utterances? (2) if the patient can modify her lung volume in the desired way, are there beneficial changes in vocal level, vocal quality, and/or phrasing? and (3) if the patient can modify her lung volume in the desired way, does she report a reduction of perceived effort when she produces speech?

Stimulability. Stimulability for modification of lung volume can be assessed by monitoring the motion of the abdominal surface during tidal breathing as described above, and, when the patient reaches end-expiration asking her to take a slightly deeper inhalation than she would for tidal breathing and begin speaking. The slightly deeper inhalation will be accompanied by a greater outward motion of the abdomen than the clinician had sensed during tidal breathing. The clinician should take care to prevent the patient from producing a too energetic inspiratory effort, and especially several such efforts in a short period of time which could result in hyperventilation. Although the procedure is inexact, an observant clinician should be able to use this procedure to determine a patient's ability to voluntarily adjust the starting lung volume for speech.

Beneficial Phonatory Changes and Reduced Sense of Effort. For those patients who can modify lung volume diagnostic questions (2) and (3) can be addressed simultaneously. The clinician will have listened to the patient's speech and already identified possible problems with vocal level, quality, and phrasing. These characteristics of the patient's speech will serve as referents for the perceptual characteristics of productions within the more efficient lung volume range. The clinician's training and experience will allow her to make a decision concerning the possible effect of the adjusted range on these characteristics. The same kind of comparison should be made for the patient's estimate of the effort involved in producing speech. When the patient is first interviewed, it is reasonable to ask her to estimate the effort involved in speech production, perhaps using a rating scale. For those patients who demonstrate an ability to modify starting lung volume for speech, and to regulate the lung volume range in which they produce utterances, it is worthwhile to ask them to rescale their sense of effort in producing speech. Patients who report a reduction of effort with a more efficient lung volume range for speech have accomplished an important clinical goal, even in the absence of significant gains in speech intelligibility.

Obviously, the assessment of starting lung volumes and lung volume ranges for speech is going to be somewhat inexact in the absence of instruments, but with a little practice the clinician should be able to identify poor and good speech breathing behaviors. One possible modification of the procedures outlined above would be to begin the stimulability assessment with lung volume adjustments but no speech production. For example, the patient could be instructed to take a slightly deeper inhalation from REL but not to phonate immediately after reaching a desired lung volume. The behavior with phonation (speech) might then be shaped from this initial, successful behavior. Whereas this is

a reasonable approach, especially if initial efforts to adjust lung volume *with speech* have proven to be very difficult for the patient, the two behaviors are not the same and success in the nonspeech adjustment may not transfer to the case of speech. Clearly, all possible approaches should be tried before concluding that a patient cannot make a desired adjustment.

The clinical procedures and steps for assessing lung volume usage for speech are summarized in Table 4–1.

Vocal Level

The assessment of speech loudness is potentially dependent on the assessment of lung volume usage because speech produced within an inefficient lung volume range may predispose a patient to produce very low P_t and, hence, low vocal loudness. The relationship between P_t and voice intensity (the latter typically measured in units of sound pressure level [SPL]), on the one hand, and between P_t and vocal loudness (the perceptual correlate of voice SPL) on the other hand, is not linear. For our purposes, however, the links can be considered to be fairly direct. As P_t increases, so does voice SPL and vocal loudness (interested readers should study the classic experiment of Ladefoged & McKinney, 1963; and see Stevens, 1998, p. 79). It is also the case, however, that the P_t-SPL-vocal loudness relationship may be complicated by laryngeal mechanisms, which can also contribute independently to the energy output of the vibrating vocal folds. The rest of this section should be read with this cautionary note in mind.

A P_t between 5 to 10 cm/H_2O has been identified as typical of conversational speech, but what do those values mean in terms of the more directly relevant clinical variable of vocal loudness? Stated otherwise,

Table 4–1. Summary of Clinical Evaluation of Lung Volume Usage

> Monitor motion of abdominal surface during rest breathing to estimate REL; REL should be at the most *inward* motion during tidal breaths:
>
> Evoke speech from patient
>
> →inflation of lungs prior to speech will be indicated by outward motion of abdominal surface; if such motion is present, *do not* treat lung volume usage
>
> →if speech is initiated close to the most inward tidal-breath motion of the abdominal surface, *treat* lung volume usage
>
> →assess stimulability for modifying starting lung volume for speech, using utterances first; if patient is not stimulable for utterances, try nonspeech breathing (control of nonspeech inhalations) and attempt to shape this behavior for utterances
>
> →if patient succeeds in modifying starting lung for speech, evaluate effects on voice level, quality, effort, and speech intelligibility

what should a clinician look for when trying to determine "normal" values of vocal loudness? This is not an easy question to answer because "normal" conversational loudness depends on a number of variables, one of which is the distance between individuals engaged in a conversation. The greater this distance, the greater the voice intensity required to maintain the same loudness (and, perhaps, an acceptable level of speech intelligibility—see immediately below). In the therapy room and in most social interactions, people engaged in conversation will be relatively close to one another—perhaps within a meter or so—and under these circumstances it is fairly easy to judge the acceptability of voice loudness. A somewhat trickier assessment has to do with a patient's ability to generate variations in voice loudness to adapt to changing acoustic environments, ranging from very quiet to extremely noisy. This raises the important question of the relationship between voice loudness and speech intelligibility.

Obviously, speech intelligibility will suffer for the patient who generates very low voice intensities, not only in noisy environments but also in some quiet situations. If the patient with a low-intensity voice is capable of increasing her output, either as a byproduct of an adjustment of lung volume range or as a result of some other manipulation, speech intelligibility should be improved. The clinician must make a qualitative judgment concerning voice loudness, using experience and common sense. It is not prudent to state an SPL value that every patient should have as a goal, for the reasons discussed above, but it certainly may be useful for a patient to monitor her efforts to achieve a reasonable voice loudness by watching a sound-level meter during clinical sessions. One ballpark goal for the patient who is attempting to achieve "normal" loudness for conversational purposes is to produce an SPL of 70 dB at a mouth-to-meter distance of 6 to 12 inches (see Baken, 1987, p. 113).

Use of the Chest Wall

As described above, the chest wall includes the rib cage, abdomen, and diaphragm; these parts of the respiratory system can create volume changes of the lungs by applying muscular and nonmuscular forces to them. For this discussion the diaphragm and abdomen are considered to be linked as one part, the diaphragm-abdomen. Footward displacement of the diaphragm will cause the ventral abdominal surface to move outward, and inward motion of the abdominal surface due to contraction of the abdominal muscles will cause the diaphragm to move upward, toward the head. Thus the three-part chest wall is reduced to two parts, the rib cage and the diaphragm-abdomen, which are capable of displacing volume to and from the lungs. In the following discussion, the diaphragm-abdomen is referred to as the abdomen.

The evaluation of chest wall behavior for speech production can be stated very simply: during an utterance, both the abdomen and rib cage should get smaller (they should both be moving inward), and during interutterance refills they should both get bigger. The evaluation of abdominal motions has already been described, and in theory the same hands-on technique could be used for the rib cage, with the understanding that the monitoring of its motions may be more difficult. This is because the motions of the rib cage during speech breathing are far more subtle than those of the abdomen.

When the rib cage and abdomen move in opposite directions during volume exchange these two parts of the chest wall are working against each other. This is called *paradoxic breathing* and is thought to be seen with some frequency among some speakers with dysarthria (Murdoch et al., 1991; Murdoch & Hudson-Tennent, 1993). For example, paradoxic speech breathing occurs when a speaker does not contract the abdominal muscles and the pressure in the thorax pushes down on the diaphragm, which in turn displaces the abdominal contents and forces the ventral abdominal wall outward. In this case, the rib cage moves inward but the abdomen moves outward during speech, the latter compromising (to varying degrees) the compressive effort of rib cage forces. The implication of paradoxic speech breathing is that the speaker will have to work harder to achieve a reasonable P_t, or will only be able to produce relatively low P_t values because of the compromising, outward abdominal motion.

Clinicians should be alert to the possibility of paradoxic chest wall motions during speech production, but such motions are not necessarily signs of neurologic disease. They are also observed during the speech of neurologically normal speakers, although the frequency of their occurrence in the normal population is thought to be low. *Chronic* paradoxic motions of the chest wall during speech production can probably be regarded as unusual and undesirable. For those patients with weak or paralyzed abdominal muscles, or who have difficulty coordinating the inward motion of the abdomen with like motion of the rib cage, simple techniques for temporary compression of the abdominal wall may improve speech breathing in particular and speech production in general. Seated patients can press a small board against their abdomen when they speak and in some cases a belt-like wrap ("abdominal binding") can be placed around the abdomen for brief intervals.

Table 4–2 summarizes possible chest wall behaviors in speech production.

Table 4–2. Summary of Possible Chest-Wall Motions (Rib Cage [RC] and Abdomen [AB]) During Speech Expirations and Interutterance Inhalations

Speech Expiration

- Both RC and AB decreasing in size: both parts working in the same direction to decrease the volume of the lungs and displace air from lungs to atmosphere (this is the "desired" behavior of the chest wall for speech)

- RC getting larger, AB getting smaller during speech: *rib cage paradoxing*, where the motion of RC increases the size of the lung while the motion of AB decreases the size of the lung; if air continues to flow from the lungs to the atmosphere the motion of the AB dominates the overall effect on lung volume change but is compromised by the opposite motion of RC

- RC getting smaller, AB getting larger during speech: *abdominal paradoxing*, where the motion of RC decreases the size of the lung while the motion of AB increases the size of the lung (via footward displacement of the diaphragm); if air continues to flow from the lungs to the atmosphere the motion RC dominates the overall effect on lung volume change but is compromised by the opposite motion of AB

Speech Inhalations

- RC and AB getting larger: both parts working in the same direction to increase the volume of the lungs and displace air from the atmosphere to the lungs (this is the "desired" behavior of the chest wall for interutterance inhalations)

- RC getting smaller, AB getting larger during inhalation: *rib cage paradoxing*, where motion of RC decreases the size of the lung while motion of AB increases size of lung (via footward displacement of the diaphragm). If air continues to flow from atmosphere to the lung the motion of the AB (via diaphragmatic contraction) dominates the overall effect on lung volume change but is compromised by the opposite motion of RC

- RC getting larger, AB getting smaller during inhalation: *abdominal paradoxing*

Readers who are interested in physical examination of chest wall structures should consult the series of papers published by Hixon & Hoit (1998, 1999, 2000).

Summary

The purpose of this chapter has been to provide a detailed account of normal speech breathing physiology, and to show why an understanding of that physiology is so critical to evaluation and management of speech breathing disorders in persons with motor speech disorders. The key concept is the relationship of the relaxation pressure at a given lung volume to the target, tracheal pressure the speaker would like to produce at that lung volume, and ultimately throughout an utterance. The speech breathing, motor control task confronting the speaker of dysarthria is to maintain a constant tracheal pressure for an utterance by creating a continuously changing muscular effort as air leaves the lungs. This motor control task can be made more difficult by a number of possible problems in speech breathing, including usage of an inefficient lung volume range, poor coordination of the chest wall parts in displacing volume, and weakness or paralysis of one of more chest wall parts. Speech breathing problems may result in weak voice, poor phrasing, and excessive muscular effort. Clinically realistic strategies for evaluation and management of speech breathing behavior in persons with motor speech disorders have been presented. The evaluation of speech breathing should be a basic step in the diagnosis phase of a motor speech disorder because some fairly simple adjustments, if successful, can have widespread effects on communication efficiency.

References

Baken, R. J. (1987). *Clinical measurement of speech and voice.* Boston: College-Hill Press.

Bunton, K. (2005). Patterns of lung volume use during an extemporaneous speech task in persons with Parkinson disease. *Journal of Communication Disorders, 38,* 331–348.

Hixon, T. J. (1973). Respiratory function in speech. In F. Minifie, T. Hixon, & F. Williams (Eds.), *Normal aspects of speech, hearing, and language* (pp. 75–125). Englewood Cliffs, NJ: Prentice-Hall.

Hixon, T. J., & Hoit, J. D. (1998). Physical examination of the diaphragm by the speech-language pathologist. *American Journal of Speech-Language Pathology, 7,* 37–45.

Hixon, T. J., & Hoit, J. D. (1999). Physical examination of the abdominal wall by the speech-language pathologist. *American Journal of Speech-Language Pathology, 8,* 335–346.

Hixon, T. J., & Hoit, J. D. (2000). Physical examination of the rib cage wall by the speech-language pathologist. *American Journal of Speech-Language Pathology, 9,* 179–196.

Hixon, T. J., & Hoit, J. D. (2005). *Evaluation and management of speech breathing disorders: Principles and methods.* Tucson, AZ: Redington Brown.

Ladefoged, P., & McKinney, N.P. (1963). Loudness, sound pressure, and subglottal pressure in speech. *Journal of the Acoustical Society of America, 35,* 454–460.

Lethlean, J., Chenery, H., & Murdoch, B. (1990). Disturbed respiratory and prosodic function in Parkinson's disease: A perceptual and instrumental analysis. *Australian Journal of Human Communication Disorders, 18,* 83–97.

Murdoch, B., Chenery, H., Bowler, S., & Ingram, J. (1989). Respiratory function in Parkinson's subjects exhibiting a perceptible speech deficit: A kinematic and spirometric analysis. *Journal of Speech and Hearing Disorders, 54,* 610–626.

Murdoch, B., Chenery, H., Stokes, P., & Hardcastle, W. (1991). Respiratory kinematics in speakers with cerebellar disease. *Journal of Speech and Hearing Research, 34,* 768–780.

Murdoch, B. E., & Hudson-Tennent, L. J. (1993). Speech breathing anomalies in children with dysarthria following treatment for posterior fossa tumors. *Journal of Medical Speech-Language Pathology, 2,* 107–119.

Murdoch, B. E., Theodoros, D. G., Stokes, P. D., & Chenery, H. J. (1993). Abnormal patterns of speech breathing in dysarthric speakers following severe closed head injury. *Brain Injury, 7,* 295–308.

Putnam, A. H. B., & Hixon, T. J. (1984). Respiratory kinematics in speakers with motor neuron disease. In M. R. McNeil, J. C. Rosenbek, & A. E. Aronson (Eds.), *The dysarthrias: Physiology, acoustics, perception, management* (pp. 37–67). San Diego, CA: College-Hill Press.

Rahn, H., Otis, A. B., Chadwick, L. E., & Fenn, W. O. (1946). The pressure-volume diagram of the thorax and lung. *American Journal of Physiology, 146,* 161–178.

Seikel, J. A., King, D. W., & Drumright, D. G. (2000). *Anatomy and physiology for speech, language, and hearing* (2nd ed.). San Diego, CA: Singular Publishing Group.

Solomon, N. P., & Hixon, T. J. (1993), Speech breathing in Parkinson's disease. *Journal of Speech and Hearing Research, 36,* 294–310.

Stevens, K. N. (1998). *Acoustic phonetics.* Cambridge, MA: MIT Press.

Thompson, E. C., & Murdoch, B. E. (1995). Respiratory function associated with dysarthria following upper motor neurone damage. *Australian Journal of Human Communication Disorders, 23,* 61–87.

Titze, I. R. (1994). *Principles of voice production.* Englewood Cliffs, NJ: Prentice-Hall.

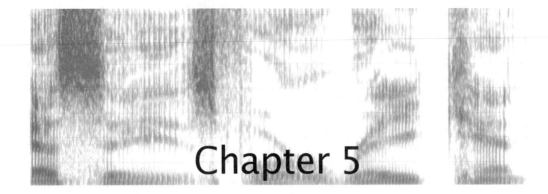

Chapter 5

VOICE PRODUCTION AND DYSFUNCTION IN MOTOR SPEECH DISORDERS

Eugene H. Buder

Introduction

The study of voice production invites us to marvel at the nature of speech as a most complex human behavior, offering for inspection levels of analysis from physics to emotional expression. There are vantages at each of these levels, presenting both basic and clinical revelations. By also viewing phonation from both basic and clinical perspectives, we can gain insights that might never have been possible from one approach alone. The complexity of this multifaceted phenomenon of voice requires great scientific humility. Yet the topic provides special scientific satisfaction to the degree to which we can patiently bring to its understanding as many interdisciplinary aspects as humanly possible. These may be among the many reasons that laryngeal function for speech has received a great deal of attention from scientists like Ray Kent, as a review of his writings on the topic finds all of the requisite scientific values in practice, and more.

Important Contributions by Kent and Colleagues

The following sampling of Kent's contributions to the topic of laryngeal function and dysfunction in speech motor disorders reveals many important themes that should profitably be considered by both basic scientists and clinical practitioners to better serve understanding and the vocal needs of people they observe. Although most of these themes are either more broad or more focused than the coverage of the chapter materials that follow, they are valuable as access points to related literature.

- Kent's work has focused on the role of the larynx as an articulator contributing to intelligibility, asking the level-headed question of how and when phonation helps or hinders a person with a motor speech disorder convey intelligible speech (R.D. Kent, 1994; R.D. Kent, Kent et al., 1989; R.D. Kent et al., 1991; R.D. Kent, Weismer, Kent, & Rosenbek, 1989; Weismer, Jeng, Laures, Kent, & Kent, 2001). This contribution is especially notable given the paucity of examinations of the intact speech signal in its real-world message-carrying context in clinical assessments and basic motor speech disorders research (Weismer, 2006), and given the ongoing need by the community to more fully incorporate the special nature of the speech motor control system in these assessment and research strategies (R.D. Kent, 2004a).

- Kent's work has always respected and incorporated individual variations in the speaker by keeping in mind such basic variables as gender and age in the design of studies and the interpretation of results. This work has revealed that laryngeal factors in intelligibility have been especially gender-specific (J. Kent et al., 1992; R.D. Kent, 1994). See also work on vocal aging for the surprising differences in male and female voices along both normal and pathologic lines (Linville, 2001, 2004). As Kent emphasized in his *The Speech Sciences* text, more work needs to be done to better incorporate age- and gender-specific knowledge in voice (R.D. Kent, 1997b, n.b. pp. 127–134), and this is particularly true in the context of motor speech disorders affecting individuals later in the life cycle.

- Kent's work has emphasized acoustics (R.D. Kent & Read, 2002), but with special care given to its interaction with perception in general (R.D. Kent, 1996), and with voice assessment in particular (R.D. Kent, Vorperian, & Duffy, 1999; R.D. Kent, Vorperian, Kent, & Duffy, 2003). Some quotations from his recent review of acoustic assessment tools in voice serve as an introduction to a theme of this chapter: "Whether voice is measured by a single dimension or by multiple dimensions, it is no simple matter to mark a single point that always divides the normal from the abnormal . . . a value deemed abnormal in one study would not necessarily be so in another" (R.D. Kent et al., 2003, p. 291). As developed somewhat further below, the bad news about norms is exacerbated by further considering the variety of strategies that speakers may adopt to accomplish vocal assessment tasks. Keeping in mind the previous point regarding individual differences, the bad news is mitigated, however, by careful consideration of individual variability that patients bring to the clinic. Ultimately, the best normative bases are the patient's own productions, and the clinical scientist's understanding of the vocal mechanism.

There are a few themes that can be carried forward from these points in attempting to gain the most from the remaining materials of this chapter: (1) the need to understand the mechanism at a functional level, (2) the need to incorporate special aspects of each individual affected voice user, beginning with the basics such as age and gender, and continuing with an exploration of their particular pathology, (3) the value of considering the acoustic signal and its physical origins, and (4) the problems, deriving specifically from the preceding three points, associated with attempting to evaluate most quantitative measures of voice behavior against any normative values.

The Vocal Mechanism

It is the first of these themes—functional understanding of the mechanism—that this chapter emphasizes, with implicit and occasionally explicit links to the other themes. In particular, because of the extensive literature, by Kent and others, relating principles of clinical neurophysiology and motor control to laryngeal function, this chapter attempts very little contribution on such principles. Rather, this chapter attempts to review: what students of the

neuromotor system should know about aspects of phonatory function that are specifically *not* under neuromotor control? Remember the basic scientific successes in understanding respiratory control, which only came about once the background mechanical system of passive forces, coupled with each other and with the active muscular forces through pleural linkage, became fully understood (see Chap-ter 4). The situation is the same, only perhaps more complicated, when we encounter the autonomous nature of *self-sustaining* vibrations of the vocal folds as a biomechanical system taking aerodynamic inputs and generating acoustic outputs.

Figure 5-1 presents a scheme that overviews the orientation of this chapter. Some typical elements of clinical and scientific assessment are listed in boxes within the descriptive domain where these elements are typically found. Given the diagnosis of a neuromuscular speech motor disorder, the observer may wish to understand the neurologic deficits to

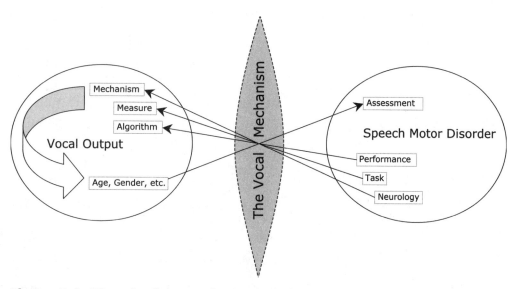

Figure 5–1. The role of the mechanism in linking vocal outputs to motor speech disorders via clinical assessment processes.

define tasks that measure vocal (phonatory) performance. However, the manners in which these tasks are elicited and performed can matter greatly. The actual vocal output, it is argued in this chapter, is refracted through the lens of the vocal mechanism, and only via deep understanding of this pathology itself may the actual neuromuscular mechanism be considered as an object of description and measured through the appropriate algorithms. The output measures must then be placed in the context of individual variables, which in addition to the pathology itself, of course, include basic considerations such as age and gender. Only through such processes can any observer arrive at an assessment of voice production.

But please note: this scheme is not a recipe for actual clinical assessment or diagnosis! See valuable texts such as Aronson (1990), Colton and Casper (1996), and Duffy (2005) for clinical and scientific guidance in the signs of motor disorders of voice. The emphasis in Figure 5-1 is more

on the central role of the vocal mechanism, which is depicted with a visual pun: the lens through which all voice reasoning must be refracted is a glottis.

Use of Vocal Function in Classifications and Assessments of Motor Speech Disorders

Considering the relative anatomic and neurologic complexity of supralaryngeal mechanisms in speech production, laryngeal behaviors and phonatory output are remarkably dominant in the classification and assessment of motor speech disorders. Table 5-1 lists those elements of motor speech ratings that are routinely used in the Mayo Clinic (derived from the classic Darley, Aronson, and Brown scales), which are specifically laryngeal or phonatory in nature: Note that these 22 descriptors represent nearly half the entire inventory of 48—see Duffy (2005, p. 90). As seen in the

Table 5–1. Ratings from Mayo Clinic Dysarthria Studies That Invoke Laryngeal Function, by Group[a]

Pitch	Loudness	Voice Quality	Respiration	Prosody/Other
Pitch level (+/−)	Monoloudness	Harsh	Inhalatory stridor	Reduced stress
Pitch breaks	Excess loudness variation	Hoarse (wet)	Grunt at end of expiration	Excess and equal stress
Monopitch	Loudness decay	Breathy (continuous)		Simple vocal tics
Myoclonus	Alternating loudness	Breathy (transient)		
Diplophonia	Overall loudness (+/−)	Strained-strangled		
		Stoppages		
		Flutter		

[a]Adapted with permission from Duffy (2005).

number of groupings in which laryngeal function appears in Table 5-1, the larynx is (almost literally) a "bottleneck" determinant of speech production, reflecting respiratory mechanisms but also articulating closely in response to segmental and suprasegmental details of speech. This central aspect of voicing in the production of speech, plus the dominance of the voice source in determining the overall amplitude of the speech (particularly in the lower frequencies at which auditory sensitivity and frequency discriminability are heightened), account for some of the clinical sensitivity to laryngeal function.

Motor speech disorders in general, and the dysarthrias in particular, have been intellectually exciting to scientists like Ray Kent who tap into the two-way flow of knowledge between clinical and basic knowledge bases (R.D. Kent, Kent, Duffy, & Weismer, 1998). The special nature of speech provides dysarthria with an especially lucid view of both neuropathology (R.D. Kent, 2004a) and normal neurophysiology of motor systems (R.D. Kent, 1990). The dysarthrias, thus, have special diagnostic value, and as already established, voice is especially prominent in supporting this value.

Following the tradition of Darley, Aronson, and Brown (1975), Duffy (2005) has compiled extensive information on the specific speech and voice characteristics by which dysarthrias can be distinguished, and Table 5-2A lists some of the voice characteristics by which the major classes of dysarthria may differ. Here, the characteristics are described in acoustic terms to emphasize that aspect of voice presentation, and apraxia of speech is not included in this table (nor reviewed in this chapter) because the disorder is not typically distinguished on phonatory characteristics (although laryngeal control is certainly

affected in this disorder, in producing voiced/voiceless consonant contrasts for example, [Seddoh et al., 1996].) Note, however, that there is substantial overlap between dysarthria types in Table 5-2A. Much of this overlap can be resolved for finer differentiation among the types if one consults additional speech characteristics and, following the Duffy (2005) text, considers whether a given characteristic is truly distinctive of the dysarthria type versus just a characteristic that may or may not be present.

However, some motor speech disorders are "mixed" as in amyotrophic lateral sclerosis (ALS) or multiple sclerosis (MS), and may progress in severity (ALS) or exhibit remitting-exacerbating cycles (MS). Others may or may not present with an accompanying tremor as in spasmodic dysphonia (SD) (Aronson & Hartman, 1981). Variations may also occur within the class of "distinguishing speech characteristic," such as tremor (this chapter returns to explore the variety of vocal modulation types in a section to follow). Table 5-2B lists the disorders of ALS, MS, and SD to overview the fact that distinguishing phonatory characteristics may, therefore, occur with so many mixtures or subtypes that simple characteristic-disorder association sets may not be the most reliable or even valid way to summarize motor dis-order-related phonatory effects (and the same is certainly true of speech characteristics as well [Weismer, 2006]).

It is beyond the scope of this chapter (indeed beyond the state of the art) to solve the problems raised in the preceding review of the tabulated information. One very important point has been emphasized by Kent and colleagues in numerous reports nonetheless, and that is to consider that speech and voice characteristics differ dramatically by "task" (R.D. Kent,

Table 5–2. Laryngeal Characteristics Used in Mayo Clinic Studies That May Distinguish Motor Speech Disorder Types[a]; (B) The Same Characteristics for Selected Disorders of Adductor Spasmodic Dysphonia (ADSD), Multiple Sclerosis (MS), and Amyotrophic Lateral Sclerosis (ALS)[b]

	Breathy	Diplo-phonic	Stridor	Harsh	Low F_0	Strained/ Strangled	F_0 breaks	SPL varies	Mono F_0	Mono SPL	Low SPL	Breaks	Tremor
A													
Flaccid	✓	✓	✓						✓	✓	✓		
Spastic				✓	✓	✓	✓		✓	✓	✓		
Ataxic							✓	✓	✓				
Hypokinetic	✓				✓				✓	✓	✓		
Hyperkinetic			✓	✓	✓	✓	✓	✓	✓			✓	✓
UUMN				✓		✓			✓		✓		
B													
ADSD		✓	✓	✓	✓	✓						✓	✓
MS			✓	✓	✓	✓			✓	✓			+wow, flutter of SPL
ALS	✓		✓	✓	✓+ high F_0	✓	✓		✓				+wow, flutter of F_0, SPL

[a]Adapted with permission from Duffy, 2005, Table 15–4

[b]Based on Hartelius et al. (1997), Strand et al. (1994), and Sapienza et al. (1999)

1997a; R.D. Kent & Kent, 2000; Ziegler, 2002). See also the chapter on neurologic disease by Ziegler and Hoole (2000) in Kent and Ball's *Voice Quality Measurement* book in which the authors find that it can be more useful to classify and understand dysphonias by "pathomechanism" than by etiology.

As a simple example of task specificity in relation to Table 5–2B, consider the "distinguishing characteristics" of voice in ALS as examined by Strand et al. (Strand, Buder, Yorkston, & Ramig, 1994). In addition to finding significant variation in the phonatory effects of ALS in four women, the report also found that fundamental frequency (F_0) variation in connected speech could be abnormally reduced (mono F_0) whereas the same parameter would show excessive variability in a sustained phonation task ("wow," which is essentially a very slow type of tremor). Also in ALS as investigated by Strand et al., and in SD as investigated by Sapienza and colleagues (Sapienza, Murry, & Brown, 1998), the variability in F_0 in a given task sometimes occurs due to "breaks." As also explored somewhat further in this chapter, a pitch break associated with a neuromuscular disorder, although still pathologic, may not necessarily reflect excessive variability in neuromuscular behavior. Instead, it may be the direct result of the predisposition for phonation to shift abruptly in vibratory "regime," simply due to nonlinearities that are necessarily part of the normally functioning vocal mechanism.

The main section of this chapter delves into the vocal mechanism in some greater detail to support assessments of vocal dysfunction in motor speech disorders that are based as much as possible on the mechanism itself, observing that the function of this mechanism may often be remarkably "autonomous," with behaviors that cannot directly be linked to neuromuscular control. These behaviors are primarily under the control of biomechanical, aerodynamic, and acoustic principles. Another reason that neuromuscular control and pathologies of phonation are not treated directly in this chapter is that many good additional texts are already available that cover the topic with a clinical scope not afforded by this chapter (e.g., Aronson, 1990; Awan, 2001; Blitzer, Brin, Sasaki, Fahn, & Harris, 1992; Boone, McFarlane, & Von Berg, 2005; Colton & Casper, 1996; Sataloff, 2005; Stemple, Glaze, & Gerdeman, 2000). Following this review, the chapter touches on some observations of voice function that are best considered in light of the autonomous nature of vocal fold vibration, some mention of task-specific variations in human performance, and a review of the multifaceted nature of voice dysfunctions like tremor, that belie easy characterization as simply "present" versus "absent" in a given task.

Outline of Phonation According to Biomechanical, Aerodynamic, and Acoustic Principles

Background Anatomy

Before delving into some of the more subtle aspects of phonation, it would be helpful to review some of the basics of laryngeal anatomy and innervation (but the reader should consult other resources for more thorough introductory details and illustrations as needed, e.g., R.D. Kent, 1997b; Titze, 1994; Zemlin, 1998). Recall that the larynx sits atop the trachea and is bounded at its superior margin by the hyoid bone. Other skeletal structures of the larynx are cartilaginous: the cricoid cartilage joins the larynx to the trachea; the thyroid cartilage is the large V-shaped structure that articulates with the cricoid and provides the anterior attachment point of the vocal folds; the arytenoids are the paired cartilages that articulate in complex ways atop the posterior surface of the cricoid, providing the posterior attachments for the vocal folds; and the epiglottis is the leaflike structure that attaches to the thyroid and helps to form the epilaryngeal tube that acoustically guides the voice source into the vocal tract (we return to this acoustic effect below). The most important muscle fibers to keep in mind for the following materials are those coursing from the arytenoid to the thyroid—the thyroarytenoid (TA), and those coursing from the cricoid to the thyroid—the cricothyroid (CT). This pair of muscles can be thought of as an agonist-antagonist pair in the sense that CT activ-

ity can lengthen the vocal folds (primarily by pulling the thyroid cartilage anteriorly), whereas TA activity can shorten the vocal folds (by pulling the thyroid cartilage posteriorly), but see the discussion of Figure 5–4 later in this chapter for further considerations.

Recall also two important aspects of the soft tissues within the larynx: (1) Ventricular, or "false," vocal folds appear just superior to the true vocal folds (as mentioned below, the false vocal folds may be muscularly drawn into play by certain motor speech disorders); and (2) the vocal folds themselves contain a muscular core (the vocalis portion of the thyroarytenoid fibers) that is surrounded by layers of connective and epithelial tissue. This layering of tissue types is the basis for the "cover-body" descriptions in vocal fold physiology and biomechanics. As depicted in Figure 5–2 below, the most fundamental

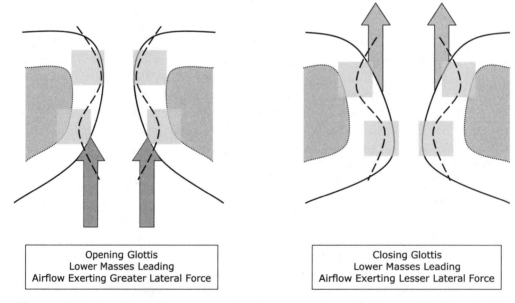

| Opening Glottis |
| Lower Masses Leading |
| Airflow Exerting Greater Lateral Force |

| Closing Glottis |
| Lower Masses Leading |
| Airflow Exerting Lesser Lateral Force |

Figure 5–2. A schematic representing the interaction of the vocal folds with the passing airstream (see arrows and textboxes), two mass model (*boxes*), mucosal wave (*dashed curves*), and cover-body distinction (*unfilled and filled portions of vocal folds, respectively*).

distinction among these layers is the dichotomy between a body portion that is less involved in vibration, and the more freely vibrating cover tissues. Note that, as just defined, this distinction is primarily mechanical in nature. As overviewed in more detail by other basic texts (R.D. Kent, 1997b; Titze, 1994), a finer three-fold physiologic distinction between mucosal, ligamental, and muscular layers can be rendered that is also important in the discussion below, as the mucosal layer carries the wavelike vibration of typical vocal fold vibration (seen in the dashed lines of Figure 5–2) and the ligamental layer can be important in understanding how muscle forces affect the fundamental frequency of vibration (reviewed in the discussion of Figure 5–4 later in this chapter). Note that there is yet a further five-fold division of basic fold layers that is primarily histologic: The mucosal layers are epithelium; the superficial layer of the "lamina propria" are connective tissues; the ligament is composed of the intermediate and deep layers of the lamina propria; and beginning at the deep lamina propria layer and underlying thyroarytenoid muscle is where the transition between cover and body aspects of typical vocal fold vibration may be drawn.

Finally, a few very basic points of information on innervation should also be kept in mind in consideration of motor speech disorders affecting phonation. Control of the respiratory musculature is discussed in Chapter 4. The larynx is supplied exclusively by cranial nerve X, the vagus, with motor cell bodies in the nucleus ambiguus. Recall also that the vagal nerve supply to the laryngeal muscles involves some complex branching: all the intrinsic muscles of the larynx are supplied by the recurrent laryngeal branch *except* the cricothyroid muscle, which is supplied by the external superior laryngeal branch. Sensory information from the larynx is carried in the internal branch of the superior laryngeal nerve (roughly, top half of larynx) and in the recurrent laryngeal nerve (roughly, bottom half of larynx).

Structural Characteristics Affecting Vibration

The biomechanical structure of the vocal folds themselves determines how they will respond to aerodynamic forces, by vibrating, to generate an acoustic signal. The primary properties of the vocal folds as vibrators are those of any vibrating system, their mass and their elasticity. Recall that the most elementary type of vibrating system is a mass-spring oscillator. In the idealized case, these elements move with no loss of energy, as would be due to friction, for example. A mass component has inertance, which is essentially a tendency to store energy as a motion that will continue in the direction with which it was imparted. An elastic component has compliance, which is essentially a tendency to store energy as a potential restoring force (opposing the direction with which it is imparted). When these mass and elastic properties are coupled (as they most definitely are in the vocal folds because they are characteristics of the tissues that make up the vocal folds), and set in motion by aerodynamic forces, they determine a simple harmonic waveform by trading off these forms of energy storage.

A simple harmonic motion has a specific natural frequency; in the vocal folds this is the fundamental frequency of vocal fold vibration, or F_0. The mass of the vocal folds has a most definite role in determining

F_0. The more massive vocal folds of a typical adult man produce a lower F_0 than an adult woman or a child. There are also many vocal fold pathologies that will add to the mass of the vocal folds (e.g., edema or neoplasm) or perhaps reduce it (e.g., atrophy associated with lower motor neuron, due to damage of the nucleus ambiguus or peripheral nerves that supply the larynx), but neurogenic motor disorders do not affect the mass in any acute postural way. It is, therefore, the property of elasticity that is of greater interest, both for normal control of F_0 but also for variations in muscle tone due to a motor disorder. For example, excessive compliance may be due to paresis, whereas excessive stiffness may be due to the spastic effects of upper motor neuron disease. Based on the simple principles of mass and compliance as determinants of natural frequency, one might expect excessive compliance to lower F_0 and excessive stiffness to raise it. Voice production is not so simple, however. Consider, for example, that excessive muscle tone in the larynx can involve all fibers of the thyroarytenoid muscles, pulling false vocal folds into a position that "loads" the vocal folds with extra mass (tending to cause a lower F_0 but also a high degree of irregularity in vocal fold vibration).

These primary aspects of mass and elasticity are important but still too crude for even a basic understanding of vocal fold biomechanics without some other aspects that might be considered secondary. Viscosity is another important characteristic of tissue, relating to the loss or dissipation of energy in vibrating systems: the more viscous a medium the more energy it absorbs. This property is mostly associated with connective tissues, but, as muscle tone may be lost due to neural degeneration and the muscle fibers revert to fat, this property may be indirectly associated with a motor dysfunction. The configuration of various connective tissues in the lamina propria of the vocal folds leads to distinctive mechanical responses involving both elasticity and viscosity. Although based on the histology of epithelial, connective, and muscular tissue types, the basic distinction between cover and body is essentially a mechanical principle. Playing a strong role in distinguishing vocal fold vibration types such as modal ("normal" vocal fold vibration, where the mucosal wave is plainly evident) versus loft (often called *falsetto*, where the vocal folds are stretched very tight, therefore eliminating the mucosal wave), the cover-body transition is controlled by characteristics of the vocalis muscle and may, therefore, be directly affected by neuromuscular dysfunction.

The geometry of the vocal fold tissue critically affects voice production, as captured by the distinction between upper and lower masses. This is again a basic biomechanical aspect of vocal fold structure that accounts for its vibratory reaction to aerodynamic forces, and this is modeled as a specific configuration of masses and elasticities (the mass elements of upper and lower vibrating medial portions of vocal fold tissues and compliance elements connecting these masses to each other and to more lateral structures). Again, it is these compliance elements that are most susceptible to muscular influence. Without sufficient freedom for the lower mass to "lead" the upper mass, the vocal fold surfaces will not be free to shift angles relative to the passing airflow and thereby draw energy from it to sustain vibration (see Figure 5-2). Very stiff vocal folds, as might be observed in a spastic or hypokinetic dysarthria, therefore, cease to vibrate.

Active Posturing Forces

Two primary muscle-controlled forces are required for normal phonation: (1) there must be a flow of air from the lungs, and (2) the vocal folds must be adducted with sufficient medial compression so as to present some impedance to this flow. These two elements are part of a very important triad of aerodynamic concepts that are related to one another in direct analogy to Ohm's law: flow encountering resistance produces pressure. The force that best encapsulates these muscular effects is, therefore, subglottal (or tracheal) pressure (P_{sg}). It is important to see that this quantity is the result of both expiratory (positive) air pressures produced by the lungs and a medial compression of the tissues at the glottis.

Pathologies producing motor speech disorders may ultimately affect the ability of the respiratory system to produce sufficient pressures for phonation (see Chapter 4). However, as a life-sustaining activity, respiration is relatively robust, and according to Duffy (2005), "[because] voice and speech are relatively resistant to respiratory disturbance . . . most neurologic voice abnormalities implicate the laryngeal mechanism rather than the respiratory system" (p. 91). So, even though voice production must always be considered to be the joint effort of the respiratory and laryngeal systems, the ongoing focus in this review is on the role of the glottis as a valve in producing subglottal pressure and working with this resource to create voice through phonation.

There are many simple measures for evaluating this pressure system and the aerodynamic valving status of the glottis, and one of the most widely used assessments, maximum duration of vowel prolongation (or MPD, standing for maximum phonation duration), was legitimized by Kent and colleagues in a survey of normative data (R.D. Kent, Kent, & Rosenbeck, 1987). Keeping in mind that MPD will be greatly determined by a patient's vital capacity, the person's ability to fully utilize this capacity, and other factors such as motivation and practice, the duration with which a patient sustains phonation can be an assessment of the status of this valve. If vocal fold flaccidity is a problem, then glottal resistance will be reduced and the MPD will be short. But following one of this chapter's themes, one has to reason based on the specific patient's overall status: Spasticity in the vocal folds, even to the degree that would lead to hyperadduction and high glottal resistance, may not yield a longer MPD if the patient is also having problems recruiting respiratory muscles, or if airway resistance is increased due to asthma or stenosis, or if lung elasticity is reduced due to aging, and so forth. Nonetheless, assessment of glottal valving can be based on MPD, especially if vital capacity is known. The "phonation quotient," for example, simply divides vital capacity by the MPD time to estimate average glottal flow, usually expressed in milliliters per second (Hirano, Koike, & von Leden, 1968).

Glottal Vibration

Self-Sustaining Dynamic Interaction of Tissue and Airflow

Ultimately, the vocal folds must modulate airflow with sufficient reliability and regularity so as to produce a harmonically rich sound source. Once again, this vocal fold vibration is a self-sustaining process, resulting from a physical interaction between tissues and airflow. Once the muscular forces tuning P_{sg} are set, phonation, as understood under the myoelastic-aerodynamic theory, can proceed with virtual autonomy. Classical textbook accounts of this theory emphasize the role of the Bernoulli effect, whereby the acceleration of air molecules rushing through a narrowing glottis facilitates glottal closure by lowering the intraglottal pressures and "sucking" the tissues shut. However, as introduced in the preceding structural description, it is actually more important to understand the wavelike motion of the vocal fold cover sections, made possible by the vertically asymmetric motions of upper and lower mass components. As depicted in Figure 5-2, the primary significance of this two-mass modeling is in the shifting configuration of the vocal fold walls relative to the passing airflow. Because this configuration shifts in phase with vocal fold motion, the tissues sustain their motion by drawing energy from the passing airstream. Through this mechanism, there is greater lateral force during the opening phase and lesser force during the closing; see Titze (1994) for further details. Figure 5-2 also depicts the fact that the body tends to be deformed considerably less than the cover during typical vocal fold vibration and that it is the mucosal cover that carries a wavelike mode of vibration. Note also that the two-mass model, schematized by two gray blocks that move in concert with the mucosal wave, is just an abstraction (a "lumped" analysis) of a motion that is actually distributed continuously through the tissues.

It is also important to avoid a misconception all too often found in introductory textbooks on speech production, which implies that a "puff of air" released during the glottal opening phase provides acous-

tic energy. It is virtually the opposite: the *cessation* of airflow at the instant of glottal closure is the acoustic event that then resonates through the vocal tract. And, even though it is the "collision" of the vocal folds that is most directly associated with voice production, this sound is not a clapping sound that might result from a collision of tissues like the hands. It is, in fact, the discontinuity of flow that results from this closure that produces the sound.

Remember that sound is best thought of as a pressure disturbance resulting from displacements of air molecules from their equilibrium distances. Here, the sudden change in flow generates such a disturbance by abruptly "holding back" flowing air molecules. To review the consequence of this for our consideration of motor control, consider that we are now at least two steps conceptually removed from muscular activity: (1) the muscle activities have only created relatively "static" background conditions by setting the respiratory system for controlled expiratory flow and setting vocal fold adduction and elasticity for a valving of that flow, and (2) the self-sustaining motion of the tissues that results from a specific dynamic system of tissue-airflow interaction generates an acoustic event that results directly only from airflow, not the tissue itself. The controlling principles are found in biomechanics and aerodynamics.

Relationships Between Acoustics and Myoelastic-Aerodynamics

Understanding how these principles translate into the acoustic components of the voice source spectrum can help us interpret this spectrum in new and valuable ways. Figure 5-3 presents a schematic drawing of an idealized voice source spectrum.

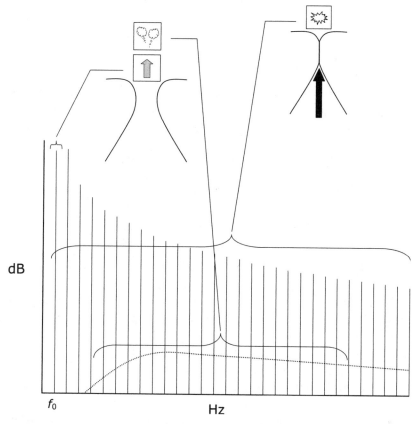

Figure 5–3. The primary elements of the glottal source spectrum (see text for details).

Note that this idealized voice source consists of a line spectrum (because it is a periodic wave that can be spectrally analyzed into pure sine wave elements). These lines represent the fundamental frequency and all of its odd and even multiples, with a slope of −12 dB/octave. The lines are the sine waves that, when summed together, would represent the exact shape of the acoustic waveform resulting from typical vocal fold vibration.

Note also that boxes depicting aerodynamic events associated with vocal fold vibration are linked in Figure 5–3 with elements of the spectrum. Somewhat simplistically, but with a lot of heuristic value, these sine waves can be thought of as follows:

the first harmonic, or H1, is the fundamental frequency, which can be associated with the entire excursion of the vocal folds as they bring the glottis through one open-close cycle. (The peak amplitude of the glottal flow is schematized in the box associated with H1 as a gray arrow.) All the higher harmonics can be associated with that abrupt discontinuity in glottal flow that occurs at the instant of glottal closure. (This is schematized by the explosion figure in a box associated with all the harmonics, but remember that this is more like an "implosion," that occurs when the flow of air is suddenly blocked by vocal fold closure.) This abrupt discontinuity is a rapid event in the time course of the glottal waveform, and that is why it is represented spectrally as higher frequency elements—higher frequencies are simply faster. (So why do they have to be at integer multiples of the fundamental? Because otherwise they would not align in time with that fundamental, and the waveform would not repeat with the fundamental periodicity.) Finally, it is important to remember that, because there is a rush of air through every vocal fold open cycle which forms a jet that may impinge on epilaryngeal structures (structures immediately superior to the vibrating vocal folds), some turbulence noise is typical in normal voices. This turbulence (schematized in a box above the open vocal folds) appears as a continuous noise in higher frequencies of the voice source spectrum. Although it is typically below the amplitude of the higher harmonics, this noise will be more intense in a breathy voice, as might occur especially when vocal fold closure is incomplete. (See the Stevens and Hanson [2004] article in Kent's *Encyclopedia of Communication Disorders* [R. D. Kent, 2004b] for further discussion of these elements of the voice spectrum.) Also consider in this light how the vocal fold "bowing" often found in the hypokinetic dysarthria of Parkinson's disease (Hanson, Gerrat, & Ward, 1984) can cause a breathy turbulence source.

Spectral interpretations of voice acoustics which are guided by the way of thinking outlined in the preceding paragraph can result in many important empirical and theoretical observations that should increasingly support our understanding of pathologic vocal fold conditions, even as influenced by motor disorders. In an article that Ray Kent, sponsored by the Acoustical Society of America, selected in 1991 to be among the nine most important papers published for the understanding of phonation, Gauffin and Sundberg (1989) established empirically that the strength of H1 (the fundamental) correlated strongly with the amplitude of the glottal airflow waveform, whereas a basic measure of the flow discontinuity at glottal fold closure (specifically, the negative peak amplitude of the differentiated flow waveform, which captures the maximum rate at which flow decelerates) correlated strongly with the overall spectral amplitude of all harmonics.

Building on both models and measures and working with Ken Stevens, Helen Hanson (H. M. Hanson, 1997; H. M. Hanson & Chuang, 1999; H. M. Hanson, Stevens, Kuo, Chen, & Slifka, 2001) established that measures of harmonic amplitudes, when adjusted for vocal tract resonance effects and calibrated to the first harmonic, effectively decompose the voice signal into factors that reflected factors such as abruptness of glottal closure and specific energy losses associated with incomplete closure. (See also the Acoustic Analysis of Voice entry [Buder, 2004a] in Kent's *Encyclopedia* for further details on spectral indicators of glottal status.) A standard treatment for spasmodic dysphonia, Botox, should reduce medial compression and allow the vocal folds to vibrate with greater amplitude. Applying relative harmonic amplitudes to assess this treatment, a recent study verified that ameliorations of muscular tension were reflected in the spectrum as increased H1 amplitude (larger vocal fold excursion) and decreased higher harmonic amplitudes (less abrupt vocal fold closing) (Cannito, Buder, & Chorna, 2005).

The most important measures of glottal efficiency can be understood in the terms developed to this point: aerodynamic input and acoustic output. Aerodynamic power is the product of both flow and pressure, acoustic power is measured in dB SPL, and because both of these concepts are in watts, the ratio of acoustic power/aerodynamic power is a simple percentage. As summarized in Titze (1994), this efficiency is typically no more than 1% (because so much of the aerodynamic power passes through the larynx as flow). It is therefore important for speakers to conserve and maximize glottal use of aerodynamic power through the right balance of flow and glottal valving of the flow. However, these considerations may tend to suggest, falsely, that the more adduction the better, as a "pressed" voice conserves aerodynamic power and generates a loud (albeit harsh) voice. It is, therefore, also important to consider the "cost" incurred by the intensity of vocal fold impact, as is taken into account in a more recent measure of vocal efficiency called the "Output-Cost Ratio" (Berry et al., 2001). Laboratory measurements such as this tend to confirm that an optimal generation of acoustic power is accomplished by a barely adducted glottal position, which yields a clinically targeted voice production mode called "resonant voice" (Verdolini, Druker, Palmer, & Samawi, 1998). This clinical goal has been addressed primarily in terms of organic voice disorders of the vocal folds themselves, such as nodules, but it has clear implications regarding normative assessment and therapeutic targets in the realm of hypo- (e.g., hypokinetic or flaccid) versus hyper- (e.g., spasmodic or spastic) adduction associated with motor speech disorders.

Interactions with the Vocal Tract

To yet more fully understand the degree to which the vocal mechanism is, at its heart, a linkage between aerodynamics and acoustics, we should also touch on aspects by which vibration of the vocal folds is affected by the airways in which they operate. One important effect that has been understood for some time is sometimes referred to as the "one-mass model." The mass in this case refers to the air trapped in the vocal tract, and such a mass has the important acoustic property of inertance. As in mechanical inertia, once this mass is set in motion, it tends to stay in motion, and when there is a flow of air through the glottis, the mass of air above and below the vocal folds is set in motion. Following Rothenberg (1981) and others, Stevens (1998) models this effect in detail to show how the glottal pulse is "skewed": the flow is somewhat delayed during the opening phase as the mass of air is set into motion, but the flow is then accelerated somewhat during the closing phase as the moving mass of air "pulls" flow through the narrowing glottis. The effect appears subtle until it is expressed in terms of an increased negative peak of the differentiated flow. Representing the rate at which flow is abruptly decelerated, the differentiated flow effect can be seen to be an important contributor to the strength of the acoustic product. The mechanics of this situation also help explain the self-sustaining nature of vocal fold vibration, and is yet another example of vocal fold behavior that is not directly controlled by any motor control system.

Another vocal tract effect on the glottal source has come to be understood more recently (Titze, 2006; Titze & Story, 1997). We are accustomed, by the pedagogy of source-filter theory, to thinking of the voice source as an acoustic generator that can be completely decoupled from the vocal tract as an acoustic resonator, but this is not actually true. Because of the morphology of the larynx immediately superior to the vocal folds, there are significant acoustic impedance effects on the vocal folds that actually facilitate their vibration by lowering the threshold pressures for oscillation. Although the literature discusses these effects primarily in terms of singing style variations, it is clear that pathologic muscular tensions and/or atrophy effects could have facilitating or deleterious effects on the ability of a patient with a motor speech disorder to shape the epilarynx for producing optimal phonation. More explorations are needed for voice disorders researchers and clinicians to absorb this fairly profound shift in thinking on the vocal mechanism. Ingo Titze, a leading expert on vocal fold vibration, is now of the view that ". . . the traditional linear source-filter theory of voice production is passé," so much so that he wishes that the traditional theory of phonation were now dubbed the "myoelastic-aeroacoustic theory of phonation" (Titze, 2006, p. v) .

Phonatory Control

Preceding sections have developed some of the principles by which we can understand the autonomous nature of vocal fold vibration, setting the stage for some appreciation of how so many aspects of phonatory control such as F_0 and intensity variation may be several steps removed from direct neuromuscular control. It is, of course, desirable for expressivity, and even valuable for intelligibility, that this sound source be controllable for sound pressure levels and fundamental frequency variations. See the review by Ramig in a book edited by R. D. Kent for discussion of how phonatory contributions to intelligibility can be especially important in hypokinetic motor speech disorders (Ramig, 1992). A series of studies from Wisconsin

have specifically demonstrated the role of F_0 variation in supporting sentence intelligibility of both normal (Laures & Weismer, 1999) and dysarthric speakers (Bunton, Kent, Kent, & Duffy, 2001), although work by Bender (2001) suggests that this intelligibility loss may be negligible when the speech and presentation conditions are optimally clear.

Intensity

The control of phonatory intensity—acoustic power—is fairly well understood to involve the role of respiratory muscles for increasing the pressures and flows with which the vocal fold system is driven (Titze, 2006). Counterintuitively, the extent of lateral excursion of the vocal folds does not increase with greater phonation intensity. Furthermore, the closed interval in the glottal cycle is actually longer for more intense phonation (Baken & Orlikoff, 2000). These observations reinforce the posturing role of adductory force in creating pressures (medial compression) for phonation. Recall once again that vocal fold motion and vocal fold impact, themselves, do not generate the primary sound of voicing, but that it is the stopping of flow that is acoustically most significant.

Fundamental Frequency

The control of fundamental frequency is more difficult to understand. Because the cricothyroid (CT) muscle is innervated by the distinctly separate branch of the vagal nerve, the external branch of the superior laryngeal nerve, it would be nice from a neuromotor point of view if it were simply this muscle that controlled vocal fold stiffness (which indeed most directly affects F_0). Recall, however, that the thyroarytenoid (TA) muscle is an antagonist to the CT, and also that a muscle stiffens when contracted. This configuration is nonlinear: when the TA muscle contracts extensively, it may retract, as the body of the vocal folds, to allow only the most superficial cover tissues to vibrate more freely and with less stiffness. The vocal ligament (intermediate and deep layers of the lamina propria), when strained, must also be considered as a stiffening element of the vocal fold system, and because subglottal (tracheal) pressure is the driving force of phonation, it can increase vibratory rate.

Titze has summarized these three factors (CT and TA activity and P_{sg}) in a plot called a muscle activation plot, or "MAP," reproduced as Figure 5–4 of this chapter. Although based on a theoretical model, most predictions emanating from its contents have been empirically validated. The plot is quite rich with information and should be consulted directly, but some es-

sential facts can be summarized verbally: (1) increasing subglottal (tracheal) pressure always raises F_0 (but note that this effect is strong only at lower frequencies); (2) increasing CT activity will raise F_0 when the TA is essentially inactive; (3) increasing TA activity will raise F_0 when the CT is essentially inactive; (4) at mid and high levels of TA activity, CT activation may initially lower F_0 but will raise it again as activation increases; and (5) at high levels of CT activation, TA activation may have no effect on F_0 or even slightly lower it.

Although these observations may seem somewhat confounding, the point is once again that complexities of the vocal mechanisms must be considered before attempting any specific diagnostic, assessment, or therapeutic predictions based on neuromuscular conditions. Use of prosodic resources can, nonetheless, be evaluated in connected speech tasks (picture description or spontaneous conversational speech) for assessment in motor speech disorders (R.D. Kent & Kent, 2000; R.D. Kent & Rosenbek, 1982). Fortuitously, shared mechanisms for SPL and F_0 control, specifically P_{sg} and TA activation, should work together in such tasks. Furthermore, because these factors may also conspire to elevate relative levels of upper harmonics, their healthy functioning supports a speaker's ability to control stress and prominence in syllabic nuclei (Sluijter & van Heuven, 1996; Strik & Boves, 1992). This aspect of phonatory control reinforces the importance of understanding and interpreting spectral correlates of voice.

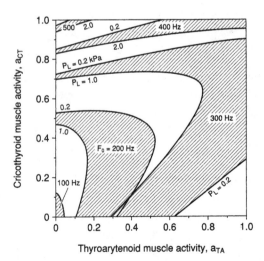

Figure 5–4. Muscle activation plot (MAP) depicting theoretical F_0 effects of lung pressure, CT muscle activation, and TA activation (reproduced with permission from the National Center for Voice and Speech from Titze [1994]).

Vibratory Regimes

The preceding section reviewed mechanisms by which F_0 and sound pressure level are ultimately under neuromotor control. These are complex mechanisms, and a full accounting of the causes of any particular F_0 or SPL output would require an understanding and measurement of many variables. Even if these measures were accessible, would the end product measures be usable for a number one clinical goal in motor speech disorders, that of "differential diagnosis"? Unfortunately not, due to the number of alternative vibratory regimes of the vocal folds. Because of nonlinear relationships among the controlling factors for vocal fold vibration there is yet another layer of complexity (again due to the autonomous nonmuscular nature of the glottis as a sound generator).

Figure 5-5 displays an extremely narrow-band spectrogram of a woman with spasmodic dysphonia sustaining the sound "ah." Even though it is generally true that the symptoms of SD are less severe in a sustained phonation like this than in connected speech, the spectrographic display reveals a multitude of "subharmonics." The intermittent but clear appearances of two or more intervening harmonics throughout this voice prolongation reflect episodes in which there is a regular alternation between shorter (usually lower amplitude) and longer (usually normal amplitude) glottal pulses. Because these alternations cause repeating chains of short-long glottal pulses the phenomenon is also called period-doubling, period-tripling (for chains of three pulses), and so forth. There is even a brief episode in this sample where there are chains of five pulses, causing four harmonics to appear in between the dominant harmonics. The perceptual quality of these episodes is a special kind of roughness. It is hard to know exactly which rating labels different

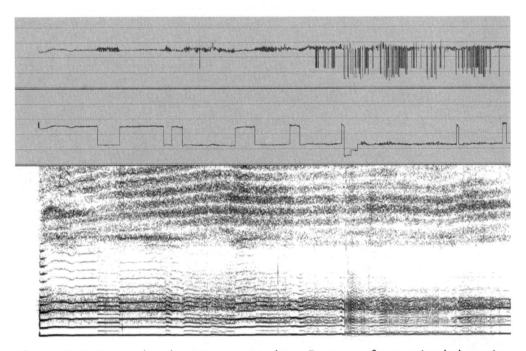

Figure 5–5. Narrow-band spectrogram and two F_0 traces of a sustained phonation by a woman with adductor spasmodic dysphonia (with permission from Michael P. Cannito for use of recording).

clinicians use for this roughness, as it seems that "harsh," "diplophonic," and "fry" might all apply, depending on the type and degree to which it occurs, the presence or absence of other qualities, and the preferences of the person doing the rating.

This phenomenon and other regime shifts such as pitch breaks, biphonation, and even chaos, have become well known to voice scientists (Herzel, Berry, Titze, & Saleh, 1994; Svec, Schutte, & Miller, 1996; Titze, Baken, & Herzel, 1993). It is increasingly clear that many types of mechanisms can cause these shifts, from slight asymmetries in the vocal folds to interactions of vocal F_0 with resonances of the vocal tract. Duffy (2005) associates diplophonia with flaccid conditions (e.g., p. 418), but in the present example the extra tones arise in a spasmodic condition. In fact, the phenomenon arises in a high proportion

of adults without any known neurologic or vocal disorders (though, intriguingly, it develops to a significantly greater degree in older women than in older men) (Buder, 2004b; Kleeman, 2002).

Figure 5–6 displays another narrow-band spectrogram in which subharmonics and other sudden voice quality changes such as pitch breaks can be seen: the speaker is a 4-month-old girl. Kent was among the first to report on the systematic occurrence of alternate phonation patterns such as seen in this spectrogram, documenting subharmonics even before it had come to be understood under the framework of nonlinear dynamics (R. D. Kent & Murray, 1982). Infants clearly explore a wide range of phonatory settings in relatively free variation, ironically revealing the possibilities that adults may unfortunately find themselves shackled

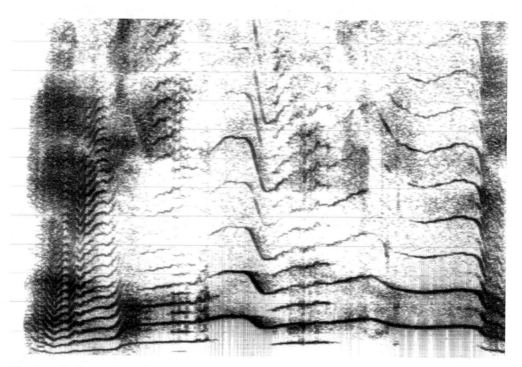

Figure 5–6. Narrow-band spectrogram of a complex phonation by a 4-month-old infant.

with due to a motor speech disorder. This example also reinforces another general point of this chapter: that aberrant phonations are, in fact, incipient within the normal mechanism.

Returning to the adult example in Figure 5–5, some measurement difficulties are presented that we may encounter in the analysis of dysfunctional phonatory samples. Two pitch traces are provided above the spectrogram. Although it is common parlance to use the psychological nomenclature "pitch" for these traces, they actually track the physical attribute of F_0 (the distinction is important in the following discussion). These are displayed in the TF32 program (Milenkovic, 2001), but they were calculated using a pitch determination algorithm implemented in the older CSpeechSP environment (Milenkovic, 1997). The algorithm tends to track a fundamental period based on the initial pulses encountered. In this respect, it is like "streaming" in the auditory system, which is a process whereby ongoing prior experience with pitch and timbre linked with a perceived source facilitates ongoing association of the sound with that source (Bregman, 1978).

In the top panel of Figure 5–5, the pitch trace has been set to follow the phonation based on the initial quality in which the speaker with SD is able to start out with a vocal output unaffected by subharmonics. Later, the medial compression due to her condition affects the voice in some way that renders it more vulnerable to the nonlinear dynamic instability of subharmonics. (It is usually of some clinical value to observe, as in this example, whether the instabilities typically "build" as persons with SD prolong such phonations, possibly due to muscle fatigue.) The pitch tracker can follow the alternating short and long periods associated with these subharmon-

ics to a point, but as they develop in severity, the tracker breaks down. However, as seen in the lower trace, the tracker can be reset to follow the doubled period, tracking the frequency that effectively drops by an octave. If cursors are set around such segments so that the ear can "track" or stream these segments in isolation, then this lower frequency may, in fact, be the dominant percept.

So we have a technical problem here: what is the "true" fundamental frequency? This matters a great deal for many reasons having to do with the nature of the motor speech disorder and its assessment in both acoustic and perceptual terms. Note, first of all, as discussed further in an entry to Kent's *Encyclopedia* (Buder, 2004a), the upper pitch trace displays quite a bit of alternation between pitch periods and would, therefore, be measured against this F_0 to have a considerable amount of pitch perturbation, or "jitter." Many, if not most, acoustic assessments of voice in motor speech disorders target jitter (Buder, 2000). The underlying mechanism that is targeted in these assessments is, hence, presumed to be neurologic, that is, due to a loss of nerve fibers (Titze, 1991) or loss of organization in neural firing (Larson, Kempster, & Kistler, 1987). Such mechanisms, and their effect in producing a "harsh" or "noisy" voice, presumably have a random influence in creating vocal fold instabilities (Baken & Orlikoff, 2000). However, these modulations of pitch period are correlated (nonrandomly alternating) and would, therefore, grossly inflate the measure of jitter as a representation of neural dysfunction. Furthermore, as listed in detail below, none of the primary mechanisms of nonlinear dynamic instabilities such as subharmonics are directly neurologic. Specifically related to the difficulties in determining a "true"

F_0, the problem can now be seen as due to a lack of clarity in the descriptive nomenclature of dysarthric voice ratings: Is the roughness of subharmonics to be classified as "harsh" voice? Is the presence of concurrent periodicities in subharmonics to be classified as "diplophonia?" Or is the alternation between higher and lower F_0s as seen in the lower pitch trace of Figure 5–5 to be classified as "pitch breaks"?

Once again, failures to understand the autonomous nature of the mechanism in general, and specifically to understand assumptions acoustic analysis algorithms make about voice, can impair correct association of vocal function measures with motor speech disorders. The pervasive nonlinearity of the vocal mechanism is, however, not to be considered as an esoteric annoyance, because it is this very nonlinearity that also predisposes the vocal mechanism to operate as a self-sustaining process in the first place, affording a good range of output frequencies, intensities, and qualities to be reliably produced over a large range of phonatory (respiratory and laryngeal) posturings. As such, this mechanism is the quintessential "quantal" device in the sense that Ken Stevens has expressed (K. Stevens, 1989), by which the acoustic "target" of voice production has a large range of robust output behaviors, in between boundary conditions of small and large subglottal pressures and medial compressions: crossing these boundaries induces voice to either initiate or cease but all values in between produce some vocal output.

It is worth summarizing these nonlinear aspects of voice by quoting and distilling points from Titze's latest text: "*a large-signal response is not simply a scaled-up version of a small-signal response, nor is the complete response a simple addition of transient and steady state responses.*

. . . The system may be very sensitive to small changes in a parameter. . . or to the initial conditions" (2006, p. 349). As summarized in the final chapter of Titze's book, there are at least eight important nonlinear relationships in the mechanisms of voice production, all of which are necessary for self-sustaining vocal fold vibration, but any one of which can cause the kind of instability that predisposes the voice to suddenly jump between vibratory regimes with very little change in neuromuscular input: (1) the relationship between pressure and flow in the glottis (compounded by wave propagation in tissue walls, a nonlinear relationship between wall displacement and flow, and the possibility of sudden detachment of the flow from the wall in the form of a jet); (2) the delayed negative feedback of the mucosal wave on itself; (3) the delayed negative feedback from the moving mass of air in vocal tract; (4) a nonlinear response of tissues (strains) to the forces that deform them (stresses); (5) tissue deformation during vocal fold collision; (6) coupling of vocal fold vibration to vocal tract resonances; (7) vocal fold asymmetries; and (8) a decrease of tissue viscosity (the aspect that damps vibration by absorbing and dissipating energy) with increasing vibration frequency.

Modulations of F_0 and SPL

The point of the preceding section on vibratory regimes was most certainly not to put off clinical or scientific studies of basic vocal parameters such as F_0 and SPL, which are exceedingly important and most certainly measurable. The point, however, was to reinforce that there are basic reasons to avoid simple summaries of these vocal parameters without consideration of various phenomena other than motor control issues that affect their behavior. At the very least, some care must be taken to inspect vocal characteristics prior to and during the extraction of these parameters so that summary measures can more truly be taken to reflect motor control, or otherwise understood to reflect the other autonomous aspects of vocal fold vibration that have been reviewed in this chapter.

Those cautions having been issued, what are the some of the motor control phenomena that may be of value to assessments in motor speech disorders (keeping in mind the desirability of tasks that focus on functional vocal control)? Kent has recognized that simple vocal modulations of F_0 and SPL during sustained vowel prolongations can, when analyzed carefully for distinct frequency domains such as wow, tremor, and flutter, help distinguish the impact of various neurologic disorders on phonatory control (R. D. Kent, Weismer, Kent, Vorperian, & Duffy, 1999, see especially Figure 2, p. 153). In a case study of severe essential tremor, Kent (Kent, Duffy, Vorperian, & Thomas, 1998) found that modulations of F_0 and SPL, when inspected closely and quantified for frequency, were quite rich in clinically significant phenomena (including observations that speech units could be entrained by the pathologic oscillations in a manner that may have helped the patient to compensate for otherwise deleterious effects of the disorder on her speech intelligibility). In the subtle and mixed dysarthrias associated with multiple sclerosis, the measurement of such modulations can help with two difficult goals: (1) the classification of subtypes of the disorder and (2) the detection of subclinical symptoms that patients may report but which clinicians do not routinely pick up (Hartelius & Buder, 1999; Hartelius, Buder, & Strand, 1997; Hartelius, Nord, &

Buder, 1995). The latter goal may be especially promising for early detection in other disorders such as Parkinson's disease for example, in which one study was able to retrospectively document a decrease in F_0 variability as early as 5 years prior to diagnosis (Harel, Cannizzaro, & Snyder, 2004).

Returning to the cautionary theme of this chapter, however, it should be noted once again that norming of vocal measures may be possible only with great care and attention to factors that have not always been thoroughly considered in traditional clinical research or practice. Exploration of modulation measures in unaffected individuals reveals that there are numerous subject and task effects that seem rarely if ever taken into account in broad clinical assessments. Consider the instructions most typically given for a sustained vowel prolongation: "take a deep breath and say 'ah' for as long and as steadily as you can, until you run out of air." Two dilemmas are posed by this question: (1) there is an inherent contradiction between "as long" and "as steadily" and (2) patients' self-selections of F_0 and SPL can have dramatic consequences on modulations in the resulting phonation (Buder, Corbin-Lewis, Coon, & Ramig, 2006). Note also that these issues themselves interact: to sustain a phonation as long as possible, a phonator should take as deep a breath as possible, almost unavoidably starting out the phonation at an atypically high F_0 and SPL, and then, to comply with the steadiness instruction, maintain these high values throughout the phonation.

These effects can be illustrated fairly directly using a technique that visualizes the modulations in a spectrogram-like representation called the "modulogram" (Buder & Strand, 2003). Instead of spectrally analyzing a sound waveform, the modulogram analyzes traces of F_0 and SPL.

Also, to accommodate the fact that very slow phenomena such as low-frequency "wows" require long spectral analysis windows whereas fast and typically transient phenomena like high-frequency "flutters" will only be visible using short windows, the modulogram analyzes wows, tremors, and flutters in three separate panels each with its own windows and bandwidths of analysis. The darkness scale of the modulogram still represents the power of a wave, but in this case, that wave is a modulation of F_0 or SPL, and the power is the depth of that modulation scaled as a percentage of the mean level.

Figures 5–7 and 5–8 present some elements from modulogram displays, showing first F_0 modulations in Figure 5–7 and then SPL modulations in Figure 5–8. The phonations were performed by the chapter author, overtly (but hopefully naturally) adopting specific strategies along the lines of differing options as might be elicited by the task instructions. In panel A of Figure 5–7, the phonation is maximally long (toward the higher end of normative results tabulated in Kent, Kent, and Rosenbek [1987]). Because the phonation starts near the top of vital capacity where passive forces exert high P_{sg}, the speaker adopts the elevated F_0 that would normally result from this high pressure and sustains it throughout (the phonation was also loud). Note that, at the beginning, there are transient wows and a fairly diffuse set of tremor frequencies that result from the difficulty of stabilizing the larynx against such high pressures once phonation begins. Then, after about 15 seconds, a typical "normal" F_0 tremor sets in around 3 to 5 Hz. This tremor is exacerbated, however, as the phonation task begins to draw on expiratory reserves, recruiting abdominal wall muscles and probably also requiring effort from TA and CT muscles to maintain glottal conditions for the ongoing "steady" F_0 and SPL with which the phonation began. These efforts result in deeper tremor, some noticeable flutter and some new wow phenomena, all elicited to the highest degree in the "last gasp." In the author's experience, most participants with less familiarity with the task (and perhaps with less motivation to prove something) become uncomfortable tapping into expiratory reserve mechanisms and sounding strained and tremulous in the process, taking the option instead to obey the "keep it steady" instruction at the expense of cutting the phonation short.

In the lower panel of Figure 5–7, the same participant has produced another phonation in which the "keep it steady" instruction was taken as the priority; the phonation begins at a lower F_0 and persists for just over half as long as the previous sample. The quantitative analysis of F_0 tremor in the phonation adopting this latter strategy yielded an average depth of modulation at the central frequency of 4 Hz of 0.59%, persisting for 45% of the time. The "long" phonation, however, had produced a significantly higher average modulation depth (although still at the same frequency of 4 Hz) of 0.67%, persisting for 60% of the time. Which would be the "correct" assessment?

An even more dramatic difference is visible in a comparison of the modulograms in Figure 5–8, which display SPL instabilities. Both of these phonations were produced with an emphasis on steady, but notice by the scales that the phonation in set (B) is nearly 10 dB quieter than in set (A). The obviously greater instability in the quieter phonation is not only due to the fact that the modulations are expressed as a percentage of the mean, therefore increasing in relative terms when the mean is lower. The absolute dB waveform

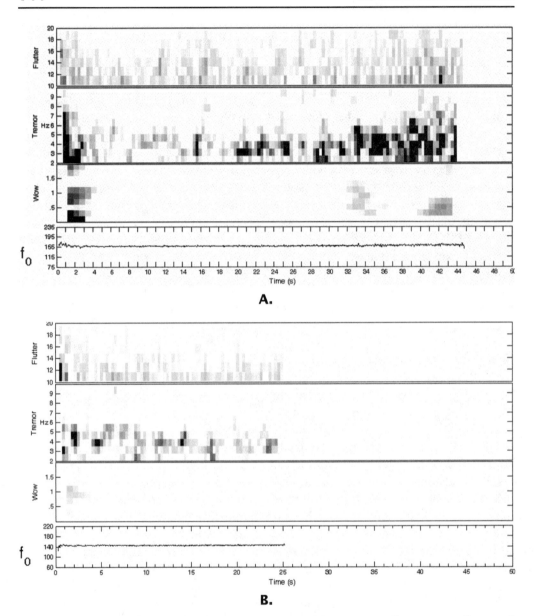

Figure 5–7. Sections of modulograms displaying F_0 wow (*lower panel in each set*), tremor (*middle panel in each set*) and flutter (*upper panel in each set*) for a neurologically unaffected adult man. Set **A.** displays a loud phonation emphasizing maximum time but attempting steadiness throughout. Set **B.** displays a comparably loud phonation emphasizing steadiness.

itself is obviously more modulated in both wow and tremor domains, and there is clear flutter as the quiet and more breathy phonation had become difficult to sustain.

There are many structural mechanisms that plausibly support phonatory stability when the speaker takes a "louder" posture and these factors are undoubtedly impor-

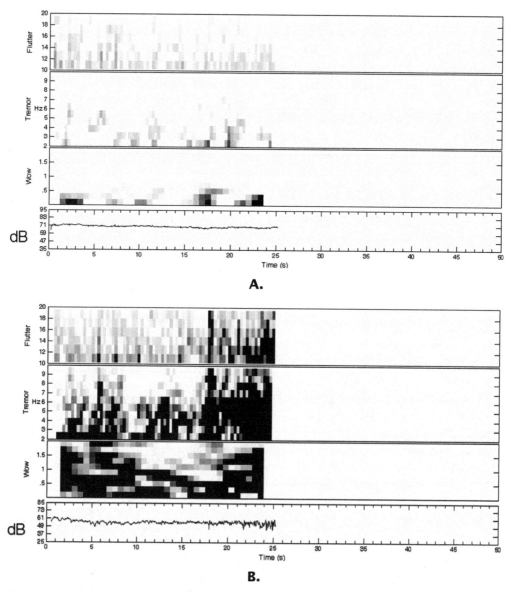

Figure 5–8. Sections of modulograms displaying SPL wow (*lower panel in each set*), tremor (*middle panel in each set*), and flutter (*upper panel in each set*) for a neurologically unaffected adult man. Set **A.** displays a loud phonation emphasizing steadiness. Set **B.** displays a comparably long phonation emphasizing steadiness, but which is very quiet.

tant in hypokinetic and flaccid dysarthrias (Dromey & Ramig, 1998). SPL modulations appear to receive less attention in the literature than F_0 modulations, but they appear to be especially important in certain motor speech disorders such as the dysarthria of MS (Hartelius et al., 1997).

These demonstrations again reinforce the fact that for the vocal mechanism, many aspects of "disordered" speech may be found as variations within the normal population, or even as secondary to task performance. Although these types of effects may not necessarily be entirely artifactual or even epiphenomenal, their interpretations must be couched within an understanding of the vocal mechanism and an allowance for variability in patients' strategies for accomplishing vocal tasks. However, this latter concern seems exacerbated when instructions are more or less self-contradictory.

Consider, in direct parallel to the sustained phonation instructions, another opposition or tradeoff in our requests for alternating motions: the requested repetitions may be either most fast or most accurate. Analyses of a large normative dataset for laryngeal DDK (repetition of "ah"s and "ha"s) reveals that unaffected participants do, in fact, trade off accuracy for speed and vice versa (Corbin-Lewis, Bassich, Buder, Baxter, & Thompson, 2005). The same normative dataset also demonstrated that gender can be a factor, that rates and accuracies differ dramatically when participants see their waveforms in real time, and even that participant variables like gender interact with visual condition (differences between men and women disappeared when visual feedback was provided). Until motivational aspects related to performance variables are taken into account, it remains inappropriate to ex-pect that any given performance by any particular individual can be directly "normed."

Summary

This chapter reviewed selected aspects of voice production that may be affected by motor speech disorders, with an emphasis on those aspects that are ironically not under direct neuromuscular control. This emphasis was not meant to discourage clinical examination of laryngeal and phonatory manifestations of motor speech disorders, but rather to encourage such examinations to take into account subtle and fascinating biomechanical, aerodynamic, and acoustic principles of voice production. It is hoped that practitioners and scientists will thereby not only feel a greater sense of wonder and respect for the mechanisms and their multifaceted dynamics, but also that they will understand more deeply why scholars like Ray Kent have exhorted us to avoid simplistic normative interpretations that could neglect to treat each voice as an individual communicative expression.

Acknowledgments. Preparation of this chapter was supported in part by grant R01DC006099 from the National Institutes of Deafness and Other Communication Disorders, and the author is grateful to Dr. Lesya B. Chorna and Jamie L. Edrington, M.A., CCC-SLP, for help with preparation of the manuscript.

References

Aronson, A. E. (1990). *Clinical voice disorders* (3rd ed.). New York: Thieme.

Aronson, A. E., & Hartman, D. E. (1981). Adductor spastic dysphonia as a sign of essential (voice) tremor. *Journal of Speech and Hearing Disorders, 46,* 52–58.

Awan, S. N. (2001). *The voice diagnostic profile: A practical guide to the diagnosis of voice disorders.* Gaithersburg, MD: Aspen.

Baken, R. J., & Orlikoff, R. F. (2000). *Clinical measurement of speech and voice.* San Diego, CA: Singular Publishing Group.

Bender, B. K. (2001). Contributions of fundamental frequency to speech intelligibility (Doctoral dissertation, The University of Memphis, 2001). *Dissertation Abstracts International, DAI-B 62/10,* 4506.

Berry, D. A., Verdolini, K., Montequin, D. W., Hess, M. M., Chan, R. W., & Titze, I. R. (2001). A quantitative output-cost ratio in voice production. *Journal of Speech, Language, and Hearing Research, 44,* 29–37.

Blitzer, A., Brin, M. F., Sasaki, C. T., Fahn, S., & Harris, K. S. (1992). *Neurological disorders of the larynx.* New York: Thieme.

Boone, D. R., McFarlane, S. C., & Von Berg, S. L. (2005). *The voice and voice therapy* (7th ed.). Boston: Allyn & Bacon.

Bregman, A. S. (1978). Auditory streaming: Competition among alternative organizations. *Perception and Psychophysics, 23,* 391–398.

Buder, E. H. (2000). Acoustic analysis of voice quality: A tabulation of algorithms 1902-1990. In R. D. Kent & M. J. Ball (Eds.), *Voice quality measurement* (pp. 119–244). San Diego, CA: Singular Publishing Group.

Buder, E. H. (2004a). Acoustic assessment of voice. In R. D. Kent (Ed.), *MIT encyclopedia of communication disorders* (pp. 3–7). Cambridge, MA: MIT Press.

Buder, E. H. (2004b). Subharmonic phonation: Measurement issue or descriptive object? *Perspectives on Voice and Voice Disorders, 14*(1), 8–12.

Buder, E. H., Corbin-Lewis, K., Coon, H., & Ramig, L. O. (2006, June). *Phonatory stability and mobility as phenotypes.* Paper presented at the 5th International Conference on Speech Motor Control, Nijmegen, The Netherlands.

Buder, E. H., & Strand, E. A. (2003). Quantitative and graphic acoustic analysis of phonatory modulations: The modulogram. *Journal of Speech, Language, and Hearing Research, 46,* 475–490.

Bunton, K., Kent, R. D., Kent, J. F., & Duffy, J. R. (2001). The effects of flattening fundamental frequency contours on sentence intelligibility in speakers with dysarthria. *Clinical Linguistics and Phonetics, 15,* 181–193.

Cannito, M. P., Buder, E. H., & Chorna, L. B. (2005). Spectral amplitude measures of adductor spasmodic dysphonic speech. *Journal of Voice, 19,* 391–410.

Colton, R. H., & Casper, J. (1996). *Understanding voice problems: A physiological perspec-tive for diagnosis and treatment* (2nd ed.). Baltimore: Williams & Wilkins.

Corbin-Lewis, K., Bassich, C. J., Buder, E. H., Baxter, A., & Thompson, N. (2005, November). *Laryngeal diadochokinesis in normal adults.* Paper presented at the annual meeting of the American Speech-Language-Hearing Association, San Diego, CA.

Darley, F. L., Aronson, A. E., & Brown, J. R. (1975). *Motor speech disorders.* Philadelphia: W. B. Saunders.

Dromey, C., & Ramig, L. O. (1998). Intentional changes in sound pressure level and rate: Their impact on measures of respiration, phonation, and articulation. *Journal of Speech, Language, and Hearing Research, 41,* 1003–1018.

Duffy, J. (2005). *Motor speech disorders: Substrates, differential diagnosis, and management* (2nd ed.). St. Louis, MO: Elsevier Mosby.

Gauffin, J., & Sundberg, J. (1989). Spectral correlates of glottal voice source waveform characteristics. *Journal of Speech and Hearing Research, 32,* 556–565. (Reprinted in Kent, R. D., Atal, B. S., & Miller, J. L. [1991]. *Papers in speech communication: Speech production* [pp. 147–156]. Woodbury, NY: Acoustical Society of America).

Hanson, D. G., Gerrat, B. R., & Ward, P. H. (1984). Cinegraphic observations on laryngeal dysfunction in Parkinson's disease. *Laryngoscope, 94,* 348–353.

Hanson, H. M. (1997). Glottal characteristics of female speakers: Acoustic correlates. *Journal of the Acoustical Society of America, 101*(1), 466–481.

Hanson, H. M., & Chuang, E. S. (1999). Glottal characteristics of male speakers: Acoustic correlates and comparison with female data. *Journal of the Acoustical Society of America, 106,* 1064–1077.

Hanson, H. M., Stevens, K. N., Kuo, H. J., Chen, M. Y., & Slifka, J. (2001). Towards models of phonation. *Journal of Phonetics, 29,* 451–480.

Harel, B., Cannizzaro, M., & Snyder, P. J. (2004). Variability in fundamental frequency during speech in prodromal and incipient Parkinson's disease: A longitudinal case study. *Brain and Cognition, 56,* 24–29.

Hartelius, L., & Buder, E. H. (1999). Phonatory characteristics in individuals with multiple sclerosis with and without cerebellar symptomatology. In H. F. Peters (Ed.), *Proceedings of the XXIVth World Congress of the International Association of Logopedics and Phoniatrics* (Vol. 2, pp. 602–605). Nijmegan, Netherlands: Nijmegan University Press.

Hartelius, L., Buder, E. H., & Strand, E. A. (1997). Long-term phonatory instability in individuals with multiple sclerosis. *Journal of Speech, Language, and Hearing Research, 40,* 1056–1072.

Hartelius, L., Nord, L., & Buder, E. H. (1995). Acoustic analysis of dysarthria associated with multiple sclerosis. *Clinical Linguistics and Phonetics, 9,* 95–120.

Herzel, H., Berry, D., Titze, I. R., & Saleh, M. (1994). Analysis of vocal disorders with methods from nonlinear dynamics. *Journal of Speech and Hearing Research, 37,* 1008–1019. (Reprinted in Sataloff, RT, & Hawkshaw, M. [Eds.], *Chaos in medicine: Source readings* [pp. 501–512]. San Diego, CA: Singular Publishing Group.)

Hirano, M., Koike, Y., & von Leden, H. (1968). Maximum phonation time and air usage during phonation. *Folia Phoniatrica, 20,* 185–201.

Kent, J., Kent, R., Rosenbek, J., Weismer, G., Martin, R., Sufit, R., et al. (1992). Quantitative description of the dysarthria in women with amyotrophic lateral sclerosis. *Journal of Speech and Hearing Research, 35,* 723–733.

Kent, R. D. (1990). The acoustic and physiologic characteristics of neurologically impaired speech movements. In W. Hardcastle & A. Marchal (Eds.), *Proceedings of the NATO conference on speech production and speech modelling* (pp. 365–401). Dordrecht, The Netherlands: Kluwer.

Kent, R. D. (1994). Laryngeal dysfunction in neurological disease: Amyotrophic lateral sclerosis, Parkinson's disease, and stroke. *Journal of Medical Speech-Language Pathology, 16,* 157–189.

Kent, R. D. (1996). Hearing and believing: Some limits to the auditory-perceptual assessment of speech and voice disorders. *American Journal of Speech-Language Pathology, 5,* 7–23.

Kent, R. D. (1997a). A speaking task analysis of the dysarthria in cerebellar disease. *Folia Phoniatrica et Logopaedica, 49,* 63–82.

Kent, R. D. (1997b). *The speech sciences.* San Diego, CA: Singular Publishing Group.

Kent, R. D. (2004a). The uniqueness of speech among motor systems. *Clinical Linguistics and Phonetics, 18,* 6–8.

Kent, R. D. (Ed.). (2004b). *The MIT encyclopedia of communication disorders.* Cambridge, MA: The MIT Press.

Kent, R. D., Duffy, J. R., Vorperian, H. K., & Thomas, J. E. (1998). Severe essential vocal and oromandibular tremor: A case report. *Phonosurgery, 1,* 237–253.

Kent, R. D., & Kent, J. F. (2000). Task-based profiles of the dysarthrias. *Folia Phoniatrica et Logopaedica, 52,* 48–53.

Kent, R. D., Kent, J. F., Duffy, J., & Weismer, G. (1998). The dysarthrias: Speech-voice profiles, related dysfunctions, and neuropathology. *Journal of Medical Speech-Language Pathology, 6,* 165–211.

Kent, R. D., Kent, J. F., & Rosenbeck, J. C. (1987). Maximum performance tests of speech production. *Journal of Speech and Hearing Disorders, 52,* 367–387.

Kent, R. D., Kent, J. F., Weismer, G., Martin, R. E., Sufit, R. L., Brooks, B. R., et al. (1989). Relationships between speech intelligibility and the slope of second-formant transitions in dysarthric subjects. *Clinical Linguistics and Phonetics, 3,* 347–358.

Kent, R. D., & Murray, A. D. (1982). Acoustic features of infant vocalic utterances at 3, 6, and 9 months. *Journal of the Acoustical Society of America, 72,* 353–365.

Kent, R. D., & Read, W. C. (2002). *The acoustic analysis of speech* (2nd ed.). Clifton Park, NY: Thomson Delmar Learning.

Kent, R. D., & Rosenbek, J. C. (1982). Prosodic disturbance and neurologic lesion. *Brain and Language, 15,* 259–291.

Kent, R. D., Sufit, R. L., Rosenbek, J. C., Kent, J. F., Weismer, G., Martin, R. E., et al. (1991). Speech deterioration in amotrophic lateral sclerosis: A case study. *Journal of Speech and Hearing Research, 34,* 1269–1275.

Kent, R. D., Vorperian, H. K., & Duffy, J. R. (1999). Reliability of the Multi-dimensional Voice Program. *American Journal of Speech-Language Pathology, 8,* 129–136.

Kent, R. D., Vorperian, H. K., Kent, J. F., & Duffy, J. R. (2003). Voice dysfunction in dysarthria: Application of the Multi-Dimensional Voice Program. *Journal of Communication Disorders, 36,* 281–306.

Kent, R. D., Weismer, G., Kent, J., & Rosenbek, J. (1989). Toward phonetic intelligibility testing in dysarthria. *Journal of Speech and Hearing Disorders, 54,* 482–499.

Kent, R. D., Weismer, G., Kent, J. F., Vorperian, H. K., & Duffy, J. R. (1999). Acoustic studies of dysarthric speech: Methods, progress, and potential. *Journal of Communication Disorders, 32,* 141–186.

Kleeman, K. M. (2002). *Gender as a factor in the occurrence of subharmonics in normal voice.* Unpublished master's thesis, The University of Memphis, Memphis, Tennessee.

Larson, C., Kempster, G., & Kistler, M. (1987). Changes in voice fundamental frequency following discharge of single motor units in cricothyroid and thyroarytenoid muscles. *Journal of Speech and Hearing Research, 30,* 552–558.

Laures, J. S., & Weismer, G. (1999). The effects of a flattened fundamental frequency on intelligibility at the sentence level. *Journal of Speech, Language, and Hearing Research, 42,* 1148–1156.

Linville, S. E. (2001). *Vocal aging.* San Diego, CA: Singular Publishing Group.

Linville, S. E. (2004). Voice disorders of aging. In R. D. Kent (Ed.), *The MIT Encyclopedia of Communication Disorders* (pp. 72–75). London: The MIT Press.

Milenkovic, P. (1997). CSpeechSP [Computer software]. Madison, WI: University of Wisconsin-Madison.

Milenkovic, P. (2001). TF32 [Computer software]. Madison, WI: University of Wisconsin-Madison.

Ramig, L. O. (1992). The role of phonation in speech intelligibility: A review and preliminary data from patients with Parkinson's disease. In R. D. Kent (Ed.), *Intelligibility in speech disorders* (pp. 119–155). Amsterdam: John Benjamins.

Rothenberg, M. (1981). Acoustic interaction between the glottal source and the vocal tract. In M. Hirano & K. N. Stevens (Eds.), *Vocal fold physiology* (pp. 305–323). Tokyo: University of Tokyo Press.

Sapienza, C. M., Murry, T., & Brown, W. S., Jr. (1998). Variations in adductor spasmodic dysphonia: Acoustic evidence. *Journal of Voice, 12,* 214–222.

Sapienza, C. M., Walton, S., & Murry, T. (1999). Acoustic variations in adductor spasmodic dysphonia as a function of speech task. *Journal of Speech, Language, and Hearing Research, 42,* 127–140.

Sataloff, R. T. (2005). *Clinical assessment of voice.* San Diego, CA: Plural Publishing Group.

Sluijter, A. M. C., & van Heuven, V. J. (1996). Spectral balance as an acoustic correlate of linguistic stress. *Journal of the Acoustical Society of America, 100,* 2471–2484.

Stemple, J. C., Glaze, L. E., & Gerdeman, B. K. (2000). *Clinical voice pathology: Theory and management.* San Diego, CA: Singular Publishing Group.

Stevens, K. (1989). On the quantal nature of speech. *Journal of Phonetics, 17,* 3–45.

Stevens, K. N. (1998). *Acoustic phonetics.* Cambridge, MA: MIT Press.

Stevens, K. N., & Hanson, H. M. (2004). Voice acoustics. In R. D. Kent (Ed.), *MIT encyclopedia of communication disorders* (pp. 63–67). Cambridge, MA: MIT Press.

Strand, E. A., Buder, E. H., Yorkston, K. M., & Ramig, L. O. (1994). Differential phonatory characteristics of four women with amyotrophic lateral sclerosis. *Journal of Voice, 8,* 327–339.

Strik, H., & Boves, L. (1992). On the relation between voice source parameters and prosodic features in connected speech. *Speech Communication, 11,* 167-174.

Svec, J. G., Schutte, H. K., & Miller, D. G. (1996). A subharmonic vibaratory pattern in normal vocal folds. *Journal of Speech and Hearing Research, 39,* 135-143.

Titze, I. R. (1991). A model for neurologic sources of aperiodicity in vocal fold vibration. *Journal of Speech and Hearing Research, 34,* 460-472.

Titze, I. R. (1994). *Principles of voice production.* Englewood Cliffs, NJ: Prentice Hall. (Reprinted, 2000, Iowa City, IA: National Center for Voice and Speech).

Titze, I. R. (2006). *The myoelastic aerodynamic theory of phonation.* Iowa City, IA: National Center for Voice and Speech.

Titze, I. R., Baken, R. J., & Herzel, H. (1993). Evidence of chaos in vocal fold vibration. In I. R. Titze (Ed.), *Vocal fold physiology: Frontiers in basic science* (pp. 143-188). San Diego, CA: Singular Publishing Group.

Titze, I. R., & Story, B. H. (1997). Acoustic interactions of the voice source with the lower vocal tract. *Journal of the Acoustical Society of America, 101,* 2234-2243.

Verdolini, K., Druker, D. G., Palmer, P. M., & Samawi, I. (1998). Laryngeal adduction in resonant voice. *Journal of Voice, 12,* 315-327.

Weismer, G. (2006). Philosophy of research in motor speech disorders. *Clinical Linguistics and Phonetics, 20,* 315-349.

Weismer, G., Jeng, J. Y., Laures, J. S., Kent, R. D., & Kent, J. F. (2001). Acoustic and intelligibility characteristics of sentence production in neurogenic speech disorders. *Folia Phoniatrica et Logopaedica, 53,* 1-18.

Zemlin, W. R. (1998). *Speech and hearing science anatomy and physiology* (4th ed.). Needham Heights, MA: Allyn & Bacon.

Ziegler, W. (2002). Task-related factors in oral motor control: Speech and oral diadochokinesis in dysarthria and apraxia of speech. *Brain and Language, 80,* 556-575.

Ziegler, W., & Hoole, P. (2000). Neurologic disease. In R. D. Kent & M. J. Ball (Eds.), *Voice quality measurement* (pp. 397-401). San Diego, CA: Singular Publishing Group.

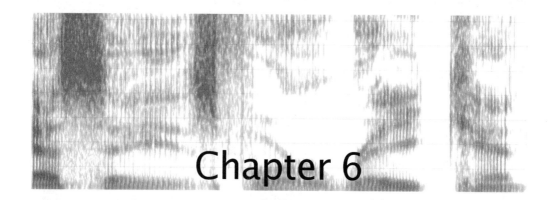

Chapter 6

SEGMENTAL ARTICULATION IN MOTOR SPEECH DISORDERS

Kris Tjaden

Introduction

Impaired articulation of speech sounds is a hallmark of motor speech disorders. In fact, it could be said that impaired speech sound articulation is a defining feature of dysarthria and apraxia of speech (AOS). For example, the classic Darley, Aronson, and Brown (1969a, 1969b) auditory-perceptual studies described in earlier chapters in this book reported imprecise consonants and distorted vowels in virtually all of the dysarthrias. Relatedly, irregular articulatory breakdown—a perceptual label that refers to unsystematic breakdown in the accuracy of speech sound production—is characteristic of many dysarthrias, including spastic, hyperkinetic, ataxic, and unilateral upper motor neuron (UUMN) dysarthria (Darley et al., 1969a; Duffy, 2005). Perceived speech sound errors in the form of consonant and vowel distortions, omissions, and substitutions also are pervasive in AOS, with distortions being the predominant error type (Odell, McNeil, Rosenbek, &

Hunter, 1990, 1991). The source of the articulatory impairment in dysarthria traditionally is attributed to disordered speech motor execution whereas the source of the articulatory impairment in AOS is attributed to disordered speech motor planning-programming. However, the effect on speech intelligibility—a measure of functional communication indexing the extent to which the acoustic signal is recovered by a listener—is broadly similar. That is, impaired articulation of speech sounds in both dysarthria and AOS contributes to reduced speech intelligibility. As elaborated in the upcoming treatment chapter (Chapter 9), the construct of speech intelligibility figures prominently in the management of motor speech disorders. Understanding the nature of the speech sound articulation impairment in dysarthria and AOS is essential for guiding these clinical decisions.

This chapter takes a different approach to the topic of segmental articulatory behavior than has been taken in other motor speech disorders texts, such as the recently updated textbook of Duffy (2005), the texts of Yorkston and colleagues (Yorkston, Beukelman, Strand, & Bell 1999; Yorkston, Miller, & Strand, 2004) or the edited texts of McNeil (1997) and Murdoch (1998). That is, rather than separately reviewing characteristics of segmental articulation for each of the dysarthrias and AOS, the current chapter more generally considers the effects of disordered speech motor execution and disordered speech motor planning-programming on speech sound articulation. This organizational scheme follows from research suggesting that different, presumed underlying pathophysiologies (i.e., spasticity, flaccidity, rigidity, incoordination) or neurologic impairments can similarly affect speech sound articulation. As one example, reduced displacement of the tongue, lips, and jaw during speech has been reported for individuals with a variety of dysarthrias as compared to neurologically normal talkers, including dysarthria secondary to Parkinson's disease, ataxic dysarthria, dysarthria secondary to amyotrophic lateral sclerosis (ALS), and dysarthria secondary to traumatic brain injury (TBI) (e.g., Forrest, Weismer & Turner, 1989; Hirose, Kiritani, & Sawashima, 1982; Jaeger, Hertrich, Stattrop, Schonle, & Ackermann, 2000; Kent, Netsell, & Bauer, 1975). The neuromotor basis of these dysarthrias or neurologic diagnoses differs, but the effect on articulatory movements and their acoustic consequences is broadly similar. That is, reduced articulatory displacements are associated with reduced acoustic contrast for vowels and consonants, which in turn is linked to reduced speech intelligibility. The current approach of more generally considering the effects of dysarthria and AOS on speech sound articulation also follows from research indicating that neurologic diseases traditionally thought to only affect speech motor

execution, such as Parkinson's disease and cerebellar ataxia, also may affect preparatory aspects of speech, another term for speech motor planning-programming (Spencer & Rogers, 2005). Relatedly, there is evidence of neuromuscular execution deficits in the speech mechanism for some persons with AOS, at least for nonspeech tasks (e.g., McNeil, Weismer, Adams, & Mulligan, 1990). Thus, AOS and dysarthria overlap in certain respects, although AOS is still considered to be a motor speech disorder distinct from dysarthria, and assessment and treatment techniques for dysarthria and AOS differ in a variety of ways (see overview of AOS in Ogar, Slama, Dronkers, Amici, & Gorno-Tempini, 2005).

It is hoped that the student-clinician will gain the following from the current chapter: (1) an understanding of the difference between segmental and suprasegmental aspects of speech, (2) an appreciation of segmental articulatory behavior in neurologically normal talkers including contemporary methods for studying segmental articulation, and (3) knowledge of the manner in which segmental articulatory behavior may be disrupted in motor speech disorders. Absent from this chapter is a detailed consideration of how motor speech disorders affect the articulatory mechanism during nonspeech orofacial tasks—commonly referred to as oral motor tasks. The role of nonspeech oral motor tasks in the management of motor speech disorders is considered elsewhere in this text, most notably in Chapter 9. The present focus on the articulatory mechanism during speech production is intended to emphasize that dysarthria and AOS are first and foremost disorders of *speech* motor control. Evidence of articulatory mechanism impairment during nonspeech oral motor tasks or tasks sensitive to nonspeech oral apraxia—in the absence of impairment during speech production—is insufficient to support a diagnosis of a motor speech disorder. Rather, dysarthria or AOS is appropriately diagnosed only when impairment in the speech mechanism is evident during the voluntary act of speaking, although a co-occurring impairment during nonspeech oral motor tasks or tasks sensitive to nonspeech apraxia often is used clinically as confirmatory evidence of dysarthria or apraxia, respectively. Even more importantly, research to date has been unable to demonstrate a convincing relationship between measures of nonspeech orofacial motor control and measures of speech production in dysarthria and AOS (Weismer, 2006). Health care providers are under increasing pressure from third party payers to use evidence-based practice guidelines to justify clinical decisions, such that assessment and treatment decisions must take into consideration the available research literature. It, therefore, would seem important that speech-language pathologists focus their clinical efforts on the speech production deficit in dysarthria and AOS, as discussed in this chapter.

Finally, although Master's level students in speech-language pathology readily recognize the importance of learning about procedures for assessment and treatment, the value of learning about the "hows and whys" of communicative disorders is not always obvious to students. The present chapter aims to demonstrate how an understanding of the nature of the articulatory impairment in motor speech disorders is invaluable for helping clinicians choose appropriate assessment tools, determine therapy goals, and select behavioral intervention techniques. Moreover, knowledge of the "hows and whys" of dysarthria and AOS differentiate a true clinician, who utilizes her knowledge of motor speech disorders to make informed management decisions on a patient-by-patient basis, from a technician, who simply carries out an assessment protocol or treatment program without understanding why a particular diagnostic procedure should be revealing of speech production impairment or why a given therapy technique should, in theory, be beneficial.

I. Segmental and Suprasegmental Properties of Speech: Definitions

The term "segmental articulation" in the title of this chapter in is perhaps best understood by contrasting segmental and suprasegmental aspects of speech. Segmental properties of speech are those attributes of speech that alter or change the identity of phonemes. These are considered in detail in the following sections. By comparison, suprasegmental properties of speech are those attributes of speech that are superimposed on individual phonemes or sequences of phonemes. Intonation, vocal intensity, and rate-rhythm are the primary suprasegmental features of speech. The terms "prosody" and "suprasegmental" are used interchangeably throughout the chapter. Although as a rule suprasegmental variables do not change the phonetic distinctions among individual speech sounds of English, adjustments in intonation, vocal intensity, and rate-rhythm can change the meaning of an utterance (Lehiste, 1996). One example is the use of intonation or voice fundamental frequency (F_0) to signal a question versus a statement. The phrase "I took my medicine" spoken with a falling F_0 contour signals a statement to listeners, whereas the same phrase spoken with a rising F_0 contour conveys a question similar to the phrase "Did I take my medicine?" Similarly, the meaning of the word "permit" differs depending on whether primary stress or emphasis—signaled by simultaneous adjustments in duration, intensity, and F_0,— is placed on the first or second syllable. Segmental properties of speech are the focus of this chapter, but prosody is frequently impaired in dysarthria and apraxia, as indicated in the chapters on speech breathing (Chapter 4) and laryngeal function (Chapter 5). Readers interested in learning more about the nature of the prosodic impairment in motor speech disorders are referred to Kent and Rosenbek's (1982) *Brain and Language* paper. This study compares the prosodic impairment in ataxic dysarthria, AOS, hypokinetic dysarthria secondary to Parkinson's disease, and right-hemisphere damage.

II. Normal Segmental Articulatory Behavior

Segmental features of speech are more or less synonymous with phonetic characteristics of speech. Phonetic properties of English primarily derive from movements of the supraglottal articulators, which for current purposes include the velum, tongue, lips, and jaw. As discussed in Chapter 5 on laryngeal function, the larynx also serves a segmental function by virtue of its role in producing the voicing distinction for obstruent consonant pairs like /p/ and /b/ or /s/ and /z/. The term "laryngeal devoicing gesture" refers to this segmental function of the larynx (Hirose, 1976). Briefly, voiced obstruents, such as the /b/ in "about," are produced with the vocal folds approximated to facilitate continuous voicing. Voiceless obstruents occur-

ring in the context of voiced phonemes, such as the /p/ in "apple," however, are produced with an abduction-adduction movement of the vocal folds—the laryngeal devoicing gesture—that is precisely timed to be initiated at the onset of supralaryngeal closure for voiceless obstruents. Appropriate timing of movements of the vocal folds also is critical for distinguishing the aspiration at the beginning of a word like "hat" as compared to "at," which does not begin with aspiration. The supraglottal articulators, however, are arguably most important for shaping the vocal tract in ways that distinguish among speech sounds. The term "vocal tract" is used here and throughout the remainder of this chapter to refer to the resonating tube formed by the oral cavity and pharynx. The vocal folds form the inferior boundary of the vocal tract, and the lips form the anterior boundary. When the velopharyngeal port is closed for production of oral consonants and vowels, the hard and soft palates demarcate the superior boundary of the vocal tract. When the velopharyngeal port is open for production of nasal consonants, however, the nasal cavity acts as the primary resonator whereas the oral and pharyngeal cavities—or vocal tract—serve as a secondary or sidebranch resonator.

The clinical phonetics text of Shriberg and Kent (2002) provides a comprehensive treatment of phonetic or segmental properties of English. The relative anterior-posterior positioning of the tongue in the oral cavity as well as the relative height of the tongue help to distinguish monopthongal vowels like /i/, /u/, /ae/, and /ɑ/. These vowels also are referred to as cardinal or corner vowels because they demarcate the acoustic extremes of the vowel quadrilateral in English. Diphthongs may be characterized as vowel-like sounds produced with a dynamic or gradually changing vocal tract shape. Lip rounding and inherent vowel duration (i.e., tense or long vowels like /i/ versus lax or short vowels like /ɪ/) also are sometimes considered segmental properties of vowels, but lip rounding and vowel duration alone do not create vowel phonemic distinctions in English. Similarly, place of articulation (e.g., labial, alveolar, palatal, velar), manner of articulation (e.g., stop, fricative, nasal) and voicing (e.g., voiced, unvoiced) are segmental features that distinguish consonants.

Before reviewing each of the supraglottal articulators in more detail, it is useful to consider methods for studying speech sound articulation. It is assumed that students will have had some exposure to this material as part of their speech science coursework. Thus, the review is highly selective and the focus is mostly on contemporary technologies. For example, strain gauges had been used since approximately 1970 to study movement characteristics of the lips, jaw, and even the velum, but these are no longer used by a number of research groups as other kinematic technologies offer broader measurement capability. Of course, it is still possible to conduct quality research using strain gauges to measure movement characteristics of supraglottal articulators, other than the tongue, during speech (e.g., Forrest et al., 1989; McHenry, 2003). Students interested in a more in-depth treatment of the topic are encouraged to consult the instrumentation chapters in McNeil's (1997) motor speech disorders text as well as the speech instrumentation text of Baken and Orlikoff (2000). Finally, although all the techniques reviewed below have been used to study segmental articulatory behavior in neurologically normal talkers, some instrumental techniques have yet to be applied to dysarthria and AOS, at least in published research reports.

Methods for Studying Segmental Articulatory Behavior

Segmental articulatory behavior has been investigated using both instrumental and auditory-perceptual methods. Some of the more commonly used instrumental methods are electromyography, kinematics, imaging, electropalatography, aerodynamics, and acoustic analyses. Researchers use both instrumental and auditory-perceptual techniques to study articulatory behavior, whereas speech-language pathologists rely on auditory-perceptual judgments and to a lesser extent acoustic analyses to make observations regarding segmental articulatory behavior. Despite the fact that speech-language pathologists do not routinely use many of the instrumental techniques reviewed below in their clinical practice, it is important for clinicians to have an appreciation of the various types of instrumentation so as to understand published research relevant to evidence-based practice.

Instrumental Techniques

Electromyography (EMG) is a record of the electrical activity generated by muscle contraction, with relatively stronger muscle contraction indicated by relatively higher amplitude of the EMG signal. Several kinds of electrodes are available for transducing the EMG signal. Surface electrodes are placed on the skin overlying a muscle whereas rigid needle and hooked-wire electrodes are embedded directly in the muscle of interest. One of the challenges in using EMG to study muscle activity in the articulatory mechanism is the relative inaccessibility of many structures and muscles, especially the velum and tongue, as well as intrinsic muscles of the larynx important for effecting the laryngeal devoicing gesture. Another difficulty in using EMG to study segmental articulatory behavior is muscle interdigitation. For example, muscle fibers in the region of the lips are intertwined making it virtually impossible to determine the specific muscle from which an electrode is recording. These statements also apply to intrinsic tongue muscles. Thus, whereas classic studies attempted to determine specific lip muscles involved in producing a given phoneme, more recent studies tend to focus on determining the synergistic nature of the perioral musculature for producing movement patterns for speech (Wohlert & Goffman, 1994; Wohlert & Hammen, 2000).

Structural movements of the articulators have been observed using a variety of kinematic technologies. Commonly reported kinematic measures include movement duration, extent or displacement, speed or rate of motion, and velocity—a directional measure of speed. The spatiotemporal index (STI), a derived kinematic measure reflecting the combined spatial and temporal stability of articulator displacement during speech, is a recently developed measure that has been reported in a number of studies, including several dysarthria studies (e.g., Kleinow, Smith, & Ramig, 2001; McHenry, 2003; Smith, Goffman, Zelaznik, Ying, & McGillem, 1995). Kinematic systems that use point-tracking operate by affixing small disks or sensors to an articulator or multiple articulators. The motion of the sensors then is tracked during speech. For example, the electromagnetic articulograph (EMA) and x-ray microbeam are used to track the motion of sensors or disks affixed to the tongue midline. EMA accomplishes fleshpoint tracking by means of magnetic fields, whereas x-ray microbeam accomplishes fleshpoint tracking using a focused x-ray beam.

Importantly, affixing small disks or sensors to the tongue does not have an appreciable effect on acoustic or perceptual measures of speech for neurologically normal talkers (Katz, Bharadwaj, & Stettler, 2006; Weismer & Bunton, 1999). At least some speakers with AOS experience reduced speech intelligibility when EMA sensors are affixed to the tongue midline, however (Katz et al., 2006). Relevant data for speakers with dysarthria are unavailable, no doubt in part due to the lack of kinematic studies investigating tongue motion during speech production for persons with dysarthria. Optotrak is another fleshpoint tracking system, but in contrast to EMA and x-ray microbeam technologies, Optotrak uses light-emitting diodes (LEDs) as sensors. Thus, Optotrak can only be used to track movements of sensors attached to externally visible articulators such as the lips and jaw.

Ultrasound is a type of imaging technology that has been used to study realtime movements of the tongue during speech (see Stone, 2005). This is accomplished by placing the ultrasound transducer in direct contact with the skin under the chin. Although ultrasound has yet to be applied to the study of segmental articulatory behavior in motor speech disorders, ultrasound has been used as a form of biofeedback in the treatment of articulation errors secondary to hearing impairment and English as a second language (Bernhardt, Gick, Bacsfalvi, & Adler-Bock, 2005). Ultrasound also has been used to characterize tongue motion of glossectomy patients during speech production (Bressman, Uy, & Irish, 2005). Magnetic resonance imaging (MRI) is another imaging technique that is widely used in clinical medicine to image soft tissues. It, therefore, might be speculated that MRI would be useful for imaging movement patterns of the lips, velum, and tongue during speech. But, the operating speed of standard MRI is too slow to capture movements of the articulators in real time. Thus, the application of standard MRI to the study of segmental articulatory behavior has largely been limited to obtaining images of static vocal tract shapes for sustained phonemes like /i/ and /s/. Vocal tract shapes obtained by MRI, then, may be related to spectral characteristics of phonetic events predicted by acoustic theory (e.g., Story, Titze, & Hoffman, 1996). Cine-MRI allows for imaging of time varying events, and, thus, may hold the most promise for the study of segmental articulatory behavior during real-time speech, especially given recent advances in microphone technology that allow for simultaneous cine-MR imaging and high-quality recording of the acoustic speech signal (NessAiver, Stone, Parthasarathy, Kahana, & Paritsky, 2006). In this manner, motions of the articulators obtained using cine-MRI might be related to the acoustic speech signal—the signal ultimately recovered by the listener.

Electropalatography (EPG) is a technique for measuring tongue-palate contact patterns during speech. A thin pseudopalate, not unlike older orthodontic retainers, is molded and fit to individual speakers. Embedded in the pseudopalate is an array of up to 96 small electrodes for sensing tongue-palate contact during speech, although a prototype, pressure-sensing EPG system also has been reported (Murdoch, Goozee, Veidt, Scott, & Meyers, 2004). Some researchers have suggested that a unique lingua-palatal contact map exists for many of the speech sounds of English, with dynamic sounds like diphthongs being characterized by movements between multiple contact patterns (e.g., Fletcher, 1989; Fletcher, McCutcheon, & Wolf, 1975).

Unlike some of the previously mentioned technologies, EPG has been used in speech production studies of both dysarthria and AOS (e.g., McAuliffe, Ward, & Murdoch, 2006; Southwood, Dagenais, Sutphin, & Garcia, 1997). One limitation of EPG is that some speech sounds are difficult to study, as some phonemes in English either do not require tongue-palate contact, such as bilabial consonants, or involve minimal tongue-palate contact, such as low and mid vowels.

Aerodynamics is the study of air pressures and flows. Although an overview of methods for studying air pressures and flows might seem better suited for inclusion in the preceding chapters on laryngeal function or speech breathing, aerodynamic studies have provided valuable information concerning velar function as well as laryngeal-supralaryngeal timing during speech (e.g., Gracco, Gracco, Löfqvist, & Marek, 1994; Müller & Brown, 1980). Common aerodynamic measures include oral and nasal airflows, oral and nasal pressures, airway resistance measures, and derived area measures reflecting either the size of the velopharyngeal port or the size of the oral constriction for consonants like /s/ (see review in Warren, Putnam, & Hinton, 1997). A pneumotachograph mask is often used to obtain airflow measures, and air pressures are recorded by means of a pressure transducer connected to a small catheter or tube that inserts into the oral or nasal cavity, depending on whether oral or nasal pressure is of interest. Thus, similar to acoustic analysis, aerodynamic analysis provides an indirect measure of segmental articulatory behavior in that the motion of a given articulator, such as the velum, is not directly tracked or imaged. Rather, aerodynamic measures allow for inferences concerning velar function and laryngeal-supralaryngeal timing during speech, as well as respiratory-laryngeal function. Because a given aerodynamic measure can be influenced by adjustments at multiple levels of the speech mechanism, however, these measures can be a challenge to interpret. For example, reduced intraoral air pressure during /p/ produced by a speaker with dysarthria could be due to factors such as velopharyngeal insufficiency (VPI), inability to achieve an adequately tight lip seal for the plosive, or even reduced respiratory support.

Segmental articulatory behavior also can be studied using acoustic analyses. A high-quality microphone, a computer equipped with a sound card, and acoustic analysis software often are the only required instrumentation, unless additional filtering of the speech signal is deemed necessary or it is desirable to record to an external device, such as a digital audiotape (DAT). There is not a strictly unique relationship between vocal tract shape and acoustic output, but general theoretical principles allow for inferences regarding underlying articulation (Fant, 1960; see also Stevens, 1999). For example, tongue advancement for vowels is directly related to the second formant frequency (F2), such that front vowels like /i/ are associated with a high F2 whereas back vowels like /u/ are associated with a low F2. Common acoustic measures of segmental articulatory behavior include sound segment durations, vowel formant frequencies, vowel formant transition characteristics such as transition slope and extent, spectral moment coefficients for obstruent consonants, and the amplitude of energy during stop gaps (see Kent, Weismer, Kent, Vorperian, & Duffy, 1999). Nasality has proven difficult to quantify using acoustic analyses, but an acoustic measure of nasality based on the amplitudes of oral and nasal formant frequencies in vowels

shows promise in this regard (see review in Chen, Stevens, Kuo, & Chen, 2000). Voice onset time (VOT)—the time period between a word-initial stop consonant release burst and the onset of periodic energy for a following vowel—also is important to mention, as VOT has been used as an acoustic index laryngeal-supralaryngeal coordination. If one is interested in measuring the time course of the laryngeal devoicing gesture for voiceless stops or fricatives, however, the duration of the entire voiceless interval—including the closure interval, burst release, and aspiration—is the appropriate measure (Weismer, 1980).

Forrest and Weismer (1997) have argued that acoustic analysis is highly desirable for a number of reasons. For example, compared to many of the other types of instrumentation previously reviewed, acoustic analysis is noninvasive and the required instrumentation is comparatively inexpensive. The acoustic signal also is unique in linking speech production and perception. That is, acoustic measures allow for inferences concerning underlying articulation and these same acoustic measures or cues are used by listeners for perceiving speech. One implication is that deviances measured in the acoustic speech stream explain or underlie listeners' perceptual errors. Finally, there is a large literature on acoustic aspects of neurologically normal speech to serve as a basis for comparison of speech disorders.

Auditory-Perceptual Analysis of Segmental Articulatory Behavior

Auditory-perceptual methods for studying segmental articulatory behavior include phonetic transcription, scaling or rating of perceptual labels such as distorted vowels, imprecise consonants, irregular articulatory breakdown and nasality, as well as intelligibility testing. Perceptual gating—a technique for studying perception of coarticulatory information in the acoustic speech stream—also is discussed, as this paradigm has been used in studies of AOS.

Both broad and narrow phonetic transcription have been used to characterize speech sound articulation. Orthographic transcription also has been used to describe segmental articulation; this is discussed below with speech intelligibility measures. Broad phonetic transcription allows for identification of phoneme substitutions and omissions, and, thus, is useful for generating confusion matrices illustrating patterns of phoneme-level perceptual errors. The majority of segmental articulation errors in AOS and dysarthria are distortions, however, which are only revealed with narrow phonetic transcription. In fact, studies employing narrow phonetic transcription indicating a preponderance of speech sound distortions in AOS were critical for clarifying that AOS is a motor disorder rather than a linguistic disorder, insofar as a linguistic disorder would be suggested by a preponderance of substitutions (Odell et al., 1990, 1991). Narrow transcription is not without problems though, as reliability is a concern and even narrow phonetic transcription may not wholly capture the nature of speech sound distortions in motor speech disorders (see Kent, 1996 for a comprehensive review of the limitations of auditory-perceptual analysis in speech and voice disorders).

Auditory-perceptual methods for studying segmental articulation also include scaling of perceptual labels such as distorted vowels, imprecise consonants, irregular articulatory breakdown, nasality, and even intelligibility. Interval scaling and direct magnitude estimation (DME) are two types of frequently used scaling techniques. In interval scaling, listeners assign a number to a given speech sample indicating the relative deviancy of a perceptual parameter. Darley et al. (1969a), for example, used a 7-point interval scale, with 1 representing normal and 7 representing severe deviation from normal. Fixed-modulus DME involves scaling a given speech sample with respect to a modulus or baseline sample. That is, listeners might judge if consonant precision for a given speech sample is half, twice, three times, and so forth, as precise as the baseline. In free-modulus DME, listeners rate a given speech sample relative to the preceding sample in a list. There are pros and cons of both DME techniques. Fixed modulus DME does not allow for cross-study comparisons, but reliability is generally good and the task is readily understood by listeners (Weismer & Laures, 2002). Free-modulus DME does allow for cross-study comparisons, but listener reliability is a concern—possibly because listeners find the task unusual (Tjaden & Wilding, 2004; Yunusova, Weismer, Kent, & Rusche, 2005). Importantly, the psychophysical properties of nasality and intelligibility, which are discussed in more detail below, are such that these constructs are poorly suited to interval scaling and should only be scaled using DME (Schiavetti, 1992; Zraick & Liss, 2000).

Intelligibility can be measured using the scaling techniques discussed above, orthographic transcription, and phonetic contrast testing (see reviews by Schiavetti [1992] and Weismer and Martin [1992]). First, however, a word about the relationship between segmental articulation and intelligibility is in order. It is widely acknowledged that integrity of speech sound articulation is the most important factor in determining intelligibility (Kent, 1992). In classic speech perception theory, consonants are viewed as the primary information-bearing elements of the acoustic speech stream (Licklider, 1951), but more recent research suggests the importance of vowels to intelligibility (e.g., Ansel & Kent, 1992; Turner, Tjaden, & Weismer, 1995). As an aside, there is growing interest in the contribution of phonatory-laryngeal variables to intelligibility in motor speech disorders. For example, Ramig (1992) hypothesized that vocal quality affects intelligibility in dysarthria, although the appropriate studies have yet to evaluate this suggestion. Sentence-level F_0 range, however, has been shown to impact intelligibility such that sentences for which the F_0 range has been synthetically flattened are associated with reduced intelligibility, both for neurologically normal talkers and at least some speakers with dysarthria (Bunton, Kent, Kent, & Duffy, 2001; Laures & Weismer, 1999). Whether the restricted sentence-level F_0 range observed in some studies of AOS contributes to reduced intelligibility for these speakers is a topic requiring further study (Cooper, Soares, Nicol, Michelow, & Goloskie, 1984; Ryalls, 1982).

Perceptual scaling techniques for quantifying intelligibility were reviewed previously. It is worth reiterating, however, that DME truly is the only appropriate scaling technique for intelligibility (Schiavetti, 1992). In addition to scaling techniques, published intelligibility tests are widely used, especially for dysarthria. The Assessment of Intelligibility of Dysarthric Speech measures single-word and sentence intelligibility (Yorkston & Beukelman, 1981). The single-word test can be scored using a multiple choice scoring format, which is essentially an identification task, or via orthographic transcription. The sentence portion of the test is scored using orthographic transcription. Intelligibility is expressed as the percentage of words correctly identified or orthographically transcribed. A computerized version of the test also is available (Yorkston & Beukelman, 1996). Kent and colleagues at the University of Wisconsin-Madison have developed a single-word phonetic contrast test for the purpose of identifying the source of reduced intelligibility in dysarthria (Kent, Weismer, Kent, & Rosenbek, 1989). The test permits evaluation of 19 segmental contrasts vulnerable to disruption by dysarthria, and the phonetic contrasts have measurable acoustic correlates. Although the test has limitations, including the fact that single-word intelligibility may not well represent intelligibility of connected speech, the test represents an important change in thinking about intelligibility testing from that of simply quantifying the severity of the speech deficit to explaining the source of the intelligibility deficit. Finally, some intelligibility studies present stimuli to listeners in multitalker babble to avoid ceiling effects, especially for speech characterized by relatively good intelligibility (e.g., Bunton, 2006; Ferguson, 2004). Multitalker babble is a type of background noise that approximates many real-world listening situations. That is, communication between a given speaker and listener frequently takes place in the midst of background noise, including other conversations—a restaurant filled with talkative diners or a cocktail party are just two examples. It might even be argued that this design provides a more ecologically valid approximation to typical listening than perceptual studies presenting stimuli in quiet.

Finally, a gating paradigm has been used to study perception of coarticulatory information in the acoustic speech stream. Coarticulation—a term Kent and Adams (1989) suggest may be used interchangeably with coordination—refers to the simultaneous adjustment of the vocal tract for two or more phonetic segments (see review in Kent & Minifie, 1977). The topic of coarticulation is considered in more detail in following sections, as incoordination has long been thought to characterize segmental articulatory behavior in both AOS and dysarthria. As will become apparent, however, there is limited empirical evidence of incoordination in motor speech disorders, at least as indicated by studies of coarticulation. In perceptual gating studies, the listener is provided with progressively longer durations or "gates" of a given stimulus, such as the consonantal portion of a consonant plus a vowel syllable, and the listener's task is to identify the vowel. Stimuli identified with greater accuracy at earlier or shorter gates are interpreted to indicate the presence of stronger anticipatory vowel coarticulation. For example, Southwood et al. (1997) reported better vowel identification at earlier gates for CVC stimuli produced by a healthy talker as compared to a talker with AOS. This finding was interpreted as evidence that the healthy talker's stimuli contained more coarticulatory information for the vowel (also Ziegler & von Cramon, 1985).

In summary, a variety of instrumental and auditory-perceptual techniques are available for characterizing segmental articulatory behavior. As will become apparent, much of what is known about speech sound articulation in motor speech disorders derives from studies employing acoustic and auditory-perceptual analyses. Before discussing the nature of the speech articulation disturbance associated with AOS and dysarthria, however, aspects of normal segmental articulatory behavior will be reviewed. The larynx will not be considered, however, so as not to duplicate information in preceding chapters.

Characteristics of Individual Articulators

The Jaw

The lower lip and jaw probably are more accurately considered a single articulator, as their anatomic connection prevents the lower lip from moving wholly independently of the jaw unless the jaw is stabilized with some type of bite block, a situation atypical of naturally produced speech. When researchers wish to study the separate movements of the lower lip and jaw, movement characteristics of the lower lip can be decoupled from movement characteristics of the jaw during postprocessing of kinematic signals (Westbury, Lindstrom, & McClean, 2002). The muscles of the jaw or mandible are similar to limb muscles in that jaw muscles have well-defined origins and insertions and are organized around a skeletal joint—which in the case of the jaw is the temporomandibular (TM) joint. During speech, jaw movement in the sagittal plane is characterized by rotation and translation (Edwards & Harris, 1990). For example, jaw opening for the /ɑ/ in "pop" involves downward rotation of the mandible as well as posterior translation. This pattern is reversed for jaw closing. The extent of jaw displacement during speech ranges from approximately 3 to 20 mm, as measured by the amount of vertical opening between the upper and lower incisors (Folkins, 1981). For comparison purposes, this range is about half the range of jaw motion for chewing. Moreover, unlike chewing, which involves reciprocal activation of muscles that open and close the jaw such that jaw opening and closing muscles are active at different times, jaw muscle activation patterns during speech production are characterized by cocontraction of antagonist muscles

(Moore, Smith, & Ringel, 1988). This is a term indicating simultaneous activity of muscles that function to open and close the jaw. The finding of cocontraction of antagonistic muscles for neurologically normal speakers was important, as earlier research with PD and AOS suggested that this pattern of muscle contraction might be a sign of neuropathology or disordered speech motor control (e.g., Fromm, Abbs, McNeil, & Rosenbek 1982; Leanderson, Meyerson, & Persson, 1972).

The Lips

In contrast to muscles of the jaw, lip or perioral muscles are not organized around a joint and vary greatly in orientation to one another resulting in interdigitation of fibers from distinct muscles. Thus, the lips are actually composed of several different muscles, although orbicularis oris superior and inferior make up the bulk of the upper and lower lips, respectively. A number of studies have attempted to examine lip muscle activation patterns during speech, but the interleaving of the various perioral muscles prevents straightforward interpretation of the data (Blair & Smith, 1986). Researchers have addressed this problem by studying muscle activity from perioral "regions" or quadrants (Wohlert & Goffman, 1994). This approach allows for conclusions regarding overall muscle activity in the upper right, upper left, lower right, and lower left perioral quadrants, but not about specific muscles in each region. Studies employing this type of methodology suggest a tight coupling of muscle activity across the four perioral quadrants during a lip protrusion or rounding task, only moderate coupling for chewing, and dissociated muscle activity across the four perioral regions during

speech (Wohlert & Goffman, 1994). Other studies have investigated the extent of lip displacement during speech. These studies indicate that, on average, the lower lip is displaced vertically about 12 mm during speech, a value about twice that of upper lip movement (Gracco, 1988; Sussman, MacNeilage, & Hanson, 1973). Some researchers have argued that the lips can be modeled as a single articulator, with the goal of controlling oral aperture or interlabial distance, whereas other researchers have argued for independent control of the upper and lower lips (see review in Smith, 1992).

The Tongue

The tongue and the jaw also are anatomically coupled, although the tongue is able to move more independently of the jaw than the lower lip. Nonetheless, the anatomic connection between muscles of the tongue—most notably the genioglossus muscle which forms the bulk of the tongue body—and the mandible results in the tongue "riding on" the jaw during speech. In fact, it has been suggested that the jaw might help compensate for a tongue that is unable to move through its full range of motion, as in dysarthria secondary to ALS, TBI, or multiple sclerosis (MS), where tongue function is disproportionately affected relative to lip or jaw function (DePaul & Brooks, 1993; Hartelius & Lillvik, 2003; Jaeger et al., 2000). Studies wishing to characterize the separate motions of the tongue and jaw during speech can mathematically decouple movements of these articulators during postprocessing of kinematic signals, as previously discussed for the jaw and lower lip (Westbury et al., 2002).

The tongue resembles the lips in that tongue muscles also are not organized around a joint and intrinsic tongue muscles interdigitate in complex ways so that it is virtually possible to determine the activity of individual muscles. Studying the muscular activity of the tongue is further complicated by the fact that electrodes are easily dislodged from the tongue during speech. Because the tongue lacks a skeletal structure, similar to an elephant's trunk, it has been suggested that the tongue might be modeled as a muscular hydrostat (Smith & Kier, 1989). A muscular hydrostat is an organ or structure composed of muscle, which in turn is composed of an incompressible liquid. An important biomechanical feature of a muscular hydrostat is that it has a constant volume such that a decrease in one dimension must be offset by an increase in another dimension. Modeling the tongue as a muscular hydrostat implies a constant interaction of both extrinsic and intrinsic tongue muscles for all movements. This contrasts with classic views of the tongue in which extrinsic tongue muscles move the tongue and intrinsic muscles modulate overall shape.

The tongue surface may be divided into functional regions. The three most anterior regions—the tongue tip, blade, and dorsum—are important for helping to create vocal tract shapes for speech sound production, whereas the tongue base has a primary role in generating pressures during the pharyngeal phase of swallowing. Barlow et al. (1997) suggest that tongue velocities for speech range from 5 to 20 cm/sec. However, this range is best considered a rough guideline, insofar as there is a great deal of speaker-to-speaker variability in tongue displacement and velocity, and these measures are affected by variables such as the speech sample being studied (e.g., Tasko & McClean, 2004).

The Velum

The velum modulates the degree of coupling between the oral and nasal cavities (see Moon & Kuehn, 2004 for a review of velar anatomy and physiology). That is, the velum is lowered for rest breathing and for production of nasal consonants and moves both superiorly and posteriorly toward the posterior pharyngeal wall for the production of oral speech sounds—the majority of the sounds of English. The lateral pharyngeal walls also move medially to assist with velopharyngeal closure, and in some individuals a bulge on the posterior pharyngeal wall—called Passavant's pad— also assists in closure. Thus, there are a variety of ways in which speakers can accomplish velopharyngeal closure (Croft, Shprintzen, & Rakoff, 1981). Furthermore, it has been suggested that the velopharyngeal mechanism might be modeled as a muscular hydrostat, similar to the tongue (Ettema & Kuehn, 1994; Moon & Jones, 1991). The pattern or degree of velopharyngeal closure varies not only among speakers but also among speech sounds. Velopharyngeal closure is complete during pressure consonants, but even neurologically normal speakers may show evidence of a small velopharyngeal port opening during oral consonants (Hoit et al., 1994). Relatedly, consonants are produced with greater velar closure forces than vowels, and high vowels tend to be produced with greater closure forces than low vowels (Kuehn & Moon, 1998). Kuehn and Moon (1994, 1995) also showed relatively low muscular activity of the levator veli palatini—the muscle responsible for velar elevation—during speech. That is, levator muscle activity for speech was only about 10 to 40% of that used for blowing. This finding is consistent with other research indicating that muscle forces generated by the supraglottal articulators during speech are only a small percentage of those generated during nonspeech, maximum performance tasks (see review in Kent, Kent, & Rosenbek, 1987).

The Big Picture: Connected Speech

As suggested in Chapter 3, speech is an enormously complex sensorimotor skill. Duffy (2005) summarizes three types of pertinent activities for speech production, including cognitive-linguistic activities, motor speech planning-programming— hereafter referred to as motor programming—and finally, neuromuscular execution. Briefly, once the intended verbal message has been identified via cognitive-linguistic activities, it must be transformed into a code that will allow for neuromuscular execution. For established or non-novel motor activities, it is generally accepted that this transformation involves the neural system retrieving and sequencing existing motor programs. A motor program can be thought of as a script for organizing motor commands that ultimately will activate muscles of the speech mechanism at the appropriately coordinated or coarticulated times. There is no consensus regarding the exact movement parameters contained in a motor program, but it has been suggested that information concerning movement duration, displacement or amplitude, acceleration, deceleration, time to peak velocity, muscle stiffness, and relative timing or coordination of movements might be specified in motor programs (McNeil, Robin, & Schmidt, 1997). Neuromuscular execution involves the neural system, appropriate structures, and muscles actually carrying out the movement param-

eters specified in the motor programs. Muscle contractions generate forces that create smooth and stable movements of the speech structures that unfold in both space and time to result in sound output.

The statement that movements of the speech mechanism result in sound output may seem obvious, but the point is not trivial because it raises the issue that speech movements are goal directed. Determining the goals of speech has long been a topic of interest and debate for speech researchers. A variety of speech goals have been proposed, including articulatory targets or postures, aerodynamic variables such as pressure and resistance, and articulator stiffness—a derived kinematic measure reflecting the ratio of movement displacement and velocity (see Kent, Adams, & Turner [1996] for a review of classes of speech production models). Although the idea is not universally accepted, a substantial body of research suggests that the goals of speech are acoustic-perceptual in nature (Perkell, Guenther, Lane, Matthies, Perrier, Vick, Wilhelms-Tricarico, & Zandipour, 2000; also Netsell, 1981, 1982). This suggestion is supported by several lines of research, including studies of motor equivalence. Motor equivalence means that the same goal can be achieved in more than one way. A common example in the speech literature is motor equivalence of the tongue and lips for production of the vowel /u/. A low second formant frequency (F2) is a critical perceptual cue for /u/, and both tongue-body raising and lip protrusion contribute to a lowering of F2. Research has shown that across repetitions of /u/, a given speaker uses differing degrees of tongue-body raising and lip protrusion to achieve the acoustic-perceptual goal of a low F2, such that there is a negative relationship between tongue-body raising and lip protrusion across repetitions of /u/ (Perkell, Matthies, Svirsky, & Jordan, 1995). In other words, tongue-body raising and lip protrusion trade off, so that when a given production of /u/ is produced with a relatively higher tongue-body position, the lips are relatively less protruded in order to accomplish the acoustic-perceptual goal of a low F2. When /u/ is produced with a relatively lower tongue-body position, however, the lips are relatively more protruded to accomplish the low F2. The idea that speakers use motor equivalence to achieve acoustic-perceptual goals for speech has clinical implications. That is, because speakers have some flexibility in achieving a particular acoustic-perceptual goal, impairment in one aspect of the articulatory mechanism, such as the tongue, might be compensated for by another part of the articulatory mechanism, such as the lips. Therapeutic efforts, therefore, may best be focused on helping patients achieve acoustic-perceptual adequacy—by whatever means, rather than requiring patients to achieve a specific articulatory position or posture for a given phoneme.

Finally, having separately reviewed characteristics of each of the articulators, it is important to emphasize that connected speech involves simultaneous movements of multiple articulators and, thus, coordination of activity across and even within some articulators, especially the tongue which is composed of distinct functional regions. This temporal and spatial overlapping of movements of the articulators to produce a sequence of phonetic events is, in essence, coarticulation. As reviewed by Kent and Minifie (1977), coarticulation may be classified as either perseveratory (left-to-right) or anticipatory (right-to-left). Perseveratory effects—such as the presence of nasalization during the vowel in "snow"—have been attrib-

uted to biomechanical constraints of the articulators or the notion that vocal tract shape change can not happen instantaneously owing to inertia. Anticipatory coarticulation occurs when articulatory adjustments for one phonetic event are anticipated during an earlier phonetic event. An example of anticipatory coarticulation is the presence of lip rounding or protrusion for the /u/ in "sue" during production of the /s/. Anticipatory coarticulation has received the most attention in the speech production literature because this type of coarticulation is thought to be revealing of the planning of upcoming speech segments. Thus, by studying anticipatory coarticulation, it may be possible to gain insight into the nature of the speech sequencing process as well as disruptions to this process caused by motor speech disorders (Katz, 2000).

Segmental Articulation in Dysarthria and AOS

The instrumental literature characterizing vocal tract function in dysarthria and AOS is fairly modest in size. In fact, students are often surprised to learn that there are perhaps only a dozen or so laboratories world-wide actively engaged in studying segmental articulatory behavior in motor speech disorders. A significant proportion of the physiologic studies investigating supraglottal function in motor speech disorders have focused on nonspeech performance of vocal tract structures (Weismer, 1997, 2006). Thus, quite a lot of what is known about segmental articulatory behavior in motor speech disorders derives from acoustic studies and, of course, perceptual studies, such as those of Darley et al. (1969a, 1969b) and Odell et al.

(1990, 1991) mentioned earlier. The advantages of acoustic analyses were previously reviewed and will not be repeated (Forrest & Weismer, 1997). It is important for students to recognize that there is no superior level of analysis or type of instrumentation for studying segmental articulatory behavior in motor speech disorders, however (for a discussion of this issue see Weismer & Liss, 1991a). Researchers may have strong preferences regarding the appropriate instrumentation or signal for analysis, but given that each instrumental technique has at least some limitations, our understanding of segmental articulatory behavior in motor speech disorders most likely will be advanced by a multifaceted approach, in which a variety of types of instrumentation or analyses are applied.

A discussion of segmental articulation in AOS and dysarthria could be approached in a variety of ways. For example, in keeping with the material on normal segmental articulation, speech-related deficits in each of the articulators might be reviewed. Although speech sound articulation does require movements of the tongue, lips, jaw, velum, and larynx, movements of individual articulators must occur in a precisely timed and coordinated fashion to effect changes in vocal tract shape that ultimately yields an acoustic signal recovered by a listener. Thus, a more global approach that is not necessarily linked to individual articulators seems more appropriate—especially in light of contemporary speech production theory suggesting that the goals of speech are acoustic-perceptual in nature (Perkell et al., 2000).

The presence of perceptually obvious speech sound inaccuracies in dysarthria and AOS is not disputed, although the localizing power and heuristic value of the Darley et al. (1969a, 1969b) perceptual classification scheme for dysarthria has been questioned, and there is not universal agreement regarding definitions of perceptual labels (Kent, 1996; Weismer, 1997, 2006). By way of review, the Darley et al. (1969a, 1969b) perceptual studies reported some degree of articulatory inaccuracy—in the form of imprecise consonants and distorted vowels—for virtually all the dysarthrias. Relatedly, irregular articulatory breakdown is characteristic of many dysarthrias, including spastic, hyperkinetic, ataxic, and unilateral upper motor neuron (UUMN) dysarthria (Darley et al., 1969a; also Duffy, 2005). Hypernasality—and less frequently hyponasality—can be perceptually prominent in some dysarthrias or neurologic diseases, such as dysarthria secondary to ALS or PD (Duffy, 2005). Perceived speech sound errors in the form of consonant and vowel distortions, omissions, and substitutions also are pervasive in AOS, with distortions predominating (Odell, McNeil, Rosenbek, & Hunter, 1990, 1991). Thus, because the existence of perceived speech sound errors is so widely acknowledged in motor speech disorders, the important question to ask seems to be what factors likely contribute to or explain perceptually obvious speech sound articulation errors or reduced intelligibility in dysarthria and AOS?

Consider Duffy's (2005) updated definition of dysarthria based on the original definition set forth by Darley et al. (1969a, 1969b, 1975). Abnormalities in the strength, tone, steadiness, speed, range, or accuracy of movements are thought to underlie the speech production impairment in dysarthria. Relatedly, McNeil et al.'s (1997) definition of AOS emphasizes intra- and interarticulator temporal and spatial segmental distortions as well as distortions of segment and intersegment transitionalization that result in prolonged phonetic events. More simply stated, the speech sound articulation impairment in AOS is one of slow and inaccurate or uncoordinated movements that result in distorted speech sounds (Kent & Rosenbek, 1983). These definitions are used below as a framework for considering segmental articulatory behavior in dysarthria and AOS. The review is necessarily selective, given the constraints of a single chapter. Readers are encouraged to consult Duffy's (2005) excellent text for a more comprehensive review (see also Weismer [1997] for a table summarizing selected studies of articulatory behavior in motor speech disorders). Finally, because relatively few studies of AOS and dysarthria have performed simultaneous instrumental and perceptual analyses, a fair amount of speculation is necessary regarding variables underlying perceived speech sound articulation errors or reduced intelligibility in motor speech disorders. Before proceeding, readers also may find it helpful to review symptoms of neuropathology presented in Chapter 3.

Muscle Strength and Tone

The notion that deficits in muscle strength have an explanatory or causal role in segmental articulation deficits in dysarthria has proven difficult to evaluate, no doubt in part due to the lack of appropriate instrumentation for measuring articulatory muscle strength or the resulting forces during speech production. For example, a device like the Iowa Oral Performance Instrument (IOPI) requires speakers to squeeze an air-filled bulb between the tongue and the roof of the mouth, and thus is only capable of measuring forces generated by the tongue during nonspeech activities (see Solomon et al. [2000] for a study using the IOPI to inves-

tigate nonspeech tongue function in Parkinson's disease). Challenges in using EMG to study muscle contraction patterns in the articulatory mechanism were previously reviewed, and include inaccessibility of certain articulators, interdigitation of muscle fibers, and studies showing that muscle contraction patterns presumed to be indicative of neuropathology also are characteristic of neurologically normal speakers.

One of the few technologies capable of providing at least an indirect measure of articulator muscle strength during speech is a miniature transducer for quantifying interlabial contact pressure. Goozee et al. (2002) found that interlabial contact pressures during a speech task did not differ for healthy controls and speakers with dysarthria secondary to TBI, although the two speaker groups did differ on a number of nonspeech measures, such as maximum interlabial contact pressure—a task requiring speakers to compress the lips as tightly as possible. The finding of similar interlabial contact pressures for speech produced by speakers with dysarthria and normal controls does not seem consistent with the idea that reductions in muscle strength help to explain speech sound articulation deficits in dysarthria. Moreover, only a fraction of the available force or muscular activity of articulatory structures—somewhere in the neighborhood of 20%—is used for connected speech (Kuehn & Moon, 1994, 1995; Müller, Milenkovic, & MacLeod, 1984). It, therefore, seems likely that significant reductions in muscle strength, perhaps in the form of a severe paresis or even paralysis, would be required for observable effects on segmental articulation.

Disturbances in muscle tone in dysarthria are thought to include variable tone, excessive tone in the form of spasticity or rigidity, and reduced tone or hypotonia. The idea that disturbances in muscle tone underlie segmental articulatory deficits in dysarthria also has been difficult to evaluate. Clark (2003) summarizes the relevant issues. Briefly, tone refers to the tendency of muscle to resist passive stretch, and can be assessed in the limbs fairly easily by passively moving a limb and judging the amount of resistance to movement offered by muscle. Muscle spindles, which are sensory organs located within muscle, play a key role in regulating muscle tone. The inaccessibility of many of the articulators prevents the sort of passive stretching used to assess tone in the limbs, however. Even more importantly, the lips, tongue, and jaw-opening muscles lack muscle spindles or an obvious stretch reflex— suggesting that neural mechanisms regulating tone in articulatory structures differ from those of the limbs. In light of these and other issues, there have been few attempts to quantitatively evaluate tone in the articulatory muscles during speech produced by persons with dysarthria. Hunker, Abbs, and Barlow (1982) developed a measure of labial tone or stiffness and reported a strong correlation between labial rigidity and lip displacement in PD, such that higher indices of labial rigidity were associated with reduced lip displacements. A follow-up study was unable to replicate this finding, however (Caliguiri, 1987). Thus, empirical support for the idea that disturbances in muscle tone in dysarthria contribute to perceived speech sound errors or reduced intelligibility is lacking.

Steadiness

Stability or steadiness of supraglottal articulatory movements has been a topic of recent interest in dysarthria, no doubt owing to the development of the spatiotemporal index or STI (Smith et al., 1995). As previously reviewed, the STI is a kinematic measure reflecting spatial and temporal stability of articulatory displacements, although some researchers have suggested that the STI is an index of coordination, which is discussed in a following section (see Fox et al., 2002 for discussion of this issue pertinent to dysarthria). The basic idea is that repeatable and, thus, highly stable articulatory displacements across multiple repetitions of an utterance should result in the movement trajectories conforming well to a single pattern. Thus, less stable movements result in poorer convergence of movement trajectories to a single pattern or template and a relatively higher STI. Movements that are more stable show good convergence to a single template and a correspondingly lower STI. The STI could be derived from the displacement signal of any articulator, but dysarthria studies to date have focused on the lower lip or the combined lower lip and jaw. Several studies have reported higher STIs for speakers with dysarthria compared to neurologically normal talkers (Kleinow et al., 2001; McHenry, 2003; see also Dromey, 2000). By way of illustration, Figure 6–1 shows movement trajectories for a speaker with idiopathic PD and a healthy speaker. Note that in the middle panel of this figure there is less "scatter" among movement trajectories for the healthy speaker as compared to the speaker with PD. This observation is supported by the lower STI for the control speaker reported in the lower panel. The relationship of the STI to perceptual impressions of dysarthria, such as intelligibility, imprecise consonants, distorted vowels, and irregular articulatory breakdown has not been studied. This is a significant limitation of this line of research because an elevated STI also

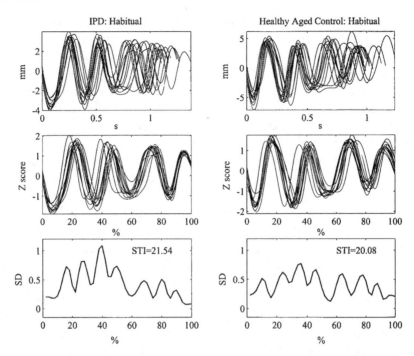

Figure 6–1. Data from an adult with IPD from the habitual rate and intensity function (*left panel*) and a healthy aged control (*right panel*). The center panel illustrates the time and amplitude and normalized waveforms. The lower panel shows the standard deviation computed at 2% intervals across the 15 normalized waveforms. The sum of these standard deviations, the STI, is shown in the upper right corner of the bottom plot. (Reproduced with permission from Kleinow, J., Smith, A., and Ramig, O. Speech motor tability in IPD: Effects of rate and loudness manipulations. *Journal of Speech, Language and Hearing, 44,* 1046. Copyright 2001 American Speech-Language-Hearing Association.)

has been reported for slower-than-normal speech produced by neurologically normal talkers, who presumably are highly intelligible and demonstrate adequate articulatory precision. Elevated STI's also have been reported for older as compared to younger healthy talkers (Kleinow et al., 2001; Wohlert & Smith, 1998).

Some years ago there was interest in measuring stability of the lips, tongue, and jaw during nonspeech, isometric fine force and position tasks. It was speculated

that fine force measures would more closely approximate the forces generated in the supraglottal mechanism during speech, as compared to maximum force tasks. However, fine force and maximum force measures share the same limitation in that both sets of measures can only be obtained during nonspeech tasks. Results of these studies indicated an overall reduction in stability during fine force and position tasks, both in dysarthria and AOS as compared to neurologically normal subjects, although the degree of instability varied across articulators (e.g., Abbs, Hunker, & Barlow, 1984; Barlow & Abbs, 1986; McNeil et al., 1990). Barlow and Abbs (1986) also reported a correlation between reduced fine-force stability and perceptual impressions of intelligibility in dysarthria, but this study has been criticized for lacking appropriate experimental controls (Weismer, 2006).

Formant frequency variability within a phoneme or segment, such as the vowel /ɑ/, also has been used to index vocal tract stability in dysarthria (e.g., Gerratt, 1983; Zwirner & Barnes, 1992). The general finding is one of increased formant frequency variability for a given phoneme or segment produced by speakers with dysarthria compared to neurologically normal talkers. For example, Zwirner and Barnes (1992) showed that speakers with dysarthria secondary to PD or Huntington's disease (HD) demonstrated greater variability of F1 during sustained /ɑ/ compared to controls. Speakers with HD also showed greater F2 variability compared to other speaker groups. However, there was no relationship between formant stability and perceived speech severity—a perceptual label that listeners are unable to judge separately from intelligibility (Weismer et al., 2000). Thus, at present, the contribution of articulatory instability to reduced intelligibility or impaired speech sound articulation in dysarthria remains unclear.

Speed and Range of Motion

Articulatory movements or changes in vocal tract shape for persons with motor speech disorders tend to be produced with abnormalities of velocity and displacement. In dysarthria, articulatory velocities and displacements tend to be reduced (e.g., Ackermann, Hertrich, & Scharf, 1995; Forrest et al., 1989; Hirose, 1986; Kent, Netsell, & Bauer 1975). Acoustically, the reduced articulatory velocities and displacements are suggested by certain formant frequency trajectory characteristics, especially for F2, as well as a compressed acoustic-phonetic working space (e.g., Kent et al., 1989; Tjaden & Wilding, 2004; Turner et al., 1995; Weismer et al., 1992; Yunusova, Weismer, Kent, & Rusche, 2005). Figure 6–2 shows the effect of dysarthria on formant trajectory characteristics. This figure shows F1 and F2 time histories or trajectories for the vowel in "sigh" produced by speakers with ALS and a group of age and gender-matched neurologically normal talkers. For the normal speakers, the F2 for the diphthong begins around 1300 Hz, and after a brief period of minimal spectral change, rapidly increases to about 2000 Hz for a total frequency excursion of about 700 Hz. There is reduced frequency excursion for F2 as well as a general "flattening" of the slowly increasing portion of F2—the F2 slope—for the speakers with ALS. This trend is most obvious for the speakers who are less than 70% intelligible. F2 slope measures in dysarthria have been shown to correlate with intelligibility, such that speakers with shallower slopes are less intelligible (Kent et al., 1989; Tjaden & Wilding, 2004; Weismer et al., 2001). Speakers with PD perceived to have more severe dysarthria, and presumably poorer intelligibility, also show a greater reduction in lip velocity during speech compared to speakers with PD perceived to have less severe dysarthria (Forrest et al., 1989).

A compression of the phonetic working space for vowels produced by speakers with dysarthria is shown by a reduction

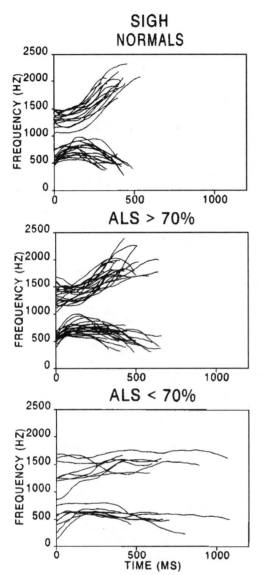

Figure 6–2. F1-F2 trajectories for the word *sigh*. (Reproduced with permission from Weismer, G., et al. Formant trajectories of males with ALS. *Journal of the Acoustical Society of America*, *91*, 1090. Copyright 1992 Acoustical Society of America.)

in the size of the vowel space area (e.g., Liss et al., 2001; Tjaden & Wilding, 2004; Turner et al., 1995; Weismer et al., 2000).

Figure 6-3 shows an example of the reduction in vowel space area for vowels in content and function words produced by speakers with ALS. Visual inspection of this figure suggests a smaller vowel quadrilateral in ALS compared to normal controls, for both content and function words. These kinds of reductions in vowel space area have been shown to correlate with intelligibility, such that speakers with smaller vowel space areas are less intelligible (McRae et al., 2002; Turner et al., 1995; Weismer et al., 2000). At least some studies of ataxic dysarthria suggest essentially normal vowel formant frequencies, however (Kent et al., 2000; also Tjaden & Wilding, 2004). It also is not entirely clear whether reduced formant frequency excursions in dysarthria, as reflected in a compressed vowel space area, are simply an index of overall severity or are a true correlate or component of speech intelligibility (Weismer et al., 2001; Yunusova et al., 2005). The distinction is clinically important, because variables that are a component of intelligibility should have direct effects on intelligiblity when modified therapeutically, whereas variables that are simply an indication of severity will not.

Reduced articulatory displacements for consonants produced by speakers with dysarthria also are suggested by a reduction in spectral contrast, as indexed by consonant first moment coefficients. Although first moment coefficients can be influenced by a number of factors, as a general rule of thumb, a more anterior constriction in the vocal tract—as for lingualveolar /s/—is associated with a higher first moment coefficient, whereas a more posterior constriction—as for linguapalatal /ʃ/—is associated with a lower first moment coefficient. Figure 6-4 shows first moment coefficients for the fricatives /s/

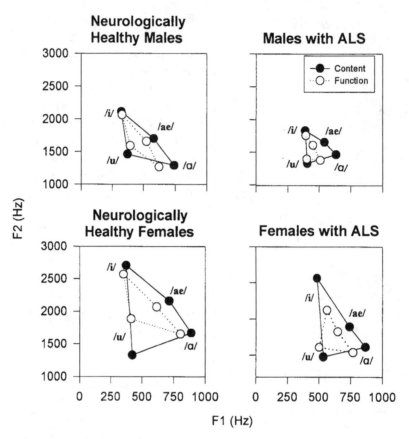

Figure 6–3. The average F1 and F2 values for vowels produced in content and function words. The data are organized by sex and group affiliations. Vowel space areas are indicated by dashed lines for function words and solid lines for content words. (Reproduced with permission from Turner, G. S., & Tjaden, K. Acoustic differences between content and function word in amyotrophic lateral sclerosis. *Journal of Speech, Language and Hearing Research, 43*, 774. Copyright 2000 by American Speech-Language-Hearing Association.)

and /ʃ/ produced in a reading passage by speakers with PD and healthy controls. Findings for several articulatory rate conditions are reported in this figure. Note the reduced distance or difference between first moment coefficients for fricatives produced by the speakers with PD as compared to the appropriate gender-matched control group. There also is evidence that reduced spectral contrast for consonants

in dysarthria is associated with reduced intelligibility or poorer consonant precision (Tjaden & Turner, 1997; Tjaden & Wilding, 2004; but for different results see McRae et al., 2002; Yunusova et al., 2005).

As an aside, it seems reasonable to assume that articulatory or syllable rate, a global temporal measure indicating the number of speech units produced per unit time excluding pauses, could be used as

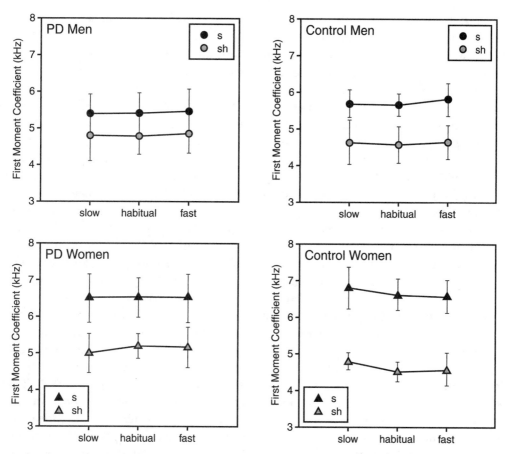

Figure 6–4. Average first moment coefficients are reported for both speaker groups as a function of gender. Vertical lines extending from the symbols indicate ± 1 standard deviation. First moment coefficient difference measures may be inferred from the space or distance in each plot between first moment coefficients for /s/ (*black triangles*) and first moment coefficients for /ʃ/ (*gray triangles*). (Reproduced with permission from McRae, P., Tjaden, K., & Schoonings, B. Acoustic and perceptual consequences of articulatory rate change in Parkinson disease, *Journal of Speech, Language and Hearing Research, 45*, 45. Copyright 2002 American Speech-Language-Hearing Association.)

an indirect measure of movement speed, such that slower articulatory rates would be associated with reduced articulatory speeds. Indeed, a slowed articulatory rate is suggested in many studies of dysarthria and AOS (e.g., Kent et al., 2000; Kent & Rosenbek, 1983; Tjaden, 2000b; Turner & Weismer, 1993; Ziegler & von Cramon, 1986), although articulatory rate is not always reduced for speakers with dysarthria secondary to PD and at least some speakers with dysarthria secondary to MS (Tjaden, 1999; Tjaden & Wilding, 2004). Acoustic studies also report lengthened segment durations in motor speech disorders, and segment-level measures typically correlate well with more global temporal measures such as articulatory rate (e.g.,

Kent & Rosenbek, 1983; Seddoh et al., 1996; Turner & Tjaden, 2000; Turner et al., 1995; Weismer et al., 2003; Ziegler & von Cramon, 1986). The relationship between articulatory speed and syllable rate is not as straightforward as it might seem, however. For example, Westbury and Dembowski (1993) compared movement characteristics of the tongue during diadochokinesis (DDK) and connected speech for a group of healthy talkers. An important finding from this x-ray microbeam study was that the tongue moved more rapidly during connected speech than DDK, as indicated by higher measures of articulator speed, but syllable rates—measured in syllables per second—were actually slower for connected speech than DDK. The implication is that measures of articulator speed and measures of syllable or articulatory rate cannot be interchanged. Taking this idea a step further, DDK syllable repetition rates—measured in syllables per second—should not be used clinically to infer speed of articulator motion.

Disturbances of articulatory velocity and displacement in AOS appear to be more complex than the simple reduction in velocity and displacement previously described for dysarthria. For example, there are reports of reduced articulatory velocities in AOS (Itoh et al., 1980) as well as normal peak velocities (McNeil et al., 1989; Robin et al,. 1989). Still other studies indicate inconsistent or variable patterns of movement velocity in AOS (Forrest et al., 1991; McNeil et al., 1989). For example, McNeil, Caliguiri, and Rosenbek (1989) reported normal peak velocities in AOS, but longer and more variable movement durations as well as frequent velocity changes, greater velocity variability, and increased displacements, a pattern opposite to that reported for dysarthria. Some

of the velocity abnormalities in AOS that have been reported could simply be a byproduct of the slower-than-normal articulatory rate typical of these speakers, however (Adams et al., 1993). Acoustically, articulatory velocity abnormalities in AOS do not seem to be well captured by F2 slope measures, as F2 slope measures are quite similar for speakers with AOS and neurologically normal talkers (McNeil et al., 1990). Relatedly, average vowel formant frequencies, such as shown in the vowel quadrilaterals in Figure 6–3, are typically normal in AOS (Kent & Rosenbek, 1983; Ryalls, 1986). Rather, formant trajectories in AOS are characterized by misdirections, prolonged steady states, and exaggerations—the latter of which would seem to support reports of increased articulatory displacements in AOS (Liss & Weismer, 1992; Weismer & Liss, 1991). As discussed in the following section, these types of qualitative observations seem to be consistent with the idea that distorted, inaccurate speech sound articulation in AOS is largely due to temporal-spatial distortions of movements or difficulties transitioning between segments rather than abnormalities of velocity of displacement per se. In other words, disturbances of velocity and displacement suggested in at least some studies of AOS more likely reflect an underlying problem with coordination.

Coordination

Incoordination is thought to characterize segmental articulatory behavior in both dysarthria and apraxia. Darley et al. (1969a) were explicit in stating that incoordination can contribute to the speech production impairment in dysarthria, although

Duffy (2005) speaks more generally of articulatory inaccuracy. In the case of AOS, a variety of terms have been used to describe incoordination including movement decomposition, segmentalization, difficulty in phasing successive speech gestures, intra- and interarticulatory spatial-temporal dyscoordinations as well as movement-timing deficits or distortions, although this list is hardly exhaustive (Katz, 2000; Kent & Rosenbek, 1983; McNeil et al., 1997). The fact that such a mish-mash of terminology has been used to describe "incoordination" in motor speech disorders should be an indication to students that there is no widely accepted definition of coordination nor is there agreement as to how coordination should be measured or quantified. Studies purporting to measure articulatory coordination generally either investigate the timing and/or extent of movements for a single speech sound—for example, timing of velar elevation for the nasal /n/—or examine the timing and/or extent of movements as a speaker transitions from one sound to another (Weismer et al., 2003). An example of this latter type of study would be research examining anticipatory vowel coarticulation in consonant plus vowel syllables, where the transition or overlap of articulatory-acoustic characteristics for the consonant and vowel are of interest.

Studies investigating coordination in dysarthria are sparse, and cross-study methodologic differences make direct comparisons difficult. Nevertheless, kinematic studies of Kent and colleagues (Kent, Netsell, & Bauer, 1975; Netsell & Kent, 1976) indicated no major disruption in the temporal sequencing of supraglottal articulatory motions for phonetic events. Similar results concerning regularity in the timing of supraglottal articulatory gestures

have been reported by Weismer et al. (2003) for dysarthria secondary to ALS or PD, although these authors suggest a trend toward subtle coordination deficits in dysarthria—especially for speakers with ALS. Relatedly, Bartle and colleagues (2006) found no group differences in tongue-jaw timing or spatial coordination for speech produced by healthy talkers and a group of talkers with TBI - most of whom presented with a perceptually-obvious dysarthria (Bartle, Goozee, Scott, Murdoch & Kuruvilla, 2006). Consistent with Weismer et al.'s (2003) findings for ALS, however, a subgroup of individuals with TBI showed evidence of articulatory incoordination (Bartle et al., 2006). Acoustic studies investigating coarticulation in dysarthria report mixed findings. Some studies suggest increased or reduced coarticulation for speakers with dysarthria compared to healthy controls, albeit quite subtle differences for controls and speakers with dysarthria (Tjaden, 1999, 2000a). Yet, other studies suggest essentially normal patterns of coarticulation in dysarthria, including studies of ataxic dysarthria as well as dysarthria secondary to PD or multiple sclerosis (Hertrich & Ackermann, 1999; Tjaden, 2003; Tjaden & Wilding, 2005). Finally, evidence of laryngeal-supralaryngeal incoordination in dysarthria is suggested by studies showing that speakers with a variety of dysarthrias have difficulty stopping vocal fold vibration at the interface of a vowel and voiceless obstruent, as for the word "up." That is, vocal fold vibration for the vowel extends inappropriately into the voiceless interval for the consonant (e.g., Tjaden & Watling, 2003; Weismer, 1984).

Given that the bulk of studies indicate mostly preserved coordination or coarticulation in dysarthria, it is not clear how incoordination might contribute to perceived articulatory imprecision, irregular articulatory breakdown, or reduced intelligibility in dysarthria. This probably is a topic in need of further study, however, given the small literature and methodologic limitations of at least some of the work to date (i.e., Tjaden, 1999). In addition, several studies reporting essentially normal coarticulation studied speakers with relatively mild dysarthria (Tjaden, 2003; Tjaden & Wilding, 2005). It is possible that coordination deficits may only be evident for speakers with more severe dysarthria, as suggested by the findings of Bartle et al. (2006).

Studies investigating coordination in AOS are more plentiful, likely because incoordination is thought to play such a large role in the segmental articulatory impairment in AOS. Students are encouraged to consult additional resources for a more comprehensive summary of the literature than that provided here (Duffy, 2005; Katz, 2000; McNeil et al., 1997). Voice onset time or VOT studies are one category of research that has added to our understanding of coordination or interarticulator timing in AOS. By way of review, word initial voiced stops have a short-lag VOT, usually on the order of 20 milliseconds (ms), whereas word initial voiceless stops have a long-lag VOT, typically 40 ms or longer. VOT studies of AOS indicate overlap of VOT values for voiced and voiceless consonants, even for stop consonant that are correctly identified or are perceived as accurate (Blumstein et al., 1977, 1980). That is, for both voiced and voiceless stops produced by speakers with AOS, acoustic measures of VOT have been shown to fall in the range of 25 to 40 ms—a value in between the ranges typical of voiced and voiceless stops. Speakers with AOS also show large variability in

VOT values for the same consonant—yet another possible sign of incoordination. The overlap of VOT values for voiced and voiceless stops coupled with observations of greater variability has been interpreted as evidence that the timing of laryngeal and supralaryngeal events in AOS is poorly coordinated. Because VOT abnormalities are so pervasive in AOS, it further has been suggested that AOS may be especially vulnerable to disruptions in timing or coordination between articulators—which in the case of VOT is the larynx and a supraglottal articulator such as the tongue or lips (Baum et al., 1990).

A study by Itoh and Sasanuma (1984) further illustrates how deficits in articulatory timing contribute to impaired speech sound articulation in AOS. These authors examined movements of the velum in a patient with AOS as well as a normal control using fiberoscopy. Fiberoscopy is not unlike FEES (fiberoptic endoscopic evaluation of swallowing)—which is used in the clinical evaluation of swallowing. The normal speaker showed regular patterns of velar displacement and duration of movements across syllable repetitions of /ten/. As an aside, the record of velar movement obtained via fiberoscopy is not unlike the displacement signals shown in Figure 6-1. The speaker with AOS, however, showed variation in the extent of velar displacement across syllable repetitions as well as variation in the duration of velar movement. For a syllable sequence such as /deenee/, the patient with AOS again showed a lot of variability in the amount and duration of velar displacement which was accompanied by a perceived phonetic change from /n/ to /d/, or more accurately a distorted /d/. This type of careful analysis of kinematic and perceptual data—even for a single speaker—helps to illustrate the presence of timing or coordination deficits in AOS as well as how those deficits might contribute to perceived speech sound errors.

The literature investigating coarticulation in AOS is fairly extensive, or at least more studies have examined coarticulation in AOS as compared to dysarthria. Katz (2000) provides a good summary of the work in this area—focusing on anticipatory coarticulation within a syllable, such as anticipation of a vowel during the fricative in a syllable like "sue." In short, about half the studies reviewed by Katz (2000) support the conclusion that coarticulation is variable in AOS, but the overall pattern is largely normal whereas about half the studies support the conclusion that coarticulation is delayed in AOS. A couple of studies suggest that coarticulation is early or excessive in AOS, however. Given such mixed findings, it is difficult to draw any strong conclusions concerning coarticulation in AOS. This is not to say that AOS is not characterized by some form of incoordination, but rather that studies of coarticulation may not be particularly sensitive to the incoordination in AOS.

Summary

To summarize, there is limited research support for the idea that deficits in muscle strength, tone, steadines, or coordination help to explain the speech sound articulation impairment in dysarthria. Rather, given the available research, it seems most likely that reductions in articulatory displacements and velocities explain perceptual impressions such as distorted vowels, imprecise consonants, and even reduced intelligibility. Relatedly, it seems most likely that the speech sound articulation impairment in AOS is related to difficulties

with coordination—not abnormalities of articulatory velocity or displacement, although studies of coarticulation do not strongly support the existence of coordination deficits in AOS.

Finally, the interaction between segmental and suprasegmental aspects of speech deserves mention. Suprasegmental aspects of speech, such as adjustments in rate or loudness, have been shown to affect segmental aspects of speech both for persons with motor speech disorders and healthy controls. Not surprisingly then, a number of therapeutic techniques for motor speech disorders use suprasegmental adjustments—such as rate reduction—to improve speech sound articulation. An example of the interaction between segmental and suprasegmental properties of speech is the expansion of the vowel acoustic working space when speakers use a slower-than-normal articulatory rate (Tjaden & Wilding, 2004; Turner et al., 1995). Not all segment types are similarly affected by these kinds of suprasegmental adjustments, however. For example, acoustic distinctiveness of vowels produced by speakers with dysarthria is more strongly influenced by rate reduction, whereas acoustic distinctiveness of stop consonants is more strongly affected by an increased vocal loudness (Tjaden & Wilding, 2004). One clinical implication is that therapeutic techniques that simultaneously stimulate a reduced rate and increased loudness—such as clear speech—may have the most promise for improving both vowel and consonant acoustic distinctiveness, and presumably intelligibility. Relatedly, there is evidence that a flattened F_0 contour compromises identification accuracy of certain vowels produced by speakers with dysarthria (Bunton, 2006). Perhaps more important was the finding that listeners' vowel identification accuracy improved when F_0 contours were synthetically enhanced or expanded, and that this improvement occurred despite the fact that vowel formant frequency measures suggested impaired segmental articulation. Although additional studies are needed, the findings are intriguing and suggest that clinical efforts to improve F_0 variation in dysarthria might yield improvements in vowel identification accuracy and, presumably, speech intelligibility. These are just a few examples of how segmental and suprasegmental properties of speech interact. The astute clinician will take note of these types of interactions and will interpret his or her judgments of segmental articulation for a given patient with respect to the overarching suprasegmental environment (i.e., what are the prevailing duration, intensity, and voice pitch characteristics being used by a given speaker).

In conclusion, speech sound articulation errors are pervasive in motor speech disorders. Because segmental articulation is so important to speech intelligibility—one of the few functional measures of communication that speech pathologists can readily measure and quantify—clinicians need to have an appreciation for the nature of the articulation impairment in motor speech disorders. Furthermore, an understanding of factors likely to explain or underlie segmental articulation errors in dysarthria and AOS, should help guide clinicians in selecting appropriate assessment tools and therapeutic techniques.

Acknowledgments. It was a privilege to have Ray as a mentor—not only as a doctoral student at the University of Wisconsin-Madison but long thereafter. I am truly honored to have been included as a contributor for this text. Certainly no individual will again have the same impact on the field of motor speech disorders, nor is anyone more deserving of a text written in his honor. (Writing of this chapter was supported by Grant R01 DC004689.)

References

Abbs, J., Hunker, C., & Barlow, S. (1983). Differential speech motor subsystem impairments in subjects with suprabulbar lesions: Neurophysiological framework and supporting data. In W. Berry (Ed.), *Clinical dysarthria* (pp. 21-56). San Diego, CA: College-Hill Press.

Ackermann, H., Hertrich, I., & Scharf, G. (1995). Kinematic analysis of lower lip movements in ataxic dysarthria. *Journal of Speech and Hearing Research, 38,* 1252-1259.

Adams, S. G., Weismer, G., & Kent, R. D. (1993). Speaking rate and speech movement velocity profiles. *Journal of Speech and Hearing Research, 36,* 41-54.

Ansel, B. & Kent, R. D. (1992). Acoustic-phonetic contrasts and intelligibility in the dysarthria associated with mixed cerebral palsy. *Journal of Speech and Hearing Research, 35,* 296-308.

Baken, R. J., & Orlikoff, R. F. (2000). *Clinical measurement of speech and voice* (2nd ed.). San Diego, CA: Singular.

Barlow, S., & Abbs, J. (1986). Fine force and position control of select orofacial structures in the upper motor neuron syndrome. *Experimental Neurology, 94,* 699-713.

Barlow, S., Finan, D., Andreatta, R., & Paseman, A. (1997). Kinematic measurement of the human vocal tract. In M. R. McNeil (Ed.), *Clinical management of sensorimotor speech disorders* (pp. 107-148). New York: Thieme.

Bartle, C. J., Goozee, J., Scott, D., Murdoch, B. E., & Kuruvilla, M. (2006). EMA assessment of tongue-jaw co-ordination during speech in dysarthria following traumatic brain injury. *Brain Injury, 20,* 529-545.

Baum, S. R., Blumstein, S. E., Naeser, M. A., & Palumbo, C. L. (1990). Temporal dimensions of consonant and vowel production: An acoustic and CT scan analysis of aphasic speech. *Brain and Language, 39,* 33–56.

Bernhardt, B., Gick B., Bacsfalvi, P., & Adler-Bock, M. (2005). Ultrasound in speech therapy with adolescents and adults. *Clinical Linguistics and Phonetics, 19,* 605–617.

Blair, C., & Smith, A. (1996). EMG recording in human lip muscles: Can single muscles be isolated? *Journal of Speech and Hearing Research, 29,* 256–266.

Blumstein, S. E., Cooper, W. E., Goodglass, H., Statlender, S., & Gottlieb, J. (1980). Production deficits in aphasia: A voice-onset time analysis. *Brain and Language, 9,* 153–170.

Blumstein, S., Cooper, W. E., Zurif, E., & Caramazza, A. (1977). The perception and production of voice-onset time in aphasia. *Neuropsychologia, 155,* 371–383.

Bressmann, T., Uy, C., & Irish, J.C. (2005). Analysing normal and partial glossectomee tongues using ultrasound. *Clinical Linguistics and Phonetics, 19,* 35, 52.

Bunton, K. (2006). Fundamental frequency as a perceptual cue for vowel identification in speakers with Parkinson's disease. *Folia Phoniatrica, 58,* 332–339.

Bunton, K., Kent, R. D., Kent, J. F., & Duffy, J. R. (2001). The effects of flattening fundamental frequency contours on sentence intelligibility in speakers with dysarthria. *Clinical Linguistics and Phonetics, 15,* 181–193.

Caliguiri, M. (1987). Labial kinematics during speech in patients with parkinsonian rigidity. *Brain, 110,* 1033–1044.

Chen, M. Y., Stevens, K. N., Kuo, H. K. J., & Chen, H. (2000). Contributions of the study of disordered speech to speech production models. *Journal of Phonetics, 28,* 303–312.

Clark, H. M. (2003). Neuromuscular treatments for speech and swallowing: A tutorial. *American Journal of Speech-Language Pathology, 12,* 400–415.

Cooper, W., Soares, C., Nicol, J., Michelow, D., & Goloskie, S. (1984). Clausal intonation after unilateral brain damage. *Language and Speech, 27,* 17–24.

Croft, C., Shprintzen, R., & Rakoff, S. (1981). Patterns of velopharyngeal valving in normal and cleft palate subjects: A multi-view videofluoroscopic and nasoendoscopic study. *Laryngoscope, 91,* 265–271.

Darley, F. L., Aronson, A. E, & Brown, J. R. (1969a). Differential diagnostic patterns of dysarthria. *Journal of Speech and Hearing Research, 12,* 246–269.

Darley, F. L., Aronson, A. E, & Brown, J. R. (1969b). Clusters of deviant speech dimensions in the dysarthrias, *Journal of Speech and Hearing Research, 12,* 462–496.

Darley, F., Aronson, A. E., & Brown, J. (1975). *Motor speech disorders.* Philadelphia: W. B. Saunders.

Dromey, C. (2000). Articulatory kinematics in patients with Parkinson disease using different speech treatment approaches. *Journal of Medical Speech-Language Pathology, 8,* 155–161.

Duffy, J. R. (2005). *Motor speech disorders: Substrates, differential diagnosis, and management* (2nd ed.). St. Louis, MO: Elsevier Mosby.

DePaul, R. & Brooks, B. (1993). Multiple orofacial indices in amyotrophic lateral sclerosis. *Journal of Speech and Hearing Research, 36,* 1158–1167.

Edwards, J., & Harris, K. (1990). Rotation and translation of the jaw during speech. *Journal of Speech and Hearing Research, 33,* 550–562.

Ettema, S. L., & Kuehn, D. P. (1994). A quantitative histologic study of the normal human adult soft palate. *Journal of Speech and Hearing Research, 37,* 303–313.

Fant, G. (1960). *Acoustic theory of speech production.* The Hague, Netherlands: Mouton.

Ferguson, S. H. (2004). Talker differences in clear and conversational speech: Vowel intelligibility for normal-hearing listeners. *Journal of the Acoustical Society of America, 116,* 2365–2373.

Fletcher, S. G. (1989). Palatometric specification of stop, affricate, and sibilant sounds. *Journal of Speech and Hearing Research, 32,* 736–748.

Fletcher, S. G., McCutcheon, & Wolf, M. B. (1975). Dynamic palatometry. *Journal of Speech and Hearing Research, 18*, 812–819.

Folkins, J. (1981). Muscle activity for jaw closing muscles during speech. *Journal of Speech and Hearing Research, 24*, 601–615.

Forrest, K., Adams, S., McNeil, M.R., & Southwood, H. (1991). Kinematic, electromyographic and perceptual evaluation of speech apraxia, conduction aphasia, ataxic dysarthria, and normal speech production. In C. A. Moore, K. M. Yorkston, & D. R. Beukelman (Eds.), *Dysarthria and apraxia of speech: Perspectives on management* (pp. 147–172). Baltimore: Paul H. Brookes.

Forrest, K., & Weismer, G. (1997). Acoustic analysis of dysarthric speech. In M. R. McNeil (Ed.), *Clinical management of sensorimotor speech disorders* (pp. 63–82). New York: Thieme.

Forrest, K., Weismer, G., & Turner, G. S. (1989). Kinematic, acoustic, and perceptual analyses of connected speech produced by Parkinsonian and normal geriatric adults. *Journal of the Acoustical Society of America, 85*, 2608–2622.

Fox, C. M., Morrison, C. E., Ramig, L. O., & Sapir, S. (2002). Current perspectives on the Lee Silverman Voice Treatment (LSVT) for individuals with idiopathic Parkinson disease. *American Journal of Speech-Language Pathology, 11*, 111–123.

Fromm, D., Abbs., J., McNeil, M. R., & Rosenbek, J. C. (1982). Simultaneous perceptual-physiological method for studying apraxia of speech. *Clinical Aphasiology, 10*, 155–171.

Gerratt, B. (1983). Formant frequency fluctuation as an index of motor steadiness in the vocal tract. *Journal of Speech and Hearing Research, 26*, 297–304.

Goozee, J., Murdoch, B. E., & Theodoros, D. G. (2002). Interlabial contact pressure exhibited in dysarthria following traumatic brain injury during speech and nonspeech tasks. *Folia Phoniatrica, 54*, 177–189.

Gracco, L. C., Gracco, V. L., Löfqvist, A., & Marek, K.P. (1994). Aerodynamic evaluation of Parkinsonian dysarthria. In J. A. Till, K. M. Yorkston, & D. R. Beukelman (Eds.), *Motor speech disorders: Advances in assessment and treatment* (pp. 65–80). Baltimore: Paul Brookes.

Hartelius, L., & Lillvik, M. (2003). Lip and tongue function differently affected in individuals with multiple sclerosis. *Folia Phoniatrica et Logopaedica, 55*, 1–9.

Hertrich, I., & Ackermann, H. (1999). Temporal and spectral aspects of coarticulation in ataxic dysarthria: An acoustic analysis. *Journal of Speech, Language, and Hearing Research, 42*, 367–381.

Hirose, H. (1976). Posterior cricoarytenoid as a speech muscle. *Annals of Otology, Rhinology and Laryngology, 85*, 334–342.

Hirose, H. (1986). Pathophysiology of motor speech disorders (dysarthria). *Folia Phoniatrica, 38*, 61–88.

Hirose, H., Kiritani, S., & Sawashima, M. (1982). Patterns of dysarthric movement in patients with amyotrophic lateral sclerosis and pseudobulbar palsy. *Folia Phoniatrica, 34*, 106–112.

Hoit, J., Watson, P., Hixon, K., McMahon, P., & Johnson, C. (1994). Age and velopharyngeal function during speech production. *Journal of Speech and Hearing Research, 37*, 295–302.

Hunker, C., Abbs, A., & Barlow, S. (1982). The relationship between parkinsonian rigidity and hypokinesia in the orofacial system: A quantitative analysis. *Neurology, 32*, 755–761.

Itoh, M., & Sasanuma, S. (1984). Articulatory movements in apraxia of speech. In J. C. Rosenbek, M. R. McNeil, & A. E. Aronson (Eds.), *Apraxia of speech: Physiology, acoustics, linguistics, management.* San Diego, CA: College-Hill Press.

Itoh, M., Sasanuma, S., Hirose, H., & Yoshioka, H., & Ushijima, T. (1980). Abnormal articulatory dynamics in a patient with apraxia of speech: X-ray microbeam observations. *Brain and Language, 11*, 66–75.

Jaeger, M., Hertrich, I., Stattrop, U., Schonle, P. W., & Ackermann, H. (2000). Speech disorders following severe traumatic brain injury: Kinematic analysis of syllable repetitions using electromagneticarticulography. *Folia Phoniatrica et Logopaedica, 42,* 187-196.

Katz, W. F. (2000). Anticipatory coarticulation and aphasia: Implications for phonetic theories. *Journal of Phonetics, 28,* 313-334.

Katz, W. F., Bharadwaj, S. V., & Stettler, M. P. (2006). Influences of electromagnetic articulography sensors on speech produced by healthy adults and individuals with aphasia and apraxia. *Journal of Speech, Language, and Hearing Research, 49,* 645-659.

Kent, R. D. (Ed.). (1992). *Intelligibility in speech disorders: Theory, measurement and management.* Amsterdam: John Benjamins.

Kent, R. D. (1996). Hearing and believing: Some limits to the auditory-perceptual assessment of speech and voice disorders. *American Journal of Speech-Language Pathology, 5,* 7-23.

Kent, R. D., & Adams, S. G. (1989). The concept and measurement of coordination in speech disorders. In S. A. Wallace (Ed.), *Perspectives on the coordination of movement* (pp. 415-449). North-Holland: Elsevier Science.

Kent, R. D., Adams, S., & Turner, G. S. (1996). Models of speech production. In N. J. Lass (Ed.), *Principles of experimental phonetics* (pp. 3-45). St. Louis, MO: Mosby-Year Book.

Kent, R. D. Kent, J. F., Duffy, J. R., Thomas, J. E., Weismer, G., & Stuntebeck, S. (2000). Ataxic dysarthria. *Journal of Speech Language and Hearing Research, 43,* 1275-1289.

Kent, R. D., Kent, J. F., & Rosenbek, J. C. (1987). Maximum performance tests of speech production. *Journal of Speech and Hearing Disorders, 52,* 367-387.

Kent, R. D., Kent, J. F., Weismer, G., Martin, R. E., Sufit, R. L., Brooks, B. R., & Rosenbek, J. C. (1989). Relationships between speech intelligibility and the slope of second-formant transitions in dysarthric subjects. *Clinical Linguistics and Phonetics, 3,* 347-358.

Kent, R. D., Kent, J. F., Weismer, G., Sufit, R. L., Rosenbek, J. C., Martin, R., & Brooks, B. (1990). Impairment of speech intelligibility in men with amyotrophic lateral sclerosis. *Journal of Speech and Hearing Disorders, 55,* 721-728.

Kent, R. D., & Minifie, F. D. (1977). Coarticulation in recent models of speech production. *Journal of Phonetics, 5,* 115-133.

Kent, R. D., & Netsell, R. (1975). A case study of an ataxic dysarthric: Cineradiographic and spectrographic observations. *Journal of Speech and Hearing Disorders, 1,* 115-134.

Kent, R. D., Netsell, R., & Bauer L. L. (1975). Cineradiographic assessment of articulatory mobility in the dysarthrias. *Journal of the Speech and Hearing Disorders, 40,* 467-480.

Kent, R. D., & Rosenbek, J. C. (1982). Prosodic disturbance and neurologic lesion. *Brain and Language, 15,* 259-291.

Kent, R. D., & Rosebenk, J.C. (1983). Acoustic patterns of apraxia of speech. *Journal of Speech and Hearing Research, 26,* 231-249.

Kent, R. D., Weismer, G., Kent, J. F., & Rosenbek, J. C. (1989). Toward phonetic intelligibility testing in dysarthria. *Journal of Speech and Hearing Disorders, 54,* 482-499.

Kent, R. D., Weismer, G., Kent, J. F., Vorperian, H. K., & Duffy, J. R. (1999). Acoustic studies of dysarthric speech: Methods, progress, and potential. *Journal of Communication Disorders, 32,* 141-186.

Kleinow, J., Smith, A., & Ramig, L. (2001). Speech motor stability in IPD: Effects of rate and loudness manipulations. *Journal of Speech, Language and Hearing Research, 44,* 1041-1051.

Kuehn, D., & Moon, J. (1994). Levator veli palatini muscle activity in relation to intraoral air pressure variation. *Journal of Speech and Hearing Research, 37,* 1260-1270.

Kuehn, D., & Moon, J. (1995). Levator veli palatini muscle activity in relation to intraoral air pressure variation in cleft palate subjects. *Cleft Palate-Craniofacial Journal, 32,* 376-381.

Kuehn, D., & Moon, J. (1998). Velopharyngeal closure force and levator veli palatini activation levels in varying phonetic contexts. *Journal of Speech, Language, and Hearing Research, 41,* 51-62.

Laures, J., & Weismer, G. (1999). The effect of a flattened F0 on intelligibility at the sentence-level. *Journal of Speech, Language, and Hearing Research, 42*, 1148-1156.

Leanderson, R., Meyerson, & Persson, A. (1972). Lip muscle function in Parkinsonian dysarthria. *Acta Otolaryngologica, 74*, 354-357.

Lehiste, I. (1996). Suprasegmental features of speech. In N. J. Lass (Ed.), *Principles of experimental phonetics* (pp. 226-244). St. Louis, MO: Mosby-Year Book.

Licklider, J. C. R. (1951). Basic correlates of the auditory stimulus. In S. S. Stevens (Ed.), *Handbook of experimental psychology* (pp. 985-1039). New York: Wiley.

Liss, J., Spitzer, S., Caviness, J., Adler, C., & Edwards, B. (2001). Lexical boundary error analysis in hypokinetic and ataxic dysarthria. *Journal of the Acoustical Society of America, 107*, 3415-3424.

Liss, J. M., & Weismer, G. (1992). Qualitative acoustic analysis in the study of motor speech disorders. *Journal of the Acoustical Society of America, 92*, 2984-2987.

McAuliffe, M. J., Ward, E. C., & Murdoch, B. E. (2006). Speech production in Parkinson's disease: II. Acoustic and electropalatographic investigation of sentence, word, and segment durations. *Clinical Linguistics and Phonetics, 220*, 19-33.

McHenry, M. A. (2003). The effect of pacing strategies on the variability of movement sequences in dysarthria. *Journal of Speech, Language and Hearing Research, 46*, 702-710.

McNeil, M. R. (Ed.). (1997). *Clinical management of sensorimotor speech disorders*. New York: Thieme.

McNeil, M. R., Caligiuri, M., & Rosenbek, J. C. (1989). A comparison of labiomandibular kinematic durations, displacements, velocities and dysmetrias in apraxic and normal adults. *Clinical Aphasiology, 17*, 173-193.

McNeil, M. R., Robin, D. A., & Schmidt, R. A., (1997). Apraxia of speech: Definition, differentiation and treatment. In M. R. McNeil (Ed.), *Clinical management of sensorimo-tor speech disorders* (pp. 311-344). New York: Thieme.

McNeil, M., Weismer, G., Adams, S., & Mulligan, M. (1990). Oral structure nonspeech motor control in normal, dysarthric, aphasic, and apraxic speakers: Isometric force and static position control. *Journal of Speech and Hearing Research, 33*, 255-268.

McRae, P. A., Tjaden, K., & Schoonings, B. (2002). Acoustic and perceptual consequences of articulatory rate change in Parkinson disease. *Journal of Speech, Language, and Hearing Research, 45*, 35-50.

Moon, J. B.. & Jones, D. (1991). Motor control of velopharyngeal structures during vowel production. *Cleft Palate-Craniofacial Journal, 28*, 58-69.

Moon, J. B., & Kuehn, D. P. (2004). Anatomy and physiology of normal and disordered velopharyngeal function for speech. In K. R. Bzoch (Ed.), *Communicative disorders related to cleft lip and palate* (5th ed., pp. 67-98). Austin, TX: Pro-Ed.

Moore, C. A., Smith, A., & Ringel, R. L. (1988). Task-specific organization of activity in human jaw muscles. *Journal of Speech and Hearing Research, 31*, 670-680.

Müller, E. M., & Brown, W. S. (1980). Variations in the supraglottal air pressure waveform and their articulatory interpretation. In N. J. Lass (Ed.), *Speech and language: Advances in basic research and practice* (Vol. 4, pp. 317-389). New York: Academic Press.

Müller, E. M., Milenkovic, P., & MacLeod, G. E. (1984). Perioral tissue mechanics during speech production. In C. DeLisi & J. Eisenfeld (Eds.), *Proceedings of the Second IMAC International Symposium on Biomedical Systems Modeling* (pp. 363-371). Amsterdam, Netherlands: North-Holland.

Murdoch, B. E. (Ed.). (1998). *Dysarthria: A physiological approach to assessment and treatment*. Cheltenham: Stanley Thornes.

Murdoch, B. E., Goozee, J., V., Veidt, M., Scott, D. H., & Meyers, I. A. (2004). Introducing the pressure-sensing palatograph—the next frontier in electropalatography. *Clinical Linguistics and Phonetics, 18*, 433-445.

NessAiver, M., Stone, M., Parthasarathy, M., Kahana, Y., & Paritsky, A. (2005). Recording high-quality speech during tagged cine-MRI studies using a fiber optic microphone. *Journal of Magnetic Resonance Imaging, 23*, 92-97.

Netsell, R. (1981). The acquisition of speech motor control: A perspective with directions for research. In R. Stark (Ed.), *Language behavior in infancy and early childhood* (pp. 127-156). New York: Elsevier.

Netsell, R. (1982). Speech motor control and selected neurologic disorders. In S. Grillner, B. Lindblom, J. Lubker, & A. Persson (Eds.), *Speech motor control* (pp. 247-261). New York: Pergamon Press.

Netsell, R., & Kent, R. D. (1976). Paroxysmal ataxic dysarthria. *Journal of Speech and Hearing Disorders, 41*, 93-109.

Odell, K., McNeil, M. R., Rosenbek, J. C., & Hunter, L. (1990). Perceptual characteristics of consonant productions by apraxic speakers. *Journal of Speech and Hearing Disorders, 55*, 345-359.

Odell, K., McNeil, M. R., Rosenbek, J. C., & Hunter, L. (1991). Perceptual characteristics of vowel and prosody production in apraxic, aphasic, and dysarthric speakers. *Journal of Speech and Hearing Research, 34*, 67-80.

Ogar, J., Slama, H., Dronkers, N., Amici, S., & Gorno-Tempini, M. L. (2005). Apraxia of speech: An overview. *Neurocase, 11*, 427-432.

Perkell, J. S., Guenther, F. H., Lane, H., Matthies, M. L., Perrier, P., Vick, J., Wilhelms-Tricarico, R., & Zandipour, M. (2000). A theory of speech motor control and supporting data from speakers with normal hearing and with profound hearing loss. *Journal of Phonetics, 28*, 233-272.

Perkell, J. S., Matthies, M., Svirsky, M., & Jordan, M. I. (1995). Goal-based speech motor control: A theoretical framework and some preliminary data. *Journal of Phonetics, 23*, 23-35.

Ramig, L. O. (1992). The role of phonation in speech intelligibility: A review and prelimi-nary data from patients with Parkinson's disease. In R. D. Kent (Ed.), *Intelligibility in speech disorders: Theory, measurement and management* (pp.119-155). Amsterdam: John Benjamins.

Robin, D., Bean, C., & Folkins, J. W. (1989). Lip movement in apraxia of speech. *Journal of Speech and Hearing Research, 32*, 512-523.

Ryalls, J. (1982). Intonation in Broca's aphasia. *Neuropsychologia, 20*, 355-360.

Ryalls, J. (1986). An acoustic study of vowel production in aphasia. *Brain and Language, 29*, 48-67.

Schiavetti, N. (1992). Scaling procedures for the measurement of speech intelligibility. In R. D. Kent (Ed.), *Intelligibility in speech disorders: Theory, measurement and man-agement* (pp. 11-35). Amsterdam: John Benjamins.

Seddoh, S., Robin, D., Sim, H., Hageman, C., Moon, J., & Folkins, J. (1996). Speech timing in apraxia of speech versus conduction aphasia. *Journal of Speech and Hearing Research, 39*, 590-603.

Shriberg, L. D., & Kent, R. D. (2002). *Clinical phonetics* (3rd ed.). Boston: Allyn & Bacon.

Smith, A. (1992). The control of orofacial movements in speech. *Critical Reviews in Oral Biology and Medicine, 3*, 233-267.

Smith, A., Goffman, L., Zelaznik, H. N., Ying, G., & McGillem, C. (1995). Spatiotemporal sta-bility and patterning of speech movement sequences. *Experimental Brain Research, 104*, 493-501.

Smith, K., K., & Kier, W. M. (1989). Trunks, tongues, and tentacles: Moving with skele-tons of muscle. *American Scientist, 77*, 29-35.

Solomon, N. P., Robin, D., & Luschei, E. (2000). Strength, endurance and stability of the tongue and hand in Parkinson disease. *Journal of Speech, Language and Hearing Research, 43*, 256-267.

Southwood, H., Dagenais, P. A., Sutphin, S. M., & Garcia, J. M. (1997). Coarticulation in apraxia of speech: A perceptual, acoustic, and electropalatographic study. *Clinical Linguistics and Phonetics, 11*, 179-203.

Spencer, K. A., & Rogers, M. A. (2005). Speech motor programming in hypokinetic and ataxic dysarthria. *Brain and Language, 94,* 347-366.

Stevens, K. N. (1999). *Acoustic phonetics.* Cambridge, MA: MIT Press.

Stone, M. (2005). A guide to analysing tongue motion from ultrasound images. *Clinical Linguistics and Phonetics, 19,* 455-501.

Story, B., Titze, I., & Hoffman, E. (1998). Vocal tract area functions for an adult female speaker based on volumetric imaging. *Journal of the Acoustical Society of America, 104,* 471-487.

Sussman, H., McNeilage, P., & Hanson, R. (1973). Labial and mandibular dynamics during the production of bilabial consonants: Preliminary observations. *Journal of Speech and Hearing Research, 16,* 397-420.

Tasko, S., & McClean, M. D. (2004). Variations in articulatory movement with changes in speech task. *Journal of Speech Language and Hearing Research, 47,* 85-100.

Tjaden, K. (1999). Can a model of overlapping gestures account for scanning speech patterns? *Journal of Speech, Language and Hearing Research, 42,* 604-617.

Tjaden, K. (2000a). An acoustic study of coarticulation in dysarthric speakers with Parkinson disease. *Journal of Speech, Language, and Hearing Research, 43,* 1466-1480.

Tjaden, K. (2000b). Exploration of a treatment technique for prosodic disturbance following stroke. *Clinical Linguistics and Phonetics, 18,* 619-641.

Tjaden, K. (2000c). A preliminary study of factors influencing perception of articulatory rate in Parkinson disease. *Journal of Speech, Language and Hearing Research, 43,* 997-1010.

Tjaden, K. (2003). Anticipatory coarticulation in multiple sclerosis and Parkinson disease. *Journal of Speech, Language, and Hearing Research, 46,* 990-1008.

Tjaden, K., & Turner, G. (1997). Spectral properties of fricatives in ALS. *Journal of Speech, Language, and Hearing Research, 40,* 1358-1372.

Tjaden, K., & Watling, E. (2003). Characteristics of diadochokinesis in multiple sclerosis and Parkinson disease. *Folia Phoniatrica et Logopaedica, 55,* 241-259.

Tjaden, K., & Wilding, G. E. (2004). Rate and loudness manipulations in dysarthria: Acoustic and perceptual findings. *Journal of Speech, Language, and Hearing Research, 47,* 766-783.

Tjaden, K., & Wilding, G. E. (2005). Effect of rate reduction and increased loudness on acoustic measures of anticipatory coarticulation in multiple sclerosis and Parkinson disease. *Journal of Speech, Language, and Hearing Research, 48,* 261-277.

Turner, G. S., & Tjaden, K. (2000). Acoustic differences between content and function words in amyotrophic lateral sclerosis. *Journal of Speech, Language and Hearing Research, 43,* 769-781.

Turner, G. S., Tjaden, K., & Weismer, G. (1995). The influence of speaking rate on vowel and space and speech intelligibility for individuals with amyotrophic lateral sclerosis. *Journal of Speech, Language and Hearing Research, 38,* 1001-1013.

Turner, G. S., & Weismer, G. (1993). Characteristics of speaking rate in the dysarthria associated with amyotrophic lateral sclerosis. *Journal of Speech and Hearing Research, 36,* 1134-1144.

Warren, D. W., Putnam, A., & Hinton, V. (1997). Aerodynamics. In M. R. McNeil (Ed.), *Clinical management of sensorimotor speech disorders* (pp. 81-106). New York: Thieme.

Weismer, G. (1980). Control of the voicing distinction for intervocalic stops and fricatives: Some data and theoretical considerations. *Journal of Phonetics, 8,* 427-438.

Weismer, G. (1984). Articulatory characteristics of parkinsonian dysarthria: Segmental and phrase-level timing, spirantization and glottal-supraglottal coordination. In M. R. McNeil, J. C. Rosenbek, & A. E. Aronson (Eds.), *The dysarthrias: Physiology, acoustics, perception, and management* (pp. 101-130). San Diego, CA: College-Hill Press.

Weismer, G. (1997). Motor speech disorders. In W. J. Hardcastle & J. Laver (Eds.), *The handbook of phonetic sciences* (pp. 191–219). Oxford: Blackwell.

Weismer, G. (2006). Philosophy of research in motor speech disorders. *Clinical Linguistics and Phonetics, 20,* 415–449.

Weismer, G., & Bunton, K. (1999). Influences of pellet markers on speech production behavior: acoustical and perceptual measures. *Journal of the Acoustical Society of America, 105,* 2882–2894.

Weismer, G., Jeng, J., Laures, J. S., & Kent, R. D. (2001). Acoustic and intelligibility characteristics of sentence production in neurogenic speech disorders. *Folia Phoniatrica et Logopaedica, 53,* 1–18.

Weismer, G., Kent, R. D., Hodge, M., & Martin, R. (1988). The acoustic signature for intelligibility test words. *Journal of the Acoustical Society of America, 84,* 1281–1291.

Weismer, G., & Laures, J. S. (2002). Direct magnitude estimates of intelligibility in dysarthria: Effects of a chosen standard. *Journal of Speech, Language, and Hearing Research, 45,* 421–433.

Weismer, G., Laures, J. S., Jeng, J., Kent, R. D., & Kent, J. F. (2000). Effect of speaking rate manipulations on acoustic and perceptual aspects of the dysarthria in amyotrophic lateral sclerosis. *Folia Phoniatrica et Logopaedica, 52,* 201–219.

Weismer, G., & Liss, J. M. (1991a). Reductionism is a dead-end in speech research: Perspectives on a new direction. In C. A. Moore, K. M. Yorkston, & D. R. Beukelman (Eds.), *Dysarthria and apraxia of speech: Perspectives on management* (pp. 15–29). Baltimore: Paul H. Brookes.

Weismer, G., & Liss, J. M. (1991b). Acoustic/perceptual taxonomies of disordered speech. In C. A. Moore, K. M. Yorkston, & D. R. Beukelman (Eds.), *Dysarthria and apraxia of speech: Perspectives on management* (pp. 245–270). Baltimore: Paul H. Brookes.

Weismer, G., & Martin, R. E. (1992). Acoustic and perceptual approaches to the study of intelligibility. In R. D. Kent (Ed.), *Intelligibility in speech disorders: Theory, measurement and management* (pp. 67–118). Amsterdam: John Benjamins.

Weismer, G., Martin, R., Kent, R. D., & Kent, J. F. (1992). Formant trajectory characteristics of males with amyotrophic lateral sclerosis. *Journal of the Acoustical Society of America, 91,* 1085–1098.

Weismer, G., Yunusova, Y., & Westbury, J. R. (2003). Interarticulatory coordination in dysarthria: An x-ray microbeam study. *Journal of Speech, Language, and Hearing Research, 46,* 1247–1261.

Westbury, J., & Dembowski, J. S. (1993). Articulatory kinematics of normal diadochokinetic performance. *Annual Bulletin of the Research Institute of Logopedics and Phoniatrics, 27,* 13–36.

Westbury, J., McClean, M., &, Lindstrom, M. (2002). Tongues and lips without jaws: Some consequences of ignoring jaw rotation. *Journal of Speech, Language and Hearing Research, 45,* 651–662.

Wohlert, A. B., & Goffman, L. (1994). Human perioral muscle activation patterns. *Journal of Speech and Hearing Research, 37,* 1032–1040.

Wohlert, A. B., & Hammen, V. L. (2000). Lip muscle activity related to speech rate and loudness. *Journal of Speech, Language and Hearing Research, 43,* 1229–1239.

Wohlert, A. B., & Smith, A. (1998). Spatiotemporal stability of lip movements in older adult speakers. *Journal of Speech Language and Hearing Research, 41,* 41–50.

Yorkston, K. M., & Beukelman, D. R. (1981). *Assessment of intelligibility of dysarthric speech.* Austin, TX: Pro-Ed.

Yorkston, K. M., & Beukelman, D. R. (1996). *Sentence Intelligibility Test.* Lincoln, NE: Tice Technologies.

Yorkston, K. M., Beukelman, D. R., Strand, E., & Bell, K. (1999). *Management of motor speech disorders in children and adults* (2nd ed., pp. 483–541). Austin, TX: Pro-Ed.

Yorkston, K., Miller, R., & Strand, E. (2003). *Management of speech and swallowing in degenerative diseases* (2nd ed.). St. Louis, MO: Mosby.

Yunusova, Y., Weismer, G., Kent, R. D., & Rusche, N. (2005). Breath-group intelligibility in dysarthria: Characteristics and underlying correlates. *Journal of Speech, Language and Hearing Research, 48,* 1294–1310.

Ziegler, W., & von Cramon, D. R. (1985). Anticipatory coarticulation in a patient with apraxia of speech. *Brain and Language, 26,* 117–130.

Ziegler, W., & von Cramon, D. R. (1986). Spastic dysarthria after acquired brain injury: An acoustic study. *Journal of Disorders of Communication, 21,* 173–187.

Zraick, R., & Liss, J. (2000). A comparison of equal-appearing interval scaling and direct magnitude estimation of nasal voice quality. *Journal of Speech, Language and Hearing Research, 43,* 979–988.

Zwirner, P., & Barnes, G. J. (1992). Vocal tract steadiness: A measure of phonatory and upper airway motor control during phonation in dysarthria. *Journal of Speech and Hearing Research, 35,* 761–768.

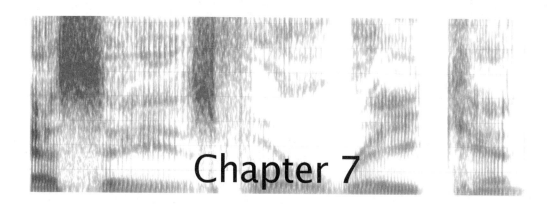

Chapter 7

THE ROLE OF SPEECH PERCEPTION IN MOTOR SPEECH DISORDERS

Julie M. Liss

"Intelligibility is as much in the ear of the listener as it is in the mouth of the speaker."
(Weismer & Martin, 1992, p. 68)

I preface this chapter with a true story from my early clinical career:

Upon meeting the patient for the first time, I asked about his illness and he began to speak. Although surely he was uttering words, I could not understand a single one of them. I then asked his name, knowing full well what it was, and I followed his labored response. I restricted the rest of my questions that day to those requiring yes and no answers and found I was able to discern them with good accuracy. I worked with him three times a week for the next month to treat his articulation and prosody deficits and noted significant and steady improvements in his intelligibility. He began to communicate with me quite effectively about his family, his favorite hobby of
bowling, and aspects of his daily routine. Our sessions became increasingly high spirited and interactive, and we both were delighted with his progress. It was, therefore, a great disappointment and surprise to me when my colleague scored the repeated intelligibility test and found absolutely no change from baseline. How could this be? If his speech production had not improved, had I just become a better listener? Did my knowledge of his life, the names of his children and bowling buddies, and his daily routine somehow help me understand what he was saying? Is it possible that I was the one who benefitted most from the 12 hours of speech therapy?

The very name *motor speech disorders* directs attention to the production aspects of this condition. Perhaps appropriately, the field has a long tradition of studying and characterizing the ways in which the neurologic damage influences speech movements and speech acoustics in motor speech disorders. Even the content of this book reveals the extent to which many aspects of speech production in motor speech disorders have been defined in great detail. However, the speech signal must be regarded as only half of the equation when it comes to matters of speech intelligibility and communication, as the preceding story portrays. The contributions of the perceiver are an integral part of the equation, as the listener actively brings to bear everything he or she knows about speech to make sense of what is being said. In this way, speech intelligibility is an emergent property of the listener's knowledge and strategies, and all the information available in the speech signal, the message, and communicative environment (Lindblom, 1990).

In this chapter, we explore the fundamental ways in which speech perception processes and phenomena must be considered in the study, diagnosis, and treatment of motor speech disorders. First, we examine how the acoustic features and abnormalities in dysarthria challenge our typical speech perception strategies. We accomplish this by considering two basic tasks in speech perception: (1) the recognition of words spoken in isolation, devoid of context, as would be the case in a single-word intelligibility test, and (2) the task of recognizing words as they occur in connected speech, with all the rich contextual information from which to draw. In the second part of this chapter, we discuss how our knowledge of speech perception strategies and constraints can be used to our advantage in the clinical domain. Specifically, we explore a novel approach

for structuring and assessing our existing interventions for motor speech disorders, and provide a rationale for the development of new ones. The overarching aim of this chapter is to equip readers with a structure for integrating their knowledge of speech perception in all their clinical practice.

The Perceptual Challenge of Dysarthric Speech

In everyday listening situations we are confronted with a spectrum of speech quality to perceive. The face-to-face exchange with a close friend takes little effort on our part, as the speech signal is clear, we are familiar with the person's voice and the words they tend to use, and there is a shared set of discussion topics and the lexicons that go with them. Move that same conversation to a cell phone exchange and the effort level necessarily increases. We must invoke more of our top-down, problem-solving skills to fill in the blanks as bits of a sentence are cut out or as the clarity of the words is obscured by noise. However, even when the quality of the acoustic signal is substantially reduced, we have a remarkable ability to extract the intended message by putting the pieces of the puzzle together in ways that make sense. This reflects the astonishing flexibility of our speech perception system to make use of all available information to land on the intended interpretation.

If our perceptual systems are so flexible and effective, why does dysarthria so often result in decreased intelligibility? To address this question, we need to focus on the critical interface between dysarthric speech signal characteristics and the cognitive-perceptual processes brought to bear on that signal by the listener. We can make the assumption that when listeners encounter dysarthric speech they deploy all their typical cognitive-perceptual processes to try to decipher it (see Bernstein & Weismer, 2001, for a discussion of the application of normal models and fundamental explanations in communication disorders). This is a reasonable assumption because we are highly practiced at dealing with degraded speech. Rarely do we have the luxury of dealing with citation-form speech, where the acoustic manifestation of a word resembles that which is produced slowly and carefully in isolation. Instead, we more often deal with conversational speech, where words can be produced as sloppy variants of their citation forms and still be understood because of the rich conversational context upon which the listener can draw.

Indeed, speech perception research has shown us that there are a variety of cognitive-perceptual processes and strategies at our disposal to deal with variable and degraded acoustic signals (Lindblom, 1990; Pisoni, 1993). Table 7-1 contains examples of these processes and strategies, including descriptions of how listeners make flexible use of whatever acoustic information is available (trading relations); how we perceptually resolve differences in speech produced by a wide variety of speakers and speaking styles (normalization and episodic memory for speech); and how our knowledge of the rules and regularities of language allows us to tolerate a significant amount of reduction and distortion of the segmental components of words (language knowledge and lexical bias). *Thus, listeners are highly accustomed to dealing with imperfect signals and to using multiple converging sources of information to decipher an utterance.*

The ultimate goal of the application of these various strategies and cognitive-perceptual processes (Table 7-1) is to figure out the semantic message that the speaker is conveying. To examine this goal with regard to motor speech disorders, we turn to two fundamental questions in the study of normal speech perception: (1) How do listeners recognize words produced in isolation and (2) How do listeners decipher connected speech? The perceptual mechanisms underlying these two tasks are somewhat different. In the task of recognizing spoken words produced in isolation, there is a close correspondence between the acoustic manifestation of the word and the lexical decision the listener renders. For the purpose of truly exploring this signal-perception relationship, we restrict our discussion of spoken word recognition to the situation in which other higher order cues (e.g., semantic, syntactic, or other contextual cues) do not come into play. In contrast, the task of deciphering connected speech allows us to consider not only segmental and suprasegmental cues, but the listener's application of top-down knowledge that affects a listener's ability to recognize the words that comprise the utterance. Throughout these sections, we speculate on how the degraded speech of dysarthria challenges the application and success of our typical perceptual strategies in these critical perceptual tasks of word recognition.

Spoken Word Recognition

Although it seems virtually effortless to recognize a word that is spoken, the modeling of this cognitive-perceptual activity continues to generate lively debate among speech perception theorists. How, specifically, does this mass of sequentially unfolding acoustic detail—detail that varies nontrivially from speaker to speaker,

Table 7–1. Selected Cognitive-Perceptual Processes and Strategies for Dealing with Reduced or Degraded Speech Signals

Processes-Strategies	Description
Trading Relations (e.g., Liberman, Cooper, Shankweiler, & Studdert-Kennedy, 1967; Mattys, White, & Melhorn, 2005; Repp, 1982; Weismer & Martin, 1992)	Speech signals are inherently highly redundant, providing multiple acoustic cues for each speech feature. Listeners are quite adept at using whatever combination of salient acoustic information is available and relatively reliable to make their perceptual decisions. This means that the full complement of acoustic cues need not be present for an accurate perception of the phoneme.
Normalization (e.g., Carre & Divenyi, 2000; Ladefoged & Broadbent, 1957; Lehiste, 1977; Miller, 1987; Miller & Lieberman, 1979)	It is remarkable that we can understand a sentence whether it is produced fast or slow, by a man, woman, or child, or even with a heavy foreign accent. This is possible because listeners have the capacity to perform *normalization processes* on the acoustic signal to accommodate many sources of variation in production. Thus, the acoustic manifestation of a word or sentence can vary widely and still be understood because the listener has the ability to "*morph*" it onto an existing mental template.
Episodic Memory for Speech (Bradlow, Nygaard, & Pisoni, 1999; Goldinger, 1996; Goldinger, Kleider, & Shelley, 1999)	In addition to the normalization process, there is evidence that listeners store detailed episodic memory traces of specific voices. These detailed memories assist listeners in perceiving the speech produced by that person on subsequent interactions. It is possible that this kind of information may be particularly useful when the speech is somehow unusual or degraded.
Knowledge of Language Rules and Regularities (e.g., Borsky, Shapiro, & Tuller, 2000; Dupoux, Pallier, Kakehi, & Mehler, 2001; Samuel, 1997; Samuel & Pitt, 2003).	Languages and the way they are produced are constrained by rules and regularities. Listeners make use of their knowledge about these rules to perceive speech. This includes knowledge of which sounds commonly and legally follow one another within a word (phonotactics); which sounds can be reduced, combined, or eliminated through phonologic processes (e.g. "jeet" produced in conversation is understood to be a reduced form of "did you eat"); semantic and syntactic constraints; prosodic structure, and so forth. This knowledge allows us to accommodate significant reductions and distortions of the speech signal.
Lexical Bias (Ganong, 1980; Samuel, 1981; Warren, 1970)	Listeners exhibit a strong tendency to perceive words as whole, even when phonemes that make up the words are absent or altered to become ambiguous in their identity. This means that listeners can tolerate a significant amount of segmental variation in the acoustic signal.

and even from token to token—converge onto the mental representation of a single word? A series of models has evolved to account for our ability to recognize a spoken word, among them the Logogen model (Morton, 1969), the Cohort theory (Marslen-Wilson & Welsh, 1978; Marslen-Wilson, 1987), the Trace model (McClelland & Elman, 1986a, 1986b), the Shortlist model (Norris, 1994), the Neighborhood Activation model (Luce & Pisoni, 1998), and the PARSYN model (Luce et al., 2000). Although a detailed comparison of these models is beyond the scope of this chapter (see Table 7–2 for a summary of each), they commonly assume that at least two fundamental processes underlie spoken word recognition: *lexical activation* and *lexical competition* (Jusczyk & Luce, 2002). When a listener encounters a spoken word, certain aspects of the acoustic signal serve to *activate* a set of possible lexical candidates. This is followed by *competition* among these candidates for the best fit with the input, and the winner of this competition is the recognized word.

Table 7–2. Selected Models and Theories of Spoken Word Recognition and Their General Descriptions

Model	Description
Logogen Model (Morton, 1969)	Words are represented in memory as "logogens" or counters. As the acoustic information from the spoken word is processed, the stimulus accumulates as evidence for the various logogens. When the evidence for a given logogen exceeds some threshold, that word is selected.
Cohort Theory (Marslen-Wilson & Welsh, 1978)	The acoustic form of the spoken word activates a cohort of lexical candidates in memory. A combination of bottom-up (acoustic-phonetic match) and top-down (syntactic and semantic context) results in the ultimate best match. The time course is largely left to right.
Trace Model (McClelland & Elman, 1986)	Acoustic input is evaluated at three interactive levels: phonetic features, phoneme, and word. Through interaction, the enhancement of a feature (e.g., voicing) will enhance phonemes and words with that feature, and will cause inhibition of candidates without that feature within a level.
Shortlist Model (Norris, 1994)	The acoustic input spurs the activation of a "short list" of word candidates that are similar to the input. These candidates compete with one another, whereby enhancement of one word inhibits surrounding words. This model attempts to tackle the issue of lexical segmentation.
Neighborhood Activation Model (Luce & Pisoni, 1998) and PARSYN (Luce et al., 2000)	Lexical activation occurs in the same way as proposed in the other models, in which the acoustic form of the word activates a cohort of lexical candidates. Competition, however, is influenced not only by the match between the input and mental templates, but also by statistical probabilities of the candidates (word frequency and neighborhood density).

Lexical Activation

The time course for lexical activation begins as soon as the first phonemes of the word are produced, such that we do not necessarily wait for the end of the word to begin our pursuit of word recognition. For example, when the speaker starts to say a word that begins with the syllable "el," we activate "elephant, elevator, elementary," and so forth (Warren & Marslen-Wilson, 1987, 1988). In this way, word-onsets play an important role in activating the initial set, or cohort, of lexical possibilities (e.g., Cole & Jakimik, 1978; Nooteboom, 1981). However, word-initial information is not the *only* contributor to lexical activation, and later occurring segments of words may be even more important for word recognition in some cases, such as to discriminate late-diverging words such as *damper* and *dampen* (see Connine, Blasko, & Titone, 1993; Connine, Titone, Deelman, & Blasko, 1997). In this way, the overall *form* of the target word—not just word-onset information—contributes to the activation of lexical items with similar phonemic composition and/or syllabic organization (e.g., the word *pat* may activate *cat*, and *beaker* may activate *speaker*) (Allopena, Magnuson, & Tanenhaus, 1998). *Thus, when a listener encounters a spoken word, a set of potential lexical candidates is activated. This pool of candidates arises from the acoustic information as it unfolds across the production of the word, as well as from the overall form of the word after it has been spoken.*

Lexical Competition

With the activation of the lexical cohort, there is *competition* among the candidates to select the word that best matches the input. This competition can be character-ized by facilitation and inhibition, such that the lexical candidates with the closest match to the input are facilitated, and those less like the input are inhibited. The competition is more than a simple goodness-of-fit matching process between input composition and candidate composition, as other factors pertaining to the macrostructure of the lexicon also have been shown to affect this process and the efficiency with which it occurs. *Lexical neighborhood density* is one such factor, and refers to the set or neighborhood of words that is similar to the target (Luce & Pisoni, 1998; Luce et al., 2000). For example, when a word has a similar form to many other words (e.g., *cat* shares a high lexical neighborhood density with all the words that are similar to it, such as *pat, kit, cap, spat, cast*, etc.), it takes more time and effort to distinguish the target from its neighbors than when a word form is relatively unique (e.g., *torque*, which has a low lexical neighborhood density). Thus, neighborhood density affects the time and effort required at the competition phase. In addition, within the members of the neighborhood, some words are more common or frequently occurring than others. Listeners take these *word frequency effects* into consideration during the competition phase, such that more common words (e.g., *big*) are facilitated over less common words (e.g., *bin*), other things being equal (Luce et al., 2000). This preference for high-frequency words facilitates target recognition when the target is common; however, the presence of high-frequency neighbors (competitors) has the opposite effect, and actually hinders target recognition.

In addition to these word-level effects of neighborhood density and word frequency, competition is affected by sublexical information as well. Listeners have been shown to attend to the finer acoustic aspects of the production of phoneme strings, such as the expected acoustic cues for coarticulation between adjacent segments (Davis, Marslen-Wilson, & Gaskell, 2002; Warren & Marslen-Wilson, 1987, 1988), as well as the probability of occurrence of phoneme sequences (Luce et al., 2000; Luce & Large, 2001). The latter aspect, called positional probabilities, or probabilistic phonotactics, simply refers to the likelihood of certain phonemes to follow one another in the words of a language. The effect of probabilistic phonotactics in the competition phase is the preference for more common phoneme sequences over uncommon or illegal sequences (e.g., the consonant string of *tbt* is illegal in words of the English language). *Thus, lexical items activated as potential candidates compete, and this competition is guided by the candidates' segmental similarity to the input, and it is affected by other lexical and sublexical factors that enhance or reduce the likelihood of a candidate to be picked. The ultimate winner of the competition is the recognized word.*

Time Course

Before we consider spoken word recognition in dysarthria, there is one more critical component to this process that must be reviewed: the time course over which spoken word recognition occurs (Mattys, 1997). There is strong evidence and a long-standing theoretical assumption that the process of word recognition occurs in a serial left-to-right manner in a time course closely aligned with the serial production of the phonemes of the word. Because of this immediate on-line processing of the word as it unfurls, word recognition sometimes can occur before the entire word

is spoken. This is possible when a word contains a *uniqueness point,* or a point before the word's end at which only one lexical candidate remains. For example, recognition of the word "spaghetti" is possible after hearing only /spag/ because no other word exists to match that sequence of acoustic-phonemic input (Grosjean, 1980; Marslen-Wilson & Welsh, 1978). Thus, the /g/ in "spaghetti" represents the uniqueness point for that word.

As it turns out, most words in the English language do not become lexically unique before their end (Luce, 1986). For example, the word *cab* cannot be recognized with certainty until sometime after the final phoneme is produced because the listener would need to rule out the possibility that the word is truly *cabin* or *cabinet* or even *cabbage*. That is, *cab* is embedded at the beginning of these longer words. Because embeddedness is more common for short than long words, and because short words tend to be high frequency in the language, this means that, in most cases, listeners are obliged to wait for the end of the word, or well into the next word in connected speech, before definitively deciding on the word's identity, lest they risk selecting the wrong lexical candidate from the activated pool (Bard, Shillock, & Altmann, 1988). This strategy of delayed commitment (see McQueen, Cutler, Briscoe, & Norris, 1995) requires that information from the beginning of the word be held in a short-term memory store until the end of the word is produced. All aspects of the word are then considered simultaneously to land on a decision. With this strategy, there is the potential for later occurring parts of the words to affect the percepts of earlier portions that are stored in short-term memory, particularly when there is something ambiguous about the early portions.

Although delayed commitment is useful for avoiding a premature and inaccurate decision, it comes with a risk, particularly if the signal is very slow or degraded: Word-initial information stored in short-term memory may fade or distort while the lexical decision process runs its course. *Thus, there is evidence for at least two forms of temporal processing in word recognition. The first is the left-to-right processing of acoustic information that is time aligned with the serial production of the phonemes that comprise the word. The second time course is the delay of a decision until the entire word has been spoken, allowing for the potential for right-to-left (retrograde) effects in the perceptual decisions. Based on the composition of the English language, it can be assumed that the latter time course represents a significant component of the processing of isolated spoken words, and particularly for words with phonemic ambiguity.*

Dysarthric Speech and Spoken Word Recognition

Now that we have reviewed some basic strategies and influences in spoken word recognition, let us turn our attention to how the nature of the speech degradation in motor speech disorders might challenge the processes of lexical activation and competition as they would occur in the recognition of isolated spoken words. Table 7–3 contains a list of the general categories of speech errors associated with motor speech disorders. For the purposes of single word recognition we focus on the segmental errors here.

Nearly all motor speech disorders are associated with some degree of segmental errors, if not stemming from frank articulatory deficits, then from those arising from incoordination among structures along the vocal tract (e.g., glottal-supraglottal coordination for voice-onset time distinctions). These errors can include omissions, substitutions, and distortions of both consonants and vowels within a word. They also manifest as disturbances in coarticulatory relationships across phoneme strings. Segmental errors in motor speech disorders will necessarily affect both the activation and competition phases in spoken word recognition. It bears stating, however, that this is not a problem unique to dysarthria, and that activation/competition problems only exist because of the structure and landscape of the lexicon, in which many words are similar and confusable (Luce & Pisoni, 1998).

Because the activation of the cohort of lexical candidates is driven primarily by the acoustic information available to the listener as the word is produced by the speaker, we can assume that segmental errors necessarily will affect the process of lexical activation. The most calamitous outcome of segmental errors is that the spoken word is not even activated as a lexical candidate because of the incompatible relationship between the acoustic form and the listener's mental template. In this scenario, there is no chance for word recognition to occur because the pattern of segmental omissions, substitutions, and distortions led the listener completely away from the target. A less dire outcome is that the segmental errors result in substantial phonemic uncertainty, such that the target word is activated, but along with a larger than necessary cohort of candidates to accommodate all possible identities of the ambiguous phonemes (Andruski, Blumstein, & Burton, 1994). This not only adds resource cost and processing time to the competition phase, but also increases the opportunity for selecting the wrong lexical candidate.

Table 7–3. Acoustic Features of Dysarthric Speech That May Affect Lexical Activation, Lexical Competition, and Lexical Segmentation

	Errors	Possible Consequences
Segmental Features	Phoneme omissions	Absent phonemes may result in the target word not being activated.
	Phoneme distortions	Distorted phonemes may introduce phonemic ambiguity or uncertainty. Activated lexical cohorts may be larger than necessary to accommodate all interpretations of the ambiguous phonemes. This may result in exceptional resource expenditure during the lexical competition phase, and increase the potential for the wrong target to be chosen as the perceived word.
	Phoneme substitutions	Phoneme substitutions may result in the target word not being activated.
Suprasegmental Features	Inappropriate syllable durations	Listeners may have difficulty applying a metrical segmentation strategy because of problems discerning strong syllables from weak ones (Liss et al., 2000, 2002).
	Inappropriate intersyllabic loudness variation	Listeners may have difficulty discerning strong and weak syllables.
	Inappropriate intersyllabic fundamental frequency variation	Flattened fundamental frequency (monotone) is associated with reductions in intelligibility (Bradlow, Torretta, & Pisoni, 1996; Laures & Bunton, 2003)
	Vowel space reduction (in particular, the reduction of strong vowels)	Vowel space reduction is associated with reduced intelligibility in single words and sentences (e.g., Bunton & Weismer, 2001; Kent et al., 1989; Liu, Tsao, & Kuhl, 2005; Turner, Tjaden, & Weismer, 1995; Weismer, Jeng, Laures, Kent, & Kent, 2001)
		Liu, Tsao, and Kuhl (2005) showed that not only did Madarin Chinese speakers with CP exhibit reduced vowel working space associated with reductions in single-word intelligibility, but that listeners had difficulty mapping these smaller working spaces onto their existing vowel percepts.

To demonstrate the possible effects of segmental errors on lexical activation and competition, let us consider an example in which a person with dysarthria produces the word *dip* with a devoiced /d/, thereby rendering it somewhat /t/-like.

As both word-initial information and overall word form information drives lexical access, we can assume that both *dip* and *tip* would be activated candidates, at least giving the distorted target a fighting chance to be selected as the perceived word. The problem, however, is that the phonemic ambiguity caused by the distortion will promote the activation of a larger than necessary lexical cohort. That is, there will be activation of all words that rhyme with *tip* and *dip*, all words in which *tip* and *dip* are embedded, and even words semantically related to each of the two (Wurm, Vakoch, & Seaman, 2004). This entire cohort will be admitted to the lexical competition phase, thereby requiring extra processing resources and increasing the opportunities for selecting a word other than *dip* as the target.

Recall that the goal of the competition phase is to distinguish the target from its competitors by assessing the acoustic similarity between the input and the lexical candidates. In this case, to what extent does *dip* produced with a devoiced /d/ match either the listener's mental templates for *dip* or *tip*? The ambiguity in this decision would need to be resolved with additional information, as neither match is perfect. In all likelihood, the weightings of subsegmental information, such as the degree of stop aspiration, would help tip the scale in the direction of one word over the other. This does not guarantee a correct choice, however, as these subsegmental cues may be faulty as well, thereby facilitating the selection of the wrong candidate in this competition (Andruski, Blumstein, & Burton, 1994). Ultimately, the recognized word, right or wrong, is related strongly to the acoustic realization of that word as it was produced by the dysarthric speaker. The lexical decision reflects the culmination of factors (acoustic and lexical) the listener considered in the competition. It is this relatively close relationship between the form of the input and the form of the recognized word that Kent et al. (1989) exploited in their single-word intelligibility test, which we discuss next. In this way, word recognition error patterns reflect the perceptually salient acoustic features of the input.

Let us now consider a practical application. In 1989, Ray Kent and his colleagues published a study entitled, "Toward phonetic intelligibility testing in dysarthria" (Kent, Weismer, Kent, & Rosenbek, 1989), which capitalized on the ways in which perceptual errors reveal the source of intelligibility deficits. This single-word intelligibility test consisted of carefully designed presentations of minimal pair sets. For example, a listener might hear the word *bad* produced by a speaker with dysarthria, and then decide from a list of four words whether the person said *bad, bet, bat,* or *mad*. Thinking back to what we have learned about spoken word recognition, we can presume that this format—selecting from a list of highly similar possibilities—constrains the lexical activation stage by ensuring the target is among the candidates. It also constrains the lexical competition process by offering confusable candidates from which the listener must select. The listener's choice reveals much about the most salient aspects of the acoustic signal. For example, if the listener incorrectly selects the word *mad*, we can attribute the error to the presence of nasal energy (hypernasality) in the acoustic signal that was sufficient to cause the listener to perceive /m/ rather than /b/ as the initial phoneme. In this way, it is possible to use these intelligibility data in an *explanatory capacity*, rather than simply as a marker of speech disorder severity. The evaluation of listener errors reveals which articulatory defects *caused* the decrements in intelligibility, suggesting that all articulatory errors and speech defects are not created equal, because some, more than others, may adversely affect a listener's ability to recover the intended word.[1] By extension, targeting those defects in therapy would then result in the most efficient and effective improvement in the speaker's intelligibility, at least for spoken single words. This test is an excellent example of using our knowledge of speech perception to sculpt meaningful assessment tools.

In summary, the speech production errors have the potential to create a situation in which the set of activated lexical candidates does not include the target word, and this is the most severe consequence to single-word intelligibility in motor speech disorders. Perhaps more often, the acoustic information is sufficient to activate the target word, along with a larger than necessary cohort of lexical candidates (due to phonemic or word form uncertainty). Extraordinary processing resources are allocated to the competition phase to consider all available information and a decision is made. The decision, right or wrong, reflects the relative importance attributed to available acoustic cues, along with lexical influences.

Deciphering Connected Speech

In the previous section, we focused on the relationship between the acoustic input and the activation, competition, and selection among lexical candidates in isolated spoken word recognition. This was useful for evaluating the close correspondence between acoustic information and lexical decisions when no complicating factors like contextual cues come into play. However, the mechanisms and details pertaining to isolated spoken word recognition cannot be applied easily to the perception of connected speech. Weismer and Martin (1992, p. 67) made the insightful prediction that, *"The explanatory principles that are emerging from the study of single-word intelligibility are likely to be quite different than those that will be discovered in the study of sentence intelligibility."*

As with our treatment of spoken word recognition, we make the assumption that listeners deploy their typical perceptual strategies as they attempt to decipher connected speech produced by someone with a motor speech disorder. What are the typical perceptual strategies used in deciphering connected speech? Just as in isolated spoken word recognition, the processes of *lexical activation* and *lexical competition* are operant in the perception of connected speech; however, their relationship changes because they are now both influenced by the speaker's message. All words in an utterance are related to one another—with some level of predictability—in a way that conveys the speaker's message. As individual words are recognized, they heighten the listener's expectation for hearing other words (i.e., *priming effect*). For example, hearing *"The student"* leads to the priming of *school* topic words, and sets up the expectation that the next word uttered will be a verb or an adverb as they typically follow nouns

---

[1]This necessarily interacts with the lexical nature of the speech target as well, recalling our discussion of neighborhood density. For example, there are areas of the lexicon that are sparse in terms of segmental confusion. For words in those areas, segmental errors may be of little consequence.

in the English language. If this turns out to be the case, as in, *"The student gave her teacher a pencil,"* perception will have been facilitated by the semantic and syntactic priming. A less semantically and syntactically predictable sequence, such as, *"The student wall appeared fresh,"* is still recognizable, but comes at additional processing costs, unless preceded by other information as in, *"In the school mural contest the teachers finished their painting weeks ago. The student wall appeared fresh."*

It is this fundamental goal of message extraction that drives word recognition in the perception of connected speech. In fact, our bias toward words as the unit of perception in connected speech allows us to tolerate significant segmental ambiguities and distortions. Perhaps one of the best known perceptual phenomena in this regard is that of *phonemic restoration*, or the auditory illusion of hearing sounds that are not actually present in the acoustic signal (Warren, 1970). Warren and Warren (1970) demonstrated this powerful effect by splicing out single phonemes in spoken sentences and replacing them with a cough. For example, they replaced /w/ in the word *wheel* in the sentence, *"It was found that the (wh)eel was on the axle."* Listeners had no trouble understanding the sentences and reported hearing all the phonemes even though one was completely eliminated. And, although they all reported hearing the coughs in the sentences, they could not confidently determine where they had occurred. This demonstrates the potent influence of context and top-down processing on speech perception as the listener's attention is focused on words rather than their phonemic constituents per se.

It makes good sense that listeners focus on words rather than phonemes in connected speech, and that these words within an utterance exert an effect on one another. After all, the goal of communication is message extraction. But how is it that we get to the words in an utterance; or rather, how do we break up the utterance into its component words? This may, at first glance, seem like a ridiculous question. As we listen to someone speak, we do not hear a continuous stream of acoustic information, instead our perception is that of hearing a sequence or string of discrete words. Yet the very fact we hear discrete words at all is remarkable when we consider the acoustic input. Unlike written sentences, in which individual words are separated by small spaces, connected speech contains very few clues to the offset of one word and the beginning of the next. This is quite apparent when we examine a spectrogram of a sentence produced without pauses (see Figure 7–1). As one can see, there is almost continuous acoustic energy in this sentence, and the brief breaks that do occur are not related to word boundaries at all, but instead to vocal tract closures associated with phonemes. The reason we hear discrete words is because of an operation called *lexical segmentation*, or the perceptual parsing of the continuous acoustic stream into word components.

Lexical segmentation is regarded as the most fundamental process in the understanding of connected speech, and lexical activation and lexical competition are both tied intimately to this task. Although the precise relationship is open to debate, one possibility is that lexical activation and competition depend on the listener's determination of word boundaries. As a word boundary is determined, a cohort of possible candidates is activated and competition among these candidates ensues. Like isolated spoken word recognition,

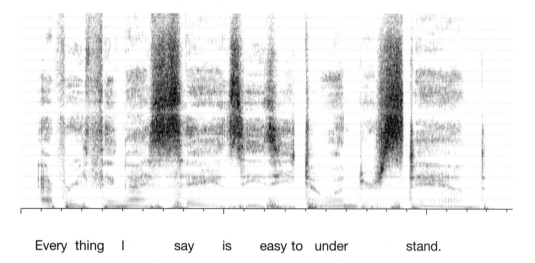

Every thing I say is easy to under stand.

Figure 7–1. Spectrogram of the sentence, "Everything I say is easy to understand." Note the rather continuous acoustic stream and the absence of obvious word boundary cues.

lexical segmentation seems that it should be a nearly impossible task, but in fact we accomplish it with amazing ease under typical circumstances. Shadowing experiments, in which listeners are required to repeat what they hear as soon as it is heard, show that this process can happen very quickly as the sentence unfolds. However, the challenge arises when we try to explain how this occurs.

Models of Lexical Segmentation: Lexically Driven Versus Sublexically Driven

Until recently there have been two approaches to explain lexical segmentation. Some theorists have claimed that speech segmentation is a byproduct of word recognition, or rather that it is a *lexically driven* process (McClelland & Elman, 1986; Norris, 1994; Norris, McQueen, Cutler, Butterfield, & Kearns, 2001). Thus, as soon as a word is recognized in the utterance it is effectively segmented from those

words around it. Lexically driven segmentation is greatly facilitated by our knowledge of the structure of language (e.g., semantic plausibility, syntactic rules) and this helps to activate very streamlined lexical cohorts. Listeners exploit the regularities of language and communication to anticipate and activate the most likely sets of lexical candidates. As stated earlier, for example, verbs usually follow nouns, and adjectives precede them; knowledge of the topic primes or enhances the activation of all words associated with that topic. *Thus, lexically driven segmentation refers to activating word forms that match various portions of the signal, and that the contextual information most highly predicts. The recognition of one word in the sentence facilitates the recognition, and hence segmentation, of the other words in that sentence.*

Other theorists have argued that speech segmentation is accomplished by a *sublexically driven* process, in which listeners scan the acoustic stream for relevant cues to let them know when one word ends and another begins. Likely candidates for these sublexical cues include prosodic or stress information, particularly the occurrence of strong syllables (Cutler & Norris, 1988; see also Textbox 7–1); phonotactic probabilities about which sounds commonly follow others within a word (McQueen, 1998; Vitevitch & Luce, 1999; Weber, 2000); allophonic variations in the way phonemes are produced in different contexts (Kirk, 2000; Nakatani & Dukes, 1977); and coarticulatory information associated with the production of phoneme sequences (Davis, Marslen-Wilson, & Gaskell, 2002; Mattys, 2004). But even within this camp, there is little agreement about which of these cues have primacy in lexical segmentation, as demonstrated by the following passage:

There is therefore now a relatively long list of cues which listeners use for segmentation and which vary among languages, including phonotactics, allophonics, and other acoustic-phonetic cues, silence, and metrical cues based on the input language's rhythmic structure. An important issue which remains to be addressed is the relative ranking of these cues: do some cues carry more weight in segmentation than others?" (McQueen & Cutler, 2001, p. 481).

Hierarchical Model of Lexical Segmentation

Although both lexically driven and sublexically driven models of speech segmentation have numerous sources of support, neither type can accommodate all patterns of findings. This has led to the call for the development of *conciliatory* or *hybrid* models, which recognize the apparent flexibility of the speech perception system to use a variety of strategies to segment the acoustic stream (McQueen & Cutler, 2001).

Recently, Mattys and his colleagues laid the groundwork for such an integrative model of speech segmentation (Mattys, White, & Melhorn, 2005). They propose that speech segmentation proceeds by both lexically *and* sublexically driven processes, depending on the quality of the acoustic signal and the richness of the contextual information in the message. Central to this model is the notion that real-world speech is composed of an array of word-boundary cues from which to choose, and that these cues converge in a complementary or confirmatory way to mark word boundaries. Listeners will use the information that is most efficient and expeditious to segment the acoustic stream. Mattys and his colleagues conceptualize a continuum, where listeners perform low-cost lexically driven segmentation whenever the signal quality and interpretive context permit, and then resort to higher-cost strategies for segmentation as necessary.

As a last resort—and most relevant to our impending discussion of dysarthric speech—listeners attend to suprasegmental information to accomplish lexical parsing when reliable segmental information is not available. Listeners scan the speech signal for strong syllables (syllables that are perceptually prominent or stressed, and that contain full vowels), which, in English, tend most often to be word onsets, and then use this information to instigate lexical access (for a more detailed account of this process, see the Metrical Segmentation Strategy in Textbox 7–1). Unlike lexically driven segmentation strategies that may proceed in a largely left-to-right fashion as the utterance unfolds, sublexically driven strategies—particularly those that use syllabic strength contrasts to predict

Textbox 7–1
Metrical Segmentation Strategy Hypothesis
(Cutler & Butterfield, 1992; Cutler & Norris, 1988)

According to the lexical segmentation model of Mattys and his colleagues (Mattys et al., 2005), listeners resort to using supraseg-mental information to make predictions about where words begin and end when the segmental information in the speech signal is ambiguous or unreliable. They base this claim on the work of Anne Cutler and her colleagues, who suggested that lexical segmentation is guided by attendance to the rhythmic structures of language (Cutler & Butterfield, 1992; Cutler & Norris, 1988). Their metrical segmentation strategy (MSS) hypothesis proposes that listeners capitalize on the juxtaposition of strong and weak syllables to identify the location of word boundaries. In particular, listeners tend to treat strong syllables as potential word onsets. Strong syllables are those that receive prosodic stress and contain a full vowel; weak syllables are unstressed and contain a reduced vowel (e.g., *table* is a strong-weak syllabic strength pattern, and *convey* is a weak-strong one). In English, listeners will be highly successful in their lexical seg-mentation if they use this strategy of treating strong syllables as potential word onsets (Cutler & Carter, 1987). This is because the majority of words in the English language begin with, or consist of, a strong syllable. Evidence in support of this hypothesis is found primarily in studies of naturally occurring *slips of the ear* and misperceptions elicited by presenting normal speech in background noise or at very low listening levels (Cutler & Butterfield, 1992; Cutler & Carter, 1987).

The evidence comes in the form of lexical boundary errors. As listeners attempt to perform lexical segmentation in degraded speech, they are apt to make errors and insert word boundaries where they do not actually exist, and delete word boundaries where they do exist. These misplacements of lexical boundaries are classified as either lexical boundary *insertions* or *deletions*. If listeners are strategically looking for strong syllables to attempt lexical segmentation, we should see insertion errors occurring more frequently before strong than before weak syllables. For example, as shown in Table 7–4, the misperception of "his pipe" for the target word "despite" is a predicted error because the listener mistakenly inserted a lexical boundary error before a strong syllable (IS, insert before strong). Likewise, the misperception "license" for the target "rice is" is predicted because a lexical boundary is erroneously deleted before a weak syllable (DW, delete before weak). Lexical boundary insertions before weak syllables (IW) and deletions before strong syllables (DS) do occur, but at a much lower rate than the predicted errors. In this way, it is possible to infer a listener's use of syllabic strength information in lexical segmentation decisions.

Table 7–4. Classification and Examples of Lexical Boundary Errors (LBE) Type and Location[a]

	Before Strong Syllable	Before Weak Syllable
INSERTION	IS	IW
Target→Error	*Despite→his pipe*	*Standard→stand her*
DELETION	DS	DW
Target→Error	*a pear→compare*	*Rice is→license*

[a]Shaded cells represent error types predicted by the Metrical Segmentation Strategy hypothesis (Cutler & Butterfield, 1992).

word onsets—necessitate a delayed commitment of lexical boundary decisions until the entire utterance has been processed (see Mattys, 1997). They also require that the listener hold in short-term memory earlier and ambiguous parts of the utterance until that information can be resolved in the final parsing solution. Thus, by their very nature, sublexically driven segmentation strategies are slower and more resource costly than lexically driven ones. The overarching idea in this model is that listeners take a systematic and hierarchical approach to lexical segmentation depending on what sort of information is available in the acoustic signal, moving from low-cost strategies to high-cost ones as necessary.

Lexical Segmentation in Dysarthria

This type of model—one that incorporates both lexically and sublexically driven segmentation strategies—does exceptionally well in accommodating how listeners might segment connected dysarthric speech. In large part, this is because dysarthria results in a variety of patterns and severities of segmental and suprasegmental degradation, sometimes even within a given speaker on a single speaking occasion. Thus, only a model that includes a flexible, context-sensitive perceptual strategy could accommodate such range of variation.

Applying this model of lexical segmentation to dysarthric speech, we can assume that listeners will default to lexically driven segmentation strategies as long as the quality of the acoustic signal and contextual predictability permit an unambiguous parsing solution. We also can assume that speech need not be in perfect form for lexically driven segmentation to occur. The listener's lexical bias and active use of contextual information can mitigate the negative effects of segmental and suprasegmental imperfections, and permit accurate lexical segmentation across some range of speech quality. However, at some level of speech signal degradation or contextual ambiguity listeners must resort to attending to sublexical information to accomplish lexical segmentation. The effectiveness of these strategies is dependent on the quality and quantity of acoustic information available. This is a problem when it comes to dysarthric speech. As shown in Table 7–3, motor speech disorders result in the disturbance of the very cues listeners use to segment the acoustic stream. It is not surprising then that part of the intelligibility deficit in motor speech disorders stems from the listener's challenge in performing lexical segmentation.

A series of experiments ongoing in our lab has shed some light on the nature of the problems that listeners face when trying to apply sublexically driven segmentation strategies—in particular attendance to syllabic strength contrasts—to different types of dysarthric speech (Cutler & Norris, 1988; Cutler & Butterfield, 1992; see also Metrical Segmentation Strategy in Textbox 7–1). Recall that strong syllables are distinguished from weak ones by the presence of a full (unreduced) vowel, and they tend to be of relatively longer duration, greater loudness, and higher pitch than those of adjacent weak syllables. There are several speech characteristics in dysarthria that we can hypothesize are especially detrimental to the distinction of strong and weak syllables. These include *monotonicity*, or the lack of fundamental frequency variation across an utterance; *equal and even* durational patterns, where weak syllables have durations similar to strong syllables; and the *reduction or centralization of strong vowels* such that their formant values are moved in the direction of a weak or neutral vowel. When present,

these speech features can blur the distinction between strong and weak syllables, thereby making it difficult to apply the metrical segmentation strategy (MSS). A lexical boundary error analysis provides evidence of this difficulty when word boundaries are not preferentially inserted before strong syllables, or deleted before weak syllables, as would be predicted by the MSS (see Textbox 7–1 for a description of lexical boundary error analysis).

In several studies, Liss et al. found evidence that listeners do attempt to apply the MSS to segment connected dysarthric speech (Liss et al., 1998, 2000, 2002). More importantly, they found that different types and severities of dysarthria offered different types of challenges to the efficient application of this strategy, presumably because of the different patterns of prosodic degradation (see Table 7–5). For example, a lexical boundary error analysis revealed that listeners were able to apply the MSS in their deciphering of speech of persons with hypokinetic dysarthria, but not of those with similar intelligibility who presented with ataxic dysarthria. Why might ataxic dysarthria prevent efficient application of this segmentation strategy? The most likely conclusion is that the listeners were not able to reliably distinguish strong and weak syllables, perhaps because they sounded alike. This was supported by acoustic measures that showed adjacent strong and weak syllables were of similar duration, and that vowels in strong syllables tended to be reduced. The key point to consider is that there was equivalent intelligibility for the ataxic and hypokinetic speech samples, but that the source of the reduced intelligibility was different for each. This series of studies provides a compelling argument for the consideration of speech perception strategies in general, and speech segmentation

Table 7–5. Patterns of Segmental and Suprasegmental Involvement Typically Associated with Various Dysarthrias

Dysarthria Type	Articulatory Imprecision	Hypophonic/ Hyperphonic	Hyper/ Hyponasal	Prosodic Disturbance	Rate Abnormalities
Flaccid					
V	jaw				
VII	labial				
IX, x		Hypo	Hypo	Monotone	
X					
XII	lingual				
Spastic	Consonant imprecision; vowel reduction	Hyper	Hypo	Monotone, monoloud	Slow
Ataxic	Irregular articulatory breakdown	Hypo(?)	Hypo(?)	Equal and excess	Slow
Spastic-Flaccid (ALS)	Consonant imprecision; vowel reduction	Hyper-Hypo	Hypo	Equal and excess	Slow
Hypokinetic	Consonant imprecision; vowel reduction	Hypo	Hypo	Monotone	Slow or fast
Hyperkinetic (chorea)	Irregular articulatory breakdown	Hyper-Hypo	Hyper-Hypo	Prosodic excess	Slow, irregular changes
Hyperkinetic (dystonia)	Irregular articulatory breakdown	Hyper-Hypo	Hyper-Hypo	Prosodic excess	Slow

Source: Adapted from Duffy, 1995; Kent, Kent, Weismer, & Duffy, 2000.

in particular, in matters of intelligibility in dysarthric speech. It is key that different patterns of dysarthria may have different effects on the way listeners are able to apply their speech perception strategies. This has significant implications for the development of interventions (see Table 7-6).

In summary, we make the assumption here that the process of lexical segmentation is mediated by a flexible, context-sensitive perceptual mechanism. Listeners will default to a lexically driven segmentation strategy as long as there is sufficient quality of the acoustic signal and a rich interpretive context. Higher cost approaches using sublexically driven segmentation strategies will be invoked when the acoustic signal is highly degraded and/or when contextual information is ambiguous. It is especially critical to recognize the contributions of different patterns and severities of dysarthria. Listeners may attempt to use syllabic strength contrasts in lexical segmentation decisions in connected dysarthric speech; however, the severity of the speech deficit and the nature of the prosodic degradation determines, in part, the success of the strategy.

Applying Our Knowledge of Speech Perception to Intervention in Motor Speech Disorders

From the preceding discussion, we can conclude that the deficits associated with dysarthric speech interfere with the fundamental processes involved in speech perception. Specifically, the abnormal speech patterns interfere with:

- activation of an optimal lexical candidate pool;
- efficient and effective competition among lexical candidates;
- and efficient and effective application of lexically and sublexically driven processes to lexically segment connected speech.

The interference with these fundamental processes is directly responsible for the compromised intelligibility and the excessive expenditure of cognitive-perceptual resources by the listener. This view represents a substantial paradigm shift from the more traditional segmental approach taken to "fix" production in speakers with dysarthria. By conceptualizing the effects of motor speech disorders in this way—that is, from the perspective of speech perception processes—we have a novel way of structuring and modifying our existing interventions, and providing motivation for new ones.

Three Concepts of Remediation

Let us begin by proposing three converging limbs of remediation, based on our knowledge of speech perception and the ways in which motor speech disorders affect speech perception strategies (see Table 7-6). The first two limbs incorporate existing intervention strategies, and the third suggests a novel one. First, we can intervene to enhance the quality of the speech signal to promote the effective and efficient application of the perceptual processes of lexical activation, lexical competition, and lexical segmentation. Second, we can delimit the lexical candidate pool for the listener by providing, in some way,

Table 7–6. Behavioral Remediation Strategies and Their Possible Effects on Perceptual Processing Strategies

Strategy	Possible Positive Effects	Possible Negative Effects
Rate control: slowing speech	If slowing speech promotes segmental quality, we can anticipate reductions in phonemic uncertainty. This would facilitate lexically driven segmentation strategies in connected speech; facilitate lexical activation of the appropriate target and optimal cohort; and facilitate lexical competition by reducing cohort size for consideration.	If listeners employ a strategy of delayed commitment until an entire utterance has been spoken, slow speech may tax short-term memory. Slowing may reduce natural strong-weak syllabic timing, which may hinder application of the MSS.
Rate control: pacing and pause insertion	Pauses after each word may facilitate lexical segmentation. Rate reductions may provide more time for lexical competition to commence.	Abnormal groupings of words (reductions in "speech naturalness") may impede the effective use of syntactic predictions in lexical access and lexical segmentation. Slow rate may tax memory load.
Increasing loudness	Loudness increase has been shown not only to affect speech audibility, but is associated also with speech rate reduction, improvements in articulation, and increases in prosodic variation. The global effects may facilitate lexically driven segmentation strategies in connected speech.	If excessive slowing results, slow speech may tax short-term memory. Increased vocal loudness may obscure strong-weak syllabic contrastivity, which may hinder application of the MSS.
Increasing prosodic variation	The use of breath groups and in contrast stressing content words through pitch and loudness may facilitate processing by focusing the listener's attention and augmenting predictions.	If the strategies are not applied in a way that approximates an appropriate range of prosodic variation, speech naturalness may suffer.
Providing topic cues, enhancing semantic and syntactic predictability; the use of alphabet and gesture cues	By constraining the size and content of the activated cohort, there is a greater opportunity for selecting the target during competition phase, and for minimizing excessive processing resources that would be incurred with larger than necessary lexical cohorts. Lexically driven segmentation strategies also are facilitated.	Some cueing strategies may tax working memory, particularly in older adults or those with impaired capacity.

Table 7–6. *continued*

Strategy	Possible Positive Effects	Possible Negative Effects
Perceptual learning training	Training facilitates the ability of the listener to map the acoustic information in the signal onto their existing mental phonologic representations. This may allow the listener to apply their perceptual strategies more effectively and efficiently because their mental representations of the speech are tuned to, or compatible with, the acoustic input.	There are no obvious negative side effects to training. Limitations may include the inability of training to extend to new but similar speakers, and the fact that only trained listeners enjoy the benefits of improved understanding of the person's speech.

semantic, syntactic, topic, or other contextual clues. By constraining the size and content of the activated cohort, there is a greater opportunity for selecting the target during competition phase, and for minimizing excessive processing resources that would be incurred with larger than necessary lexical cohorts. Lexically driven segmentation strategies also are facilitated this way. Finally, it is the case that intelligibility of dysarthric speech is reduced but listeners are flexible and over short periods of time can learn to utilize the available acoustic information in a way that improves word recognition. It is possible to train the listeners to become better processors of the degraded speech through a mechanism of *perceptual learning*. Through systematic exposure and training, speaker-specific and/or dysarthria-specific speech properties are learned and internal phonologic maps and phonemic representations can be altered to accommodate their patterns of speech. This perceptual training facilitates efficient lexical activation and competition by reducing phonemic uncertainty; facilitates lexically driven segmentation strategies; and may provide for a more efficient use of segmental

and suprasegmental information in sublexically driven segmentation. Each of these remediation limbs is addressed in turn.

Modification of the Speech Signal

Without question, the vast majority of treatment in motor speech disorders is behavioral in nature. We teach the speaker with dysarthria to talk differently—slower, louder, or clearer—in ways that presumably affect intelligibility or speech quality. This certainly makes intuitive sense, but these presumptions, by and large, have not been evaluated in any systematic way from the standpoint of listener needs. Even when behavioral treatments are shown to improve intelligibility, we still do not know *why* those perceptual benefits are accrued.

Selecting a Target for Remediation

With a speech perception-based intervention structure, speech signal modifications should be undertaken with specific goals in mind, namely to facilitate the processes of lexical access, lexical competition, and/ or lexical segmentation. Optimally, it would be possible to choose speech remediation targets based on their well-documented effects on perceptual processes, but until research has provided such evidence we still can use listener needs as a guidepost for our interventions. We simply need to ask: *What changes to the speech signal will have the most beneficial impact on the listener's ability to effectively apply their perceptual strategies?*

The answer to this question is a fairly straightforward one when it comes to isolated spoken word recognition, because of the close correspondence between the acoustic signal and the listener's decisions. Explanation-based single-word tests such at that of Kent et al. (1989) provide precisely the type of information necessary to select a target for remediation that will facilitate the processes of lexical activation and competition in single-word recognition. Unfortunately, there is little reason to expect that the remediation of speech errors identified in single-word intelligibility tests will offer the same degree of benefit to the processing of connected speech. Because of listeners' lexical bias and their routine application of higher level knowledge sources, certain segmental errors may be of little consequence in the perception of connected speech, even when the errors are damaging to isolated spoken word recognition. For example, recall our production of *dip* with the devoiced /d/ as uttered by a speaker with dysarthria. If the word is produced in isolation, with no additional contextual cues, the listener may very well mistakenly recognize the word as *tip*. However, if the word is produced in a sentence, such as, "*The dip*

was made with sour cream," the segmental error probably will not even be noticed. Thus, the effect of segmental errors on the recognition of words in connected speech is less straightforward than their effects on isolated spoken word recognition because of the contributions of higher level knowledge to perception.

Furthermore, the mere presence of speech errors and aberrant acoustic features in dysarthric speech does not mean they are the cause of the intelligibility decrements. This is exemplified in a study by Weismer, Jeng, Laures, Kent, and Kent (2001). They examined an explanation for intelligibility deficits in sentential speech by evaluating speaking rate, vowel space, and second formant slope measures in speakers with ALS and PD. Although significant correlations were found between many of their acoustic measures and speech intelligibility, they concluded that these measures might be better conceptualized as an index of severity rather than component features of the intelligibility deficit. That is to say, it may not be the reduced vowel space, per se, that causes reduced intelligibility, but that both the reductions in vowel space and intelligibility reflect the level of speech impairment severity. This is an important distinction because it suggests that treatment aimed at modifying vowel working space, for example, may not result in commensurate improvements in intelligibility.

This brings us back to our original question: *What changes to the speech signal will have the most beneficial impact on the listener's ability to effectively apply his or her perceptual strategies?* When it comes to connected speech, it may be misguided to focus on segmental quality (articulatory integrity) in lieu of utterance or phrase level quality because of the way listeners process connected speech. This observation actually squares well with the majority of behavioral treatments commonly applied in clinical practice. Global modifications of speaking rate, vocal loudness, and prosodic variation have the benefit of promoting segmental quality while offering other processing benefits to listeners. We now consider, from the perspective of speech perception strategies, the common remediation targets of speaking rate, vocal loudness, and speech prosody.

Reducing Speaking Rate

A common practice for improving the intelligibility of dysarthric speech is to slow down, by increasing articulation time and/or pause time (see Yorkston, Beukelman, Strand, & Bell, 1999 for an excellent description of rate control techniques and their application in various forms of dysarthria). Patients are either taught to slow their speech volitionally, or they are provided with external cues such as pacing boards to attain slower speech. The benefits of slowing are presumed to be twofold. First, even though much dysarthric speech tends already to be slow, additional slowing may promote articulatory accuracy by allowing more time for articulators to reach their targets. The evidence for this claim is not abundant (see, for example, Tjaden, Rivera, Wilding, & Turner, 2005; Turner, Tjaden, & Weismer, 1995). However, if articulation is improved, it may account for a portion of the intelligibility gain offered by slowed speech, where phoneme identification is enhanced because of a closer correspondence between the acoustic signal and the listener's mental phonemic templates. Second, overall slowing of speaking rate is

thought to give the listener more time to process the acoustic information. As we described earlier, sublexically driven segmentation strategies are higher cost with regard to their loads on short-term memory and processing resources than are lexically driven ones. It would make sense that a slower rate of speech might benefit the application of lexical segmentation strategies, at least at the phrase or short sentence level, as long as the slowing did not reduce or eliminate the natural alternation of strong-weak (long-short) syllables in speech rhythm. Longer utterances spoken slowly actually may be more difficult to process because of the excessive amount of information that must be retained and manipulated in working memory while the listener tests out predictions of lexical boundary locations. Though this is only a hypothesis, it is a testable one that could be addressed by an investigation of the tradeoff between slowed speaking rate benefits and working memory load in the perception of dysarthric speech.

Because volitional slowing is difficult to achieve and maintain, external cuing devices frequently are necessary. Pacing boards are one form of a rigid rate control device, where speakers produce one word with each finger tap on the board. This technique effectively eliminates the lexical segmentation problem because physical pauses are inserted between all words. The listener's task, then, is to use higher level knowledge sources to facilitate lexical activation and competition for each word in the utterance. Although rigid techniques have been reported to be highly effective at increasing intelligibility in many cases, they are usually regarded as a last resort in the clinical armamentarium because they disrupt speech naturalness. According to

Yorkston and her colleagues, *"By encouraging a one-word-at-a-time style with pauses between each word, they disrupt the breath group units that are important in normal speech prosody. Rigid rate control techniques also may be perceived as being unnatural because they encourage a disproportionate amount of pause time"* (Yorkston et al., 1999, p. 422). Such an observation is highly consistent with consideration of the perceptual needs of the listener. Even though intelligibility gains can be made with rigid rate control techniques, they affect perceptual processing strategies in a way that is both noticeable and objectionable to the listener. For this reason, rate control techniques that preserve prosody may be preferred.

Speaking Louder

Significant gains in speech intelligibility have been reported in many studies evaluating the systematic increase in speaking intensity and effort by way of the Lee Silverman Voice Treatment approach (LSVT; see Fox, Morrison, Ramig, & Sapir, 2002, for a review of this literature). The goal of LSVT is to up-regulate the habitual loudness of speech produced by people with dysarthria through a series of maximum effort therapy sessions. In addition to the obvious audibility benefits incurred by such treatment, speaking loudly has been shown to produce global effects in both segmental and suprasegmental features of speech. By increasing vocal loudness and effort, it has been reported that speaking rate slows, articulatory integrity improves, and utterance-level prosodic variation is enhanced. From the standpoint of speech perception, all these things should directly facilitate lexical activation, lexical competition, and lexical segmentation. It can be further hypothesized that speech modified by LSVT facilitates lexically driven speech segmentation strategies.

Prosody

Nearly all dysarthric speech is associated with some degree of prosodic defect in stress patterning, intonation contours, and/or speech rate and rhythm (see Table 7–5). Interestingly, only recently has prosody become regarded as a first-line target for speech remediation. Historically, and even in some more recent texts, clinicians are encouraged to consider prosody as the "icing on the cake" that should be addressed after other production parameters have been repaired (e.g., Dworkin, 1991). In contrast, Yorkston and her colleagues suggest an early attention to prosody, stating that, *"By using prosody to signal important words and syntactic junctions, their listeners are provided important information to decode the speaker's messages . . . prosodic features that signal stress patterns and syntactic boundaries may improve intelligibility . . . (and) attention to prosody may improve the naturalness of speech and be important in reducing the handicap"* (Yorkston et al., 1999, p. 461).

Yorkston's rationale for addressing prosody is precisely in line with a speech perception perspective. Suprasegmental information facilitates processing of connected speech in a number of ways: (1) providing syllabic strength cues for explicit metrical segmentation, (2) demarcating syntactic processing units within which listeners can apply their knowledge of rules and regularities of language, and (3) perceptually highlighting content words to facilitate lexically driven segmentation strategies. As such, the speech perception perspective would promote prosody as a first-line target for remediation.

A number of strategies are used clinically to enhance prosody in motor speech disorders. Speakers with dysarthria are instructed on the use of *breath groupings* to consolidate phrases into temporal units. This technique is often employed when speakers habitually produce one or two words per breath. Although listeners may benefit in terms of lexical segmentation from the abnormal pattern (e.g., one word per breath), there appears to be an additional processing load that affects intelligibility and message extraction (recall the downside of rigid rate control techniques). Another remediation strategy for prosody involves *contrastively stressing* words within an utterance. Speakers are instructed to emphasize a content word by making it louder and higher in pitch than the words around it. Although difficult to generalize to spontaneous speech, this strategy gives perceptual prominence to the content word, facilitating lexical segmentation and lexical access.

To date, syllabic strength contrastivity has not been the target of remediation, per se. However, the results of the work on lexical boundary errors in the perception of dysarthric speech, and the apparent dysarthria-specific nature of these problems, suggest that such a remediation target may be warranted (Liss et al., 1998, 2000, 2002). The goal of this intervention would be to modify the speech signal in ways that would facilitate the listener's ability to use syllabic strength to lexically segment the dysarthric speech. Global approaches of rate reduction or increasing speech loudness may well have the desired effect, particularly if they enhance syllabic strength contrastivity cues such as strong vowel formant patterns, fundamental frequency variation, and syllabic duration contrasts. Of course, it is conceivable that global approaches may, under some circumstances, serve to reduce the contrast between strong and weak syllables, thereby undermining the goal of that intervention. Speech targets for syllabic contrastivity will become more specific as we learn about the ways in which dysarthria form and severity influence lexical segmentation.

Activation of Optimal Lexical Candidate Pool

The second limb of remediation includes strategies to promote the activation of an optimal lexical candidate pool, which would be effective either in single word or connected speech perception in motor speech disorders. The goal of this approach is to delimit lexical activation in ways that will reduce the resource cost of the lexical competition phase. Recalling the model of Mattys et al. (2005), a high-quality interpretive context (rich contextual information) can promote successful lexical segmentation in the face of a degraded acoustic signal (see also Lindblom, 1990). Simply stated, the more listeners know about the topic and content of the message, the better they can predict and anticipate the lexical items that comprise the message (i.e., contextual priming).

Interestingly, the idea of promoting intelligibility and communicative effectiveness by providing the listener with information to enhance perceptual processing has appeared primarily in one domain of speech-language pathology: augmentative and alternative communication. This makes sense because AAC devices usually are reserved for people who have severe production impairments and who are very difficult to understand. These people have little chance of significantly changing the quality of their speech output by behavioral means. By manipulating signal-independent information (see Lindblom, 1990) such as semantic and syntactic content of the message or alphabet and gesture cues, listener processing benefits can be incurred with minimal additional effort on the part of the speaker. Benefits to intelligibility can be immediate and significant.

One of the most comprehensive accounts of such an approach is provided by Katherine Hustad, contributing author to this book and a former student of Ray Kent (her chapter, Optimizing Communicative Effectiveness, appears in Yorkston et al., 1999). In this chapter, specific suggestions are made for conveying information to the listener about the message topic and the identity of the words in the message, much of it based on the results of prior research (see Table 12-2 in Yorkston et al., 1999). Examples of these techniques include:

- providing the topic, context, or semantic cues
- providing a syntactic template or structure
- creating semantically and syntactically predictable utterances
- using supplementary cues such as first-letter, word-class cues, or gestures.

All these techniques serve a similar function: By constraining the size and content of the activated cohort, there is a greater opportunity for selecting the target during competition phase, and for minimizing excessive processing resources that would be incurred with larger than necessary lexical cohorts. Lexically driven segmentation strategies also are facilitated.

Although none of these techniques has been evaluated specifically with regard to their effects on perceptual processing, this promises to be a fruitful domain of inquiry.

Data from such investigations would serve to refine strategies and determine their most efficient application. Already there is evidence that certain listener characteristics may affect the utility of signal-independent cues. For example, a number of studies have shown that listener age may be a consideration (e.g., Drager & Reichle, 2001; Garcia & Hayden, 1999; Gordon-Salant & Fitzgibbons, 1997; Jones, Mathy, Azuma, & Liss, 2004). This might be expected because attention and working memory are detrimentally affected by normal aging (Campbell & Charness, 1990; Kirasic, Allen, Dobson, & Binder, 1996), and these cognitive resources are necessary for the efficient and effective application of signal-independent information. Other studies have suggested that different disability patterns associated with dysarthria also affect the utility of signal-independent cue strategies (Garcia & Dagenais, 1998). Finally, there is growing evidence that different types of cues provide varying levels of benefit. For example, Hustad, Auker, Natale, and Carlson (2003) showed variable benefits of using a topic cue (speaker points to topic on a communication board before speaking), or an alphabet cue (speaker points to a letter on an alphabet board before speaking) to enhance intelligibility in the dysarthria of ALS. However, the greatest intelligibility benefits were accrued when the topic and alphabet cues were combined, such that the combined cues resulted in a 40% improvement in intelligibility over the no-cue condition.

In summary, it can be hypothesized that this limb of remediation directly influences the efficiency and effectiveness with which listeners apply their typical speech perception strategies. Much remains to be learned about speaker and listener characteristics that affect cue administration and use. Also, much remains to be discovered about the specific benefits of various sources of signal-independent information. Nonetheless, this approach promises to be a powerful tool in the treatment of motor speech disorders.

Perceptual Training

The final limb of remediation has as its treatment target the listener. Numerous studies have shown that perceptual training with a degraded speech signal can facilitate the subsequent processing of that signal. This has been shown with electronically time-compressed speech (e.g., Dupoux & Green, 1997; Sebástián-Gallés, Dupoux, Costa, & Mehler, 2000); synthetic speech (e.g., Greenspan, Nusbaum, & Pisoni, 1988; Reynolds, Isaacs-Duvall, & Haddox, 2002); and non-native language speech (e.g., Clarke & Garrett, 2004). The variables of listener experience and familiarity with a specific speaker or type of speaker have been addressed in motor speech disorders (see, for example, DePaul & Kent, 2000; Flipsen, 1995) however the perceptual training aspect has received less attention with this population (Liss et al., 2002; Tjaden & Liss, 1995a, 1995b). The precise mechanisms underlying the benefits of this exposure or training are not completely understood, but it is likely that training facilitates the ability of the listener to map the acoustic information in the signal onto their existing mental phonologic representations. In this way, the perceptual training allows the listeners to apply their perceptual strategies more effectively and efficiently because their mental representations of the speech are tuned to, or compatible with, the acoustic input.

We typically do not think of listeners as the focus of treatment, but in many ways this makes excellent sense: The perceptual benefits can be rapid and significant, and the speaker is not required to make any modification whatsoever to his or her speech. This is an important consideration because behavioral modifications require exceptional effort on the part of the speaker, who already is motorically taxed by the disease or illness. And because so many individuals with motor speech disorders suffer impairments that limit their social exposure, training a spouse or caregiver may be sufficient to greatly improve the majority of communicative interactions in the person's life.

As this limb represents a novel remediation strategy, there is no well-supported protocol for its implementation. However, the speech perception literature contains numerous studies that suggest the important characteristics of a training paradigm to achieve the desired outcome. This evidence falls under the categories of (1) training material, (2) feedback type and frequency, and (3) training regimen and intensity.

A recent example of a perceptual training paradigm provides us with some important guidelines for training material, feedback, and regimen. Davis and colleagues compared different types of training material for listeners exposed to vocoded (synthesized) speech designed to emulate speech heard by cochlear implant users (Davis, Johnsrude, Hervais-Adelman, Taylor, & McGettigan, 2005). They discovered that listeners benefitted more from training on real-speech sentences than they did from training on nonsense speech strings (containing no real words), "jabberwocky" speech (in which content words are replaced by nonsense words in the sentence), or syntactic prose (real words presented in a syntactically correct string, but not making semantic sense). It also was found to be essential that listeners be given feedback about the identity of the utterance to gain perceptual training benefits. It was of note that the feedback could be of either spoken (acoustic) form or written form. As long as the listener knew the lexical targets, they were able to extract the salient information from the signal to tune their perceptual systems. Results were interpreted to mean that the adjustment of segmental categorization (phonologic maps, for example) is affected by higher-level, top-down, lexical influences (see also Bowers & Davis, 2004; Kraljic & Samuel, 2005; Norris, McQueen, & Cutler, 2003). Therefore, to make these perceptual adjustments about segmental patterns, the segmental features must be presented as produced in a word. Training effects also occurred relatively quickly, with benefits enjoyed after only about 20 minutes of training, and exposure to 30 to 40 sentence tokens. They also found evidence for generalization to nontrained words, suggesting that this procedure allows listeners to apply their knowledge to novel material. There is some evidence that benefits gained from perceptual training on a single speaker can be successfully applied to a class of speakers with similar speech characteristics (see, however, Eisner & McQueen, 2005).

Taking such results into consideration, a perceptual training protocol designed for use in a clinical setting might be the systematic exposure to real sentential speech produced by a person with dysarthria. The speech sample should contain a reasonable representation of the range of variance typically produced by the speaker. The listener would receive feedback about the speech, minimally in the form of a written transcript. Learning could be tracked by probes presented at intervals in the training processes, whereby listeners would be asked to transcribe novel sentences produced by the speaker. Training could proceed until an asymptote in performance is achieved, and may extend across a single session or multiple sessions as the performance data warrant.

Summary

This chapter has examined the fundamental ways in which the processes of speech perception must be considered in accounts of intelligibility deficits in motor speech disorders, and other speech defects for that matter. Segmental and suprasegmental errors in motor speech disorders provide varying degrees of challenge to the listener's application of their typical perceptual strategies. By understanding the ways in which these challenges occur, it is possible to justify three converging limbs of remediation. These limbs can be conceptualized as three routes to affect that critical interface between the signal characteristics and signal-independent factors, which is the point of intelligibility.

Acknowledgments. This work was supported, in part, by a grant from the National Institutes of Health (NIH NIDCD R01DC006859). Special thanks are extended to Dr. Sven Mattys for his insightful comments on previous versions of this chapter, and for providing the framework and impetus for the ideas expressed herein.

References

Allopena, P. D., Magnuson, J. S., & Tanenhaus, M. K. (1998). Tracking the time course of spoken word recognition using eye movements: Evidence for continuous mapping models. *Journal of Memory and Language, 38*, 419–439.

Andruski, J. E., Blumstein, S. E., & Burton, M. (1994). The effect of subphonetic differences on lexical access. *Cognition, 52*, 163–187.

Bard, E. G., Shillcock, R. C., & Altmann, G. T. M. (1988). The recognition of words after their acoustic offsets in spontaneous speech: Effects of subsequent context. *Perception and Psychophysics, 44*, 395–408.

Bernstein, L. E., & Weismer, G. (2001). Basic science at the intersection of speech science and communication disorders. *Journal of Phonetics, 28*(2), 225–232.

Borsky, S., Shapiro, L. & Tuller, B. (2000) The temporal unfolding of local acoustic information and sentence context. *Journal of Psycholinguistic Research, 29*(2), 155–168.

Bowers, J. S., & Davis, C. J. (2004). Is speech perception modular or interactive? *Trends in Cognitive Sciences, 8*, 3–5.

Bradlow, A. R., Nygaard, L. C., & Pisoni, D. B. (1999). Effects of talker, rate, and amplitude variation on recognition memory for spoken words. *Perception and Psychophysics, 61*, 206–219.

Bradlow, A. R., Torretta, G. M., & Pisoni, D. B. (1996). Intelligibility of normal speech I: Global and fine-grained acoustic-phonetic talker characteristics. *Speech Communication, 20*, 255–272.

Bunton, K., & Weismer, G., (2001) The relationship between perception and acoustics for a high-low vowel contrast produced by speakers with dysarthria. *Journal of Speech, Language, and Hearing Research, 44*, 1215–1228.

Campbell, J. I. D., & Charness, N. (1990). Age related declines in working memory skills: Evidence from a complex calculation task. *Developmental Psychology, 26*(6), 879–888.

Carre, R. & Divenyi, P. L. (2000). Modeling and perception of "gesture reduction." *Phonetica, 57*(2–4), 152–169.

Clarke, C. M., & Garrett, M. F. (2004). Rapid adaptation to foreign-accented English. *Journal of Acoustical Society of America, 116*, 3647–3658.

Cole, R. A., & Jakimik, J. (1978). Understanding speech: how words are heard. In G. Underwood (Ed.), *Strategies of information processing.* London: Academic Press.

Connine, C. M., Blasko, D. G., & Titone, D. (1993). Do the beginnings of spoken words have a special status in auditory word recognition? *Journal of Memory and Language, 32*, 193–210.

Connine, C. M., Titone, D., Deelman, T., & Blasko, D. (1997). Similarity mapping in spoken word recognition. *Journal of Memory and Language, 37*, 463–480.

Cutler, A., & Butterfield, S. (1992). Rhythmic cues to speech segmentation: Evidence from juncture misperception. *Journal of Memory and Language, 31*, 218–236.

Cutler, A., & Carter, D. M . (1987). The predominance of strong initial syllables in the English vocabulary. *Computer Speech and Language, 2*, 133–142.

Cutler, A., & Norris, D. G. (1988). The role of strong syllables in segmentation for lexical access. *Journal of Experimental Psychology: Human Perception and Performance, 14*, 113–121.

Davis, M. H., Johnsrude, I. S., Hervais-Adelman, A., Taylor, K., & McGettigan, C. (2005). Lexical information drives perceptual learning of distorted speech: Evidence from the comprehension of noise-vocoded sentences. *Journal of Experimental Psychology: General, 134*, 222–241.

Davis, M. H., Marslen-Wilson, W. D., & Gaskell, M. G. (2002). Leading up the lexical garden-path: Segmentation and ambiguity in spoken word recognition. *Journal of Experimental Psychology: Human Perception and Performance, 28*, 218–244.

DePaul, R., & Kent, R. D. (2000). A longitudinal case study of ALS: Effects of listener familiarity and proficiency on intelligibility judgments. *American Journal of Speech-Language Pathology, 9*, 230–240.

Drager, K. D. R., & Reichle, J. E. (2001). Effects of discourse context on the intelligibility of synthesized speech for young adult and older adult listeners: applications for AAC. *Journal of Speech, Language, and Hearing Research, 44*, 1052-1057.

Duffy, J. R. (1995). *Motor speech disorders: Substrates, differential diagnosis, and management.* St. Louis, MO: Mosby-Yearbook.

Dupoux, E., & Green, K. (1997). Perceptual adjustment to highly compressed speech: Effects of talker and rate changes. *Journal of Experimental Psychology: Human Perception and Performance, 23*, 914-927.

Dupoux, E., Pallier, C., Kakehi, K., & Mehler, J. (2001) New evidence for prelexical phonological processing in word recognition. *Language and Cognitive Processes, 16*, 491-505.

Dworkin, J. P. (1991). *Motor speech disorders: A treatment guide.* St. Louis, MO: Mosby-Yearbook.

Eisner, F., & McQueen, J. M. (2005). The specificity of perceptual learning in speech processing. *Perception and Psychophysics, 67*, 224-238.

Flipsen, P. (1995). Speaker-listener familiarity: Parents as judges of delayed speech intelligibility. *Journal of Communication Disorders, 28*, 3-19.

Fox, C. M., Morrison, C. E., Ramig, L. O., & Sapir, S. (2002). Current perspectives on the Lee Silverman Voice Treatment (LSVT) for individuals with idiopathic Parkinson disease. *American Journal of Speech-Language Pathology, 11*, 111-123.

Ganong, W. F. (1980) Phonetic categorisation in auditory word perception. *Journal of Experimental Psychology: Human Perception and Performance, 6*, 110-125.

Garcia, J. M., & Dagenais, P. A. (1998). Dysarthric sentence intelligibility: Contribution of iconic gestures and message predictiveness. *Journal of Speech, Language, and Hearing Research, 41*, 1282-1293.

Garcia, J. M., & Hayden, M. (1999). Young and older listener understanding of a person

with severe dysarthria. *Journal of Medical Speech-Language Pathology, 7*, 109-112.

Goldinger, S. D. (1996). Words and voices: Episodic traces in spoken word identification and recognition memory. *Journal of Experimental Psychology: Learning, Memory, and Cognition, 22*, 1166-1183.

Goldinger, S. D., Kleider, H. M., & Shelley, E. (1999) The marriage of perception and memory: creating two-way illusions with words and voices. *Memory and Cognition, 27*(2), 328-338.

Gordon-Salant, S., & Fitzgibbons, P. J. (1997). Selected cognitive factors and speech recognition performance among young and elderly listeners. *Journal of Speech, Language, and Hearing Research, 40*(2), 423-431.

Greenspan, S. L., Nusbaum, H. C., & Pisoni, D. B. (1988). Perceptual learning of synthetic speech produced by rule. *Journal of Experimental Psychology: Learning, Memory, and Cognition, 14*, 421-433.

Grosjean, F. (1980). Spoken word recognition processes and the gating paradigm. *Perception and Psychophysics, 28*, 267-283.

Hustad, K. C., Auker, J., Natale, N., & Carlson, R. (2003). Improving intelligibility of speakers with profound dysarthria and cerebral palsy. *Augmentative and Alternative Communication, 19*, 187-198.

Jones, W., Mathy, P., Azuma, T., & Liss, J. (2004). The effect of aging and synthetic topic cues on the intelligibility of dysarthric speech. *Augmentative and Alternative Communication, 20*, 22-29.

Jusczyk, P., & Luce, P. A. (2002). Speech perception and spoken word recognition: Past and present. *Ear and Hearing, 23*, 1-40.

Kent, R. D., Kent, J. F., Weismer, G., & Duffy, J. R. (2000). What dysarthrias can tell us about the neural control of speech. *Journal of Phonetics, 28*, 273-302.

Kent, R. D., Weismer, G., Kent, J. F., & Rosenbek, J. C. (1989). Toward phonetic intelligibility testing in dysarthria. *Journal of Speech and Hearing Disorders, 54*, 482-489.

Kirasic, K. C., Allen, G. L., Dobson, S. H., & Binder, K. S. (1996). Aging, cognitive resources, and declarative learning. *Psychology and Aging, 11*, 658-670.

Kirk, C. (2000). Syllabic cues to word segmentation. In A. Cutler, J. M. McQueen, & R. Zondervan (Eds.), *Spoken word access processes* (pp. 131-134). Nijmegen, The Netherlands: Max-Planck Institute for Psycholinguistics.

Kraljic, T., & Samuel, A. G. (2005). Perceptual learning for speech: Is there a return to normal? *Cognitive Psychology, 51*(2), 141-178.

Ladefoged, P., & Broadbent, D. E. (1957). Information conveyed by vowels. *Journal of the Acoustical Society of America, 29*(1), 98-104.

Laures, J. S., & Bunton, K. (2003). Perceptual effects of a flattened fundamental frequency at the sentence level under different listening conditions. *Journal of Communication Disorders, 36*, 449-464.

Lehiste, I. (1977). Isochrony reconsidered. *Journal of Phonetics, 5*, 253-63.

Liberman, A. M., Cooper, F. S., Shankweiler, D. P., & Studdert-Kennedy, M. (1967). Perception of the speech code. *Psychological Review, 74*, 431-461.

Lindblom, B. (1990). Explaining phonetic variation: A sketch of the H and H theory. In W. Hardcastle & A. Marchal (Eds.), *Speech production and speech modeling,* (pp. 403-439). Dordrecht, The Netherlands: Kluwer Academic Publishers.

Liss, J. M., Spitzer, S. M., Caviness, J. N., & Adler, C. (2002). The effects of familiarization on intelligibility and lexical segmentation in hypokinetic and ataxic dysarthria. *Journal of the Acoustical Society of America, 112*, 3022-3030.

Liss, J. M., Spitzer, S., Caviness, J. N., Adler, C., & Edwards, B. (1998). Syllabic strength and lexical boundary decisions in the perception of hypokinetic dysarthric speech. *Journal of the Acoustical Society of America, 104*, 2457-2466.

Liss, J. M., Spitzer, S. M., Caviness, J. N., Adler, C., & Edwards, B. W. (2000). Lexical boundary error analysis in hypokinetic and ataxic dysarthria. *Journal of the Acoustical Society of America, 107*, 3415-3424.

Liu, H. M., Tsao, F. M., & Kuhl, P. K. (2005). The effect of reduced vowel working space on speech intelligibility in Mandarin-speaking young adults with cerebral palsy. *Journal of the Acoustical Society of America, 117*(6), 3879-3889.

Luce, P. A. (1986). *Neighborhoods of words in the mental lexicon.* Unpublished doctoral dissertation, Indiana University, Bloomington.

Luce, P. A., Goldinger, S. D., Auer, E. T., & Vitevitch, M. S. (2000). Phonetic priming, neighborhood activation, and PARSYN. *Perception and Psychophysics, 62*, 615-625.

Luce, P. A., & Large, N. R. (2001). Phonotactics, density, and entropy in spoken word recognition. *Language and Cognitive Processes, 16*, 565-581.

Luce, P. A. & Pisoni, D. B. (1998). Recognizing spoken words: The neighborhood activation model. *Ear and Hearing, 19*, 1-36.

Marslen-Wilson, W. D. (1987). Functional parallelism in spoken word-recognition. *Cognition, 25*, 71-102.

Marslen-Wilson, W. D., & Welsh, A. (1978). Processing interactions and lexical access during word recognition in continuous speech. *Cognitive Psychology, 10*, 29-63.

Mattys, S. L. (1997). The use of time during lexical processing and segmentation: A review. *Psychonomic Bulletin and Review, 4*, 310-329.

Mattys, S. L. (2004). Stress versus coarticulation: towards an integrated approach to explicit speech segmentation. *Journal of Experimental Psychology: Human Perception and Performance, 30*, 397-408.

Mattys, S. L., Pleydell-Pearce, C. W., Melhorn, J. F., & Whitecross, S. E. (2005). Detecting silent pauses in speech: A new tool for measuring on-line lexical and semantic processing. *Psychological Science, 16*(12), 958-964.

Mattys, S. L, White, L., & Melhorn, J. F. (2005). Integration of multiple speech segmentation cues: A hierarchical framework. *Journal of Experimental Psychology: General, 134*(4), 477-500.

McClelland, J. L., & Elman, J. L. (1986). The TRACE model of speech perception. *Cognitive Psychology, 18*, 1-86.

McQueen, J. M. (1998). Segmentation of continuous speech using phonotactics. *Journal of Memory and Language, 39*, 21-46.

McQueen, J. M., & Cutler, A. (2001). Spoken word access processes: An introduction. *Language and Cognitive Processes, 16*, 469-490.

McQueen, J. M., Cutler, A., Briscoe, T., & Norris, D. (1995). Models of continuous speech recognition and the contents of the vocabulary. *Language and Cognitive Processes, 10*(3), 309-331.

Miller, J. L. (1987). Rate-dependent processing in speech perception. In A. Ellis (Ed.), *Progress in the psychology of language* (pp. 119-157). Hillsdale, NJ: Lawrence Erlbaum.

Miller, J. L., & Liberman, A. M. (1979). Some effects of later-occurring information on the perception of stop consonant and semivowel. *Perception and Psychophysics, 25*(6), 457-465.

Morton, J. (1969). Interaction of information in word recognition. *Psychological Review, 76*, 165-178.

Nakatani, L. H., & Dukes, K. D. (1977). Locus of segmental cues for word juncture. *Journal of the Acoustical Society of America, 62*(3), 714-719.

Norris, D. (1994). Shortlist: A connectionist model of continuous speech recognition. *Cognition, 52*, 189-234.

Norris, D., McQueen J. M., & Cutler, A. (2003). Perceptual learning in speech. *Cognitive Psychology, 47*, 204-238.

Norris, D., McQueen, J. M., Cutler, A., Butterfield, S., & Kearns, R. (2001). Language universal constraints on speech segmentation. *Language and Cognitive Processes, 16*, 637-660.

Nooteboom, S. G. (1981). Lexical retrieval from fragments of spoken words: Beginnings vs. endings. *Journal of Phonetics, 9*, 407-424.

Pisoni, D. B. (1993). Long-term memory in speech perception: Some new findings on talker variability, speaking rate, and perceptual learning. *Speech Communication, 13*, 109-125.

Repp B. H. (1982). Phonetic trading relations and context effects: New experimental evidence for a speech mode of perception. *Psychological Bulletin, 92*(1), 81-110.

Reynolds, M., Isaacs-Duvall, C. & Haddox, M. (2002). A comparison of learning curves in natural and synthesized speech comprehension. *Journal of Speech, Language and Hearing Research, 45*, 802-810.

Samuel, A. G. (1981). Phonemic restoration: Insights from a new methodology. *Journal of Experimental Psychology: General, 110*, 474-494.

Samuel, A. G. (1997). Lexical activation produces potent phonemic percepts. *Cognitive Psychology, 32*, 97-127.

Samuel, A. G., & Pitt, M. A. (2003). Lexical activation (and other factors) can mediate compensation for coarticulation. *Journal of Memory and Language, 48*, 416-434.

Sebástián-Gallés N, Dupoux E, Costa A, & Mehler J. (2000). Adaptation to time-compressed speech: Phonological determinants. *Perceptual Psychophysiology, 62*, 834-842.

Tjaden, K. K., & Liss, J. M. (1995a). The role of listener familiarity in the perception of dysarthric speech. *Clinical Linguistics and Phonetics, 9*, 139-154.

Tjaden, K. K., & Liss, J. M. (1995b). The influence of familiarity on judgments of treated speech. *American Journal of Speech-Language Pathology, 4*(1), 39-47.

Tjaden, K., Rivera, D., Wilding, G., & Turner, G. S. (2005). Characteristics of the lax vowel space in dysarthria. *Journal of Speech, Language, and Hearing Research, 48*(3), 554-566.

Turner, G. S., Tjaden, K., & Weismer, G. (1995). The influence of speaking rate on vowel space and speech intelligibility for individuals with amyotrophic lateral sclerosis. *Journal of Speech and Hearing Research, 38*, 1001-1013

Vitevitch, M. S., & Luce, P. A. (1999). Probabilistic phonotactics and neighborhood activation in spoken word recognition. *Journal of Memory and Language, 40,* 374-408.

Warren, R. M. (1970). Perceptual restoration of missing speech sounds. *Science, 167,* 392-393.

Warren, R.M. & Warren, R.P. (1970). Auditory illusions and confusions. *Scientific American, 223,* 30-36.

Warren, P., & Marslen-Wilson, W. D. (1987). Continuous uptake of acoustic cues in spoken word-recognition. *Perception and Psychophysics, 41,* 262-275.

Warren, P., & Marslen-Wilson, W. D. (1988). Cues to lexical choice: Discriminating place and voice. *Perception and Psychophysics, 43,* 21-30.

Weber, A. (2000). Phonotactic and acoustic cues for word segmentation in English. In B. Yuan, T. Huang, & X. Tang (Eds.), *Proceedings of the 6th International Conference on Spoken Language Processing* (Vol. 3, pp. 782-785). Beijing.

Weismer, G., Jeng, J-Y, Laures, J., Kent, R. D., & Kent, J. F. (2001). Acoustic and intelligibility characteristics of sentence production in neurogenic speech disorders. *Folia Phoniatrica et Logopaedica, 53,* 1-18.

Weismer, G., & Martin, R. (1992). Acoustic and perceptual approaches to the study of intelligibility. In R. D. Kent (Ed.), *Intelligibility in speech disorders: Theory measurement and management* (pp. 67-118). Amsterdam: John Benjamin.

Wurm, L. H., Vakoch, D. A., & Seaman, S. R. (2004). Recognition of spoken words: Semantic effects in lexical access. *Language and Speech, 47,* 175-204.

Yorkston, K. M., Beukelman, D. R., Strand, E. A., & Bell, K. R. (1999). *Management of motor speech disorders in children and adults.* Austin, TX: Pro-Ed.

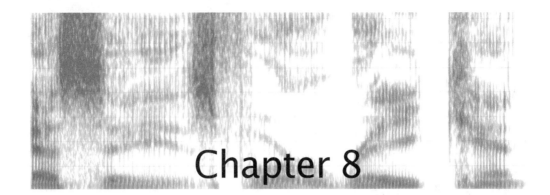

Chapter 8

DYSPHAGIA IN PATIENTS WITH MOTOR SPEECH DISORDERS

John C. Rosenbek and Harrison N. Jones

Readers may be surprised to find a chapter on swallowing tucked in behind seven chapters on speech in a book on motor speech disorders. However, Ray Kent's lifetime of contributions to speech-language pathology includes seminal publications on swallowing. With a colleague, he wrote two papers on normal swallowing in the 1980s (Kennedy & Kent, 1985, 1988). Those two papers and subsequent publications (Tasko, Kent, & Westbury, 2002) helped to establish Kent's influence in swallowing, just as dozens of papers referenced elsewhere in this volume have established his primacy in motor speech disorders (among dozens of topics). This chapter's inclusion is also appropriate for clinical and research reasons. Speech and swallowing are both highly complex sensorimotor functions. The classical speech subsystems of the respiratory structures, larynx, velopharynx, and orofacial mechanism also comprise the critical components of the oropharyngeal swallowing mechanism, although their interactions differ during performance of these two activities.

In addition, normal speech and swallowing depend upon nervous system integrity from the cortex to the peripheral nerves responsible for innervating these structures and the contributions of these areas may be similar for the sensorimotor activities of speech and swallowing. One suspects, however, that the neural networks underlying speech and swallowing may differ in important ways. As a result, patients with motor speech disorders often, but not inevitably, present with coexisting swallowing difficulties, called *dysphagia*. Consequently, speech-language pathologists who evaluate and treat motor speech disorders must also be prepared to provide comprehensive dysphagia services. It can even be argued that narrow specialization in one or the other can reduce one's clinical effectiveness, although specialization is the norm in research.

The main purpose of this chapter is to provide an overview of swallowing disorders in patients with motor speech disorders. More specifically, this chapter provides the reader with the following:

(1) definitions of normal and abnormal swallowing, (2) an overview of swallowing anatomy and physiology, (3) a discussion of the neural control of swallowing, (4) a review of techniques to evaluate swallowing function, (5) a survey of the signs of dysphagia, (6) classification and pathophysiology of dysphagia, (7) descriptions of the swallowing abnormalities in a variety of neurologic disorders associated with motor speech disorders, (8) concepts and methods in treatment, and (9) future directions.

Definitions of Normal and Abnormal Swallowing

Normal swallowing is defined as the efficient and safe transfer of liquid, including saliva, and food from the mouth into the stomach. Swallowing begins in utero and continues throughout a person's lifetime unless damage or disruption occurs to the responsible structures and nervous system components. The historical reference to the swallow as a reflex has been replaced by the notion that the swallow is a highly patterned response capable of variable degrees of volitional control. The structures and nervous system components critical to this patterned response are described in a subsequent section. Abnormal swallowing or *dysphagia* is defined as inefficient or unsafe transfer of material from the mouth to the stomach. It is traditional to divide dysphagia into three types—oral, pharyngeal, and esophageal. The oral and pharyngeal stages are intricately related and, therefore, oropharyngeal swallow function is often assessed and treated in an integrative manner. *Oropharyngeal dysphagia*, this chapter's emphasis, is defined as inefficient or unsafe transfer of material

from the mouth through the pharynx and into the upper portion of the esophagus. *Esophageal dysphagia* is inefficient or absent movement of material through the esophagus and into the stomach. Esophageal dysphagia remains the nearly exclusive providence of physicians, particularly gastroenterologists. Oropharyngeal dysphagia, on the other hand, is within the scope of practice of the speech-language pathologist (SLP), usually as part of an interdisciplinary team composed of physicians, surgeons, occupational therapists, dieticians, nurses, dentists, and other health care professionals. Managing that shared responsibility requires the SLP to understand the anatomy and physiology of normal swallowing.

Normal Swallowing Anatomy and Physiology

Swallowing is traditionally divided into three stages: oral, pharyngeal, and esophageal. Activities of the three stages can overlap, especially if one or more of the stages are abnormal, as can happen in neurologic disease. For example, if a patient has difficulty moving food and drink through the mouth in a coordinated and timely fashion, this may negatively influence pharyngeal stage function. Indeed, it has been argued that the oral and pharyngeal stages are so intricately related that separating them into two stages is artificial (Martin-Harris, Michel, & Castell, 2005). Nonetheless, it simplifies learning swallowing anatomy and physiology to divide the interactive act of swallowing into phases and that division is preserved in this chapter. Color Plate 1 details the structures involved in oropharyngeal swallowing discussed in the following sec-

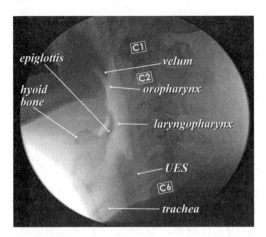

Figure 8–1. Lateral x-ray image of pharyngeal and laryngeal structures involved in swallowing.

tions. Figure 8–1 is a close-up from a lateral x-ray image of pharyngeal and laryngeal structures.

Oral Stage

The oral stage of swallowing, which Kennedy and Kent (1988) call the horizontal system, has a primary function of transporting foods and liquids to the pharynx for ingestion. The oral stage is primarily under volitional control and its activities are more variable than pharyngeal stage activities (Kennedy & Kent, 1985) due to bolus factors such as temperature, texture, and taste, and personal factors such as hunger and level of consciousness (Erktekin & Aydogdu, 2003). Kent and colleagues (Tasko, Kent, & Westbury, 2002) have highlighted the large variability of oral stage function, especially tongue and jaw movements, among normal swallowers, leading them to conclude that it is "surprisingly difficult to provide a . . . quantitative description of the tongue kinematics during liquid swallowing" (p. 137). Nonethe-

less, it is safe to say that multiple structures and muscles are involved with oral stage function. The jaw-closing muscles of the mandible assist in jaw stabilization and mastication. The suprahyoid and infrahyoid muscles, which connect the hyoid bone in the neck to the jaw above and the larynx below, reposition the hyoid and larynx superiorly. The intrinsic and extrinsic muscles of the tongue move the bolus and propel it posteriorly. The lip and cheek muscles provide the anterior seal often required during the oral stage (Miller, 1999). Miller (1999) describes oral stage function:

> Early in swallowing, the lips are sealed and the tongue . . . is positioned so that its anterior tip makes contact with the hard palate. This seals the oral cavity anteriorly. The hyoid bone raises during this time. Next, the intrinsic muscles of the tongue . . . propel the bolus into and through the pharynx (p. 8).

Omitted from this description is the velum, which elevates to close off the mouth from the nose so that material does not pass into the nose during swallowing. The velum rises to perform this protective function early in the swallow sequence.

Pharyngeal Stage

The oral stage ends and the pharyngeal phase begins with the initiation of the pharyngeal swallow. The posterior thrust of the tongue heralds initiation of the pharyngeal phase (Miller, 1999). This thrust is the main propulsive force acting on the bolus as it enters the pharynx and esophagus (Erktekin & Aydogdu, 2003). Respiration and swallowing must be coordinated during the pharyngeal stage and an apneic period during which breathing is suspended and the larynx is closed by approximating the vocal folds occurs for airway protection (Martin-Harris, Brodsky, Michel, Ford, Walters, & Heffner, 2005; Martin-Harris, Brodsky, Price, Michel, & Walters, 2003). Laryngeal elevation occurs through the activity of suprahyoid and submental muscles to facilitate closing of the laryngeal vestibule and repositioning of the larynx anterosuperiorly under the base of tongue. This action also helps open the upper esophageal sphincter (UES), which is here assumed to be part of the pharyngeal stage. This mechanical action on the UES is facilitated by UES relaxation. Progressive top to bottom contraction of the pharyngeal constrictors occurs to shorten the pharynx and clear remaining material into the esophagus (Erktekin & Aydogdu, 2003). When all these actions occur with the proper timing and force, even large boluses can pass through the pharynx and into the esophagus quickly and safely. Variability is present in the pharyngeal stage, but not to the same degree as in the oral stage.

Esophageal Stage

The esophageal stage transports foods and liquids through the UES toward the lower esophageal sphincter (LES) and into the stomach. The esophageal stage begins with entry of the bolus into the upper esophagus. The major muscular component of the UES, the cricopharyngeus, remains actively contracted, except during activities such as swallowing, belching, and vomiting, in order to control the flow of contents between the esophagus and upper airway (Miller, 1999). A peristaltic wave propels the bolus caudally toward the LES, which relaxes to allow

entry of foods and liquids into the stomach (Logemann, 1998; Miller, 1999). The greatest automaticity of control occurs in the esophageal phase.

Neural Control of Swallowing

Swallowing's complexity is managed by a nervous system network extending across all levels of the neuroaxis from the myoneural junction where nervous system and muscle join to the cortex. The interested reader should consult Corbin-Lewis, Liss, and Sciortino's (2004) book-length discussion of swallowing anatomy and physiology. The complexity of this system is simplified for this chapter.

Higher Nervous System Control

Martin and Sessle (1993) reviewed the extant literature on cortical and subcortical contributions to swallowing. Areas seemingly important to swallowing even when it is automatic as opposed to willed include what they describe as the lateral pericentral and perisylvian cortex, anterior cingulate cortex, and right insula. They originally described the contributions of these regions as involving initiation and modulation of the swallow response. Subsequently, Martin and colleagues (2004) have refined their conclusions about cortical and subcortical involvement. While admitting the need for further research, they conclude that swallowing involves the left lateral precentral, postcentral, and supramarginal gyri, anterior cingulate cortex, right frontal and parietal opercula, and the insula, among other areas. Although activation is present in both left and right hemispheres, the left hemisphere is more active than the right, suggesting the same lateralization for swallowing as for language. However, this lateralization is more variable from person to person than is it is for language. Given the multiple areas of involvement, these authors speculate that cortical and subcortical regions contribute sensory processing and motor programming and planning that contribute to the activity of the central pattern generator (CPG) in the brainstem.

Martin et al.'s (2004) notions about cortical asymmetry have been posited by others. For example, Hamdy and colleagues (1996) also reported that swallowing demonstrates bilateral but asymmetric cortical representation. Furthermore, Hamdy and colleagues (1998) state that damage to the more dominant hemisphere for swallowing may be associated with increased risk for dysphagia and that recovery of swallowing function is associated with cortical reorganization in the intact hemisphere.

Mosier and colleagues (Mosier & Bereznaya, 2001; Mosier, Liu, Maldjian, Shah, & Modi, 1999) have collected data from functional brain imaging interpreted as demonstrating that the multiple cortical and subcortical regions critical to swallowing are organized into what they call interacting modules. As but one example of their elegant set of notions about nervous system organization for swallowing, they identify a module involving the primary motor and sensory cortices, the supplementary motor area, and the cingulate gyrus. They assign to this module primary responsibility for planning and executing the sequence of movements necessary to normal swallowing.

What students need to understand is that the complexity of swallowing requires an extensive neural network of cortical and subcortical structures for its normal execution. The implications of this network for clinical and research activities are multiple. As pointed out by Hamdy and colleagues (1998), recovery may be influenced by site of lesion. More importantly, it means that a variety of nervous system diseases involving a variety of nervous system regions can cause swallowing impairment. The truth of this last observation is amply supported in a subsequent section when patterns of swallowing impairment in a variety of neurologic conditions are surveyed.

Cranial Nerves

Sensory information from the muscles and joints whose activity is responsible for swallowing is transported to the brainstem along sensory branches of cranial nerves V, VII, IX, and X. Cranial nerves I and II also supply sensory information involved in eating—smell and vision, respectively (Murray & Musson, 2005). Motor commands are supplied from higher cortical areas to the swallowing muscles via the motor branches of cranial nerves V, VII, IX, X, XI and XII (see Plate 2) and to the diaphragm by the phrenic nerve. All 12 of the cranial nerves are shown in Plate 3.

Swallowing depends in part on the integrity of the aforementioned nerves. Sensory and motor information, however, must be integrated for complex swallowing events to unfold normally. The first level of this integration occurs in the sensory and motor networks of the bilateral brainstem central pattern generator (CPG).

Central Pattern Generator

The presently popular conceptualization of a swallowing CPG is due in large part to the work of Arthur Miller, a physiologist at the University of California in San Francisco (Miller, 1999). CPGs are critical to the orderly sequencing of events, such as those especially required in the pharyngeal and esophageal stages of swallowing. According to Miller, a variety of sensory signals generated by, for example, taste, touch, and temperature converge on the nucleus tractus solitarius and surrounding reticular activating system in the medulla. This nucleus and associated reticular activating system comprise the sensory portion of the CPG. In Miller's view, this component is important in triggering a sequence of signals necessary to the orderly sequence of events in the pharyngeal and esophageal swallow. Nucleus ambiguus and the surrounding reticular activating system comprise the motor portion of the CPG with output to the muscles controlling the face, tongue, larynx, pharynx, and velum. It is through this component of the CPG that signals go to the various structures in a pattern of sequential excitation.

The bilateral CPGs are critical to normal swallowing but do not operate in isolation. Instead, their activity is influenced by higher portions of the nervous system. The sensory (nucleus tractus solitarius) and motor (nucleus ambiguus) components of the swallowing CPG are shown in Plate 4.

Evaluation of Swallowing

Evaluation of swallowing typically begins with a clinical swallowing examination. The traditional components are a history; an oral motor exam, often with sensory testing; a focused physical examination to assess items such as voice quality, strength of cough, and palpation of laryngeal excursion with swallowing; and observation of how a variety of liquids and solids are swallowed. During this last part, the clinician provides a variety of materials to be swallowed and then closely observes for signs of dysphagia such as drooling, coughing, throat clearing, and changes in vocal quality. In the hands of an experienced clinician, this examination is useful in quickly determining whether a person has a swallowing disorder. Because the health consequences of swallowing disorders can be so serious, especially if it results in aspiration or passage of material into the lungs, the clinical examination is often followed by an instrumental examination.

A variety of instrumental examinations have been used to study normal and abnormal swallowing. Foremost among them is a radiologic procedure called a *videofluoroscopic swallowing evaluation (VFSE)*. This method allows for a moving x-ray image of the oropharyngeal swallowing mechanism during swallows of barium, a radio-opaque substance. During a VFSE, swallowing is assessed in the lateral (from the side) and anterior-posterior (front to back) planes while an individual is swallowing a variety of substances, such as thin and thick barium, barium paste or pudding, and a solid item such as a quarter of a plain cookie coated with barium. During the VFSE, if swallowing abnormalities are detected, strategies to improve swallowing function may be attempted. The benefit of these strategies can then be determined during the VFSE, which is typically videotaped to allow for further review and analysis. Figure 8–2 is a still frame of a swallow of thin liquid during VFSE in the lateral position. Note the dark appearance of the barium as it moves through the pharynx. Also visible on this film are many of the key structures involved in swallowing: the jaw, lips, teeth, tongue, soft palate, larynx, hyoid, epiglottis, and upper esophageal sphincter. Figure 8–3 is a still frame of a swallow of thin liquid in the anterior-posterior position.

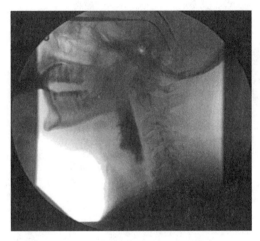

Figure 8–2. Lateral image from VFSE during swallowing of a thin liquid.

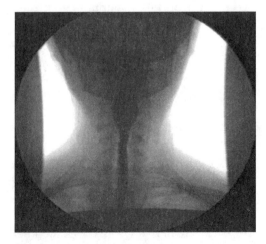

Figure 8–3. Anterior-posterior image from VFSE during swallowing of a thin liquid.

VFSE allows for a detailed assessment of swallow function, determines the cause of the swallowing disorder, if one is present, and provides additional information for the clinician to make appropriate recommendations with regard to oral intake, therapeutic intervention, and consultations to other health care professionals (Martin-Harris, Logemann, McMahon, Schleicher, & Sandidge, 2000).

Another increasingly common method for evaluating the swallow is called *fiberoptic endoscopic evaluation of swallowing (FEES)* (Langmore, Schatz, & Olsen, 1988). During this procedure, a small diameter endoscope is passed through the nose into the pharynx just above the larynx. Plate 5 is an illustration, which that demonstrates the position of the endoscope, whereas Figure 8–4 shows a lateral x-ray image of an endoscope in position during a FEES study.

In contrast to the VFSE, a FEES study allows for direct visualization of many of the structures of the larynx and pharynx. Plate 6 illustrates many of the pharyngeal and laryngeal structures that are visible during FEES; Plate 7 is a still image of a similar view during a FEES study.

The clinician performing the study typically first evaluates the appearance of the laryngeal structures at rest and with movement, such as may be elicited with phonation and coughing. The presence and severity of secretions can be assessed during FEES. Plate 8 shows clear "bubbly" secretions throughout the larynx. Secretions are not typically able to be visualized during VFSE.

A variety of liquids and foods similar as to those used with videofluoroscopy are utilized during FEES. However, barium is not used during FEES. Rather, liquids and foods are dyed blue or green to contrast the colors of the pharynx and larynx. During the study, the clinician

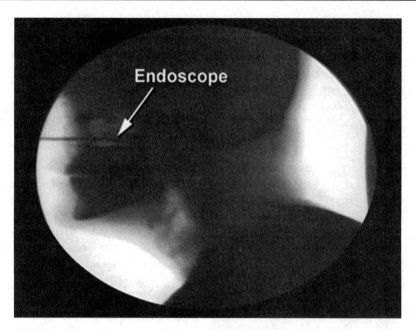

Figure 8–4. Position of the endoscope during FEES as seen under fluoroscopy. (Reprinted with permission from the Department of Veterans Affairs, Veteran Health Administration, from J. Murray & N. Musson, 2005, *Understanding Dysphagia*, CD [Version 1.0].)

observes movements before the swallow is completed and then examines the larynx and pharynx for evidence of swallowing adequacy after the swallow. If material has entered the larynx and/or trachea, it will be visible after the swallow. Material that was not completely swallowed and remains in the pharynx will also be visible. During the swallow, FEES does not allow for visualization of the swallow due to a period called the "white out" during pharyn-geal constriction.

FEES is generally a well-tolerated procedure and is considered safe with few reported serious complications (Aviv, Murry, Zschommler, Cohen, & Gartner, 2005). Much like videofluoroscopy, FEES allows a skilled clinician to assess the integrity of the oropharyngeal swallowing mechanism, determine the biomechanical abnormalities of the swallowing disorder if one is present, assess the benefit of swallowing strategies and techniques, and make appropriate recommendations. More recently, FEES has been coupled with sensory testing in a procedure called FEESST, which delivers air pulse stimuli to the larynx via the endoscope to assess laryngeal sensation (Aviv et al., 1998).

Signs of Dysphagia

The most commonly identified signs of dysphagia are derived from the perceptual or computer-assisted evaluation of a video-fluoroscopic swallowing examination. The signs can be classified into one of three

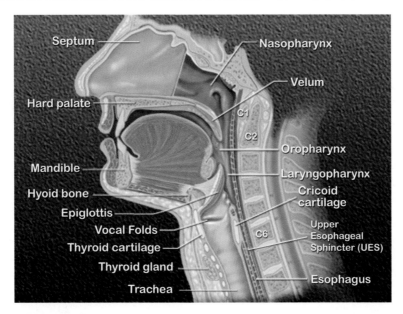

Plate 1. Illustration of structures involved in swallowing. (Reprinted with permission from the Department of Veterans Affairs, Veteran Health Administration, from J. Murray & N. Musson, 2005, *Understanding Dysphagia*, CD [Version 1.0].)

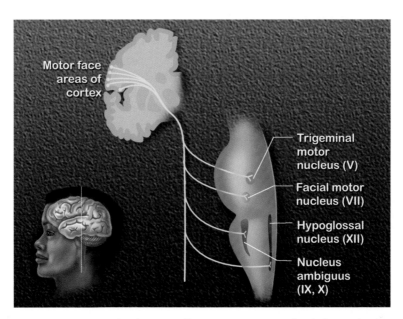

Plate 2. Motor commands for swallowing are supplied from higher cortical area via the motor branches of cranial nerves V, VII, X, XI, and XII. (Reprinted with permission from the Department of Veterans Affairs, Veteran Health Administration, from J. Murray & N. Musson, 2005, *Understanding Dysphagia*, CD [Version 1.0].)

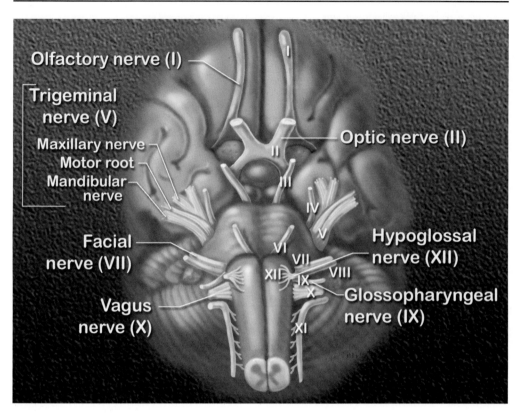

Plate 3. The 12 cranial nerves are illustrated. Multiple cranial nerves are involved in sensory and motor aspects of swallowing including V, VII, IX, X, and XII. (Reprinted with permission from the Department of Veterans Affairs, Veteran Health Administration, from J. Murray & N. Musson, 2005, *Understanding Dysphagia*, CD [Version 1.0].)

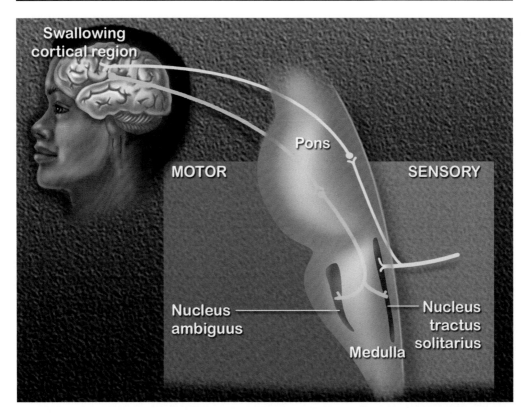

Plate 4. The sensory (nucleus tractus solitarius) and motor (nucleus ambiguus) components of the CPG. (Reprinted with permission from the Department of Veterans Affairs, Veteran Health Administration, from J. Murray & N. Musson, 2005, *Understanding Dysphagia*, CD [Version 1.0].)

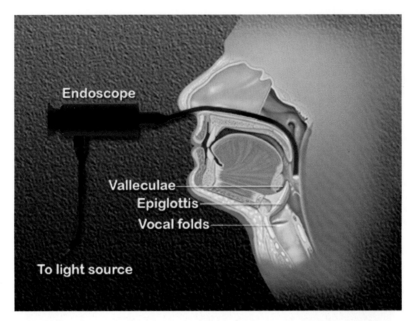

Plate 5. Position of the endoscope during FEES. (Reprinted with permission from the Department of Veterans Affairs, Veteran Health Administration, from J. Murray & N. Musson, 2005, *Understanding Dysphagia*, CD [Version 1.0].)

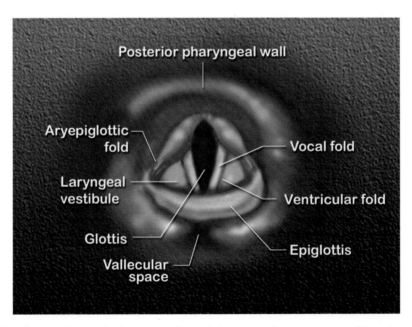

Plate 6. Illustration of pharyngeal and laryngeal structures. (Reprinted with permission from the Department of Veterans Affairs, Veteran Health Administration, from J. Murray & N. Musson, 2005, *Understanding Dysphagia*, CD [Version 1.0].)

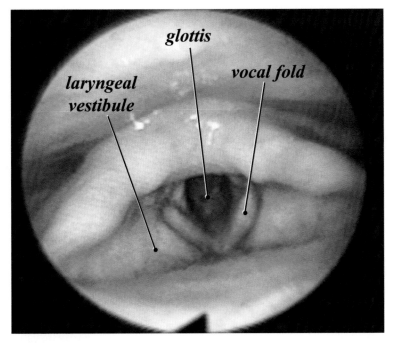

Plate 7. Video still image demonstrating the view of laryngeal and pharyngeal structure during FEES.

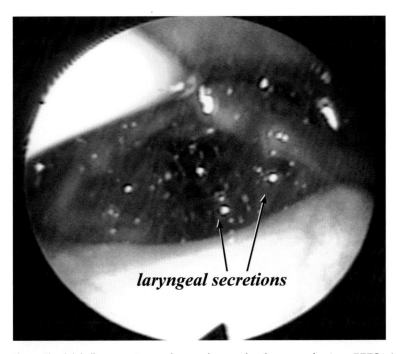

Plate 8. Clear "bubbly" secretions throughout the larynx during FEES. A feeding tube can also be observed.

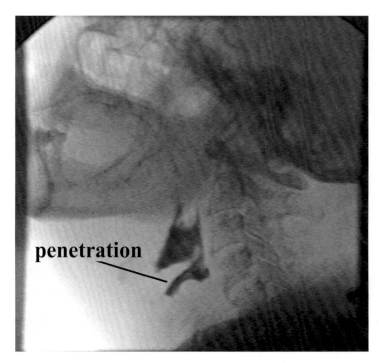

Plate 9. Penetration, or entry of material into the larynx but not into the trachea, during VFSE.

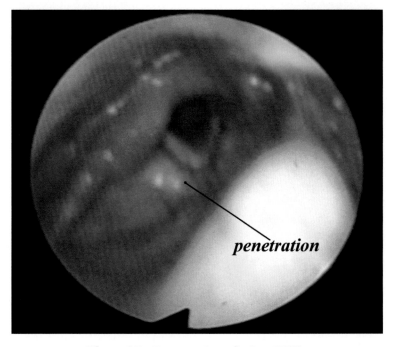

Plate 10. Penetration during FEES.

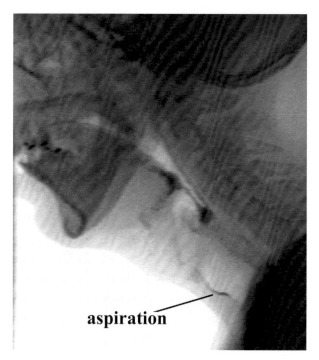

Plate 11. Aspiration, or entry of material into the trachea, during VFSE.

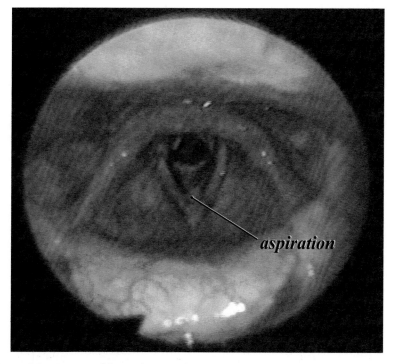

Plate 12. Entry of liquid into the trachea (aspiration) during FEES.

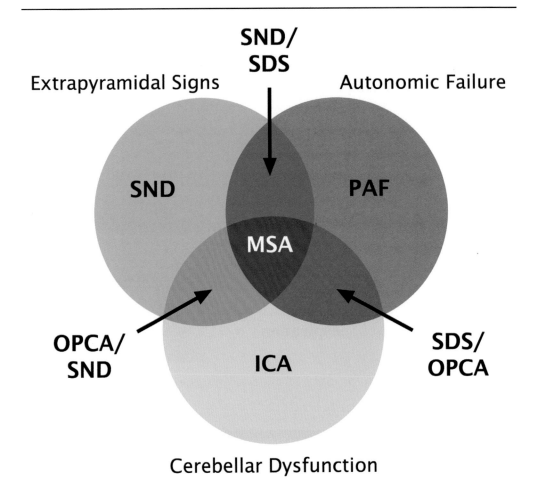

Plate 13. The relationship between MSA and related neurodegenerative diseases. (Reprinted with permission of McGraw-Hill Companies, from "Multiple System Atrophy," by L. M. Shulman, A. Minager, and W. J. Weiner. 2004. Multiple system atrophy. In R. L. Watts & W. C. Koller [Eds.], *Movement Disorders: Neurogenic Principles and Practice*, p. 359.)

groups based on measurement of bolus flow and structure movement.

The first broad class of measures is concerned with the *timing of events* during swallowing. These measures of timing relate the movement of the bolus in relationship to the position and movement of structures. For example, a common measure is oral transit time. This measure is calculated as the time that elapses between the moment the bolus begins to move backward in the mouth and the moment its leading edge reaches the posterior ramus of the mandible. Clearly, to make these and related measures, the clinician has to have a keen eye and knowledge of anatomy.

The second broad class of measures involves measurement of the *completeness of bolus flow* with swallowing. Incomplete bolus flow in which material is left behind in the mouth or pharynx results in what is often called residue or residual. It is common then for the clinician to note residual in the mouth, the vallecular space, and the piriform sinuses, as shown in Figure 8–5.

The third broad class of measures involves *direction of bolus flow*. The most frequently employed of these direction measures are penetration and aspiration, both of which have very specific meanings. *Penetration* occurs when material enters the larynx but does not pass into the trachea. Penetration during a VFSE is shown in Plate 9; Plate 10 shows penetration during FEES.

Aspiration is defined as material passing through the larynx and into the trachea, as shown during VFSE in Plate 11 and during FEES in Plate 12.

Both kinds of events can be measured with the penetration-aspiration (PA) scale, an 8-point scale to quantitatively measure

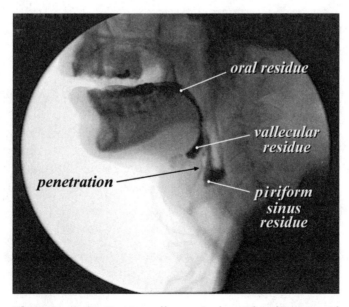

Figure 8–5. Postswallow oral and pharyngeal residue is exhibited during the VFSE. Residue is seen on the tongue, in the valleculae, and in the piriform sinuses. Penetration can also be observed.

the depth of airway entry and whether or not the material is expelled (Rosenbek, Robbins, Roecker, Coyle, & Wood, 1996). Although originally designed for use with VFSE, recent data suggest the PA scale can be used with FEES as well (Colodny, 2002) The penetration-aspiration scale is shown in Table 8–1. Both penetration and aspiration are especially alarming to clinicians because of their potential negative effect on health.

Classification and Pathophysiology

The dysarthrias were originally classified into types based on hypotheses about the underlying neurologic condition com-

monly called the pathophysiology (Darley, Aronson, & Brown 1969a, 1969b, 1975). Dysphagia clinicians, many of whom learned about the dysarthrias before learning about dysphagia, applied the same approach to swallowing disorders. For example, certain signs such as increased vallecular residue are hypothesized to result from lingual weakness. In addition, attempts have been made to identify distinctive clusters of dysphagia signs in certain disorders paralleling the posited distinctive speech signs. Applying these approaches to speech disorders has prompted generations of debate as has been abundantly discussed in previous chapters. The attempts are only a little less controversial in dysphagia, primarily because there was no concerted effort in the dys-

Table 8–1. The Penetration-Aspiration (PA) Scale*

PA Score	Description
1	Material does not enter the airway
2	Material enters the airway, remains above the vocal folds, and is ejected from the airway
3	Material enters the airway, remains above the vocal folds, and is not ejected from the airway
4	Material enters the airway, contacts the vocal folds, and is ejected from the airway
5	Material enters the airway, contacts the vocal folds, and is not ejected from the airway
6	Material enters the airway, passes below the vocal folds, and is ejected into the larynx or out of the airway
7	Material enters the airway, passes below the vocal folds, and is not ejected from the trachea despite effort
8	Material enters the airway, passes below the vocal folds, and no effort is made to eject

*Reprinted with kind permission of Springer Science and Business Media, from J. C. Rosenbek, J. A. Robbins, E. B. Roecker, J. L. Coyle, & J. L. Wood. 1996. A penetration-aspiration scale. *Dysphagia, 11*, p. 94, Table 2.

phagia community to popularize a classification system.

Understanding the pathophysiology is important, however, given that clinicians are being prodded to base treatments on the nature of the underlying deficit (Huckabee & Pelletier, 1998). For example, muscle strengthening exercises may make the most sense for those who have a swallowing abnormality resulting from weakness. As another example, signs resulting from discoordination may be posited to require skill training in the form of systematic repetition of swallowing movements of increasing complexity.

Classification in dysphagia is rudimentary. As will be obvious from the subsequent review of signs in a variety of neurologic disorders, the signs of swallowing abnormality across a wide variety of disorders are similar and their variability among persons with any of these neurologic diagnoses can be substantial. This means that two people with the same disease may have entirely different signs. Therefore, in the following descriptions of swallowing signs in a variety of diseases, the emphasis will be on those most frequently occurring as identified in the literature and in our clinical experience. The reader is reminded that a person may have the disease and have no dysphagia, or one that is not described in the summary below.

Dysphagia in Neurologic Disease

What follows are descriptions of the swallowing abnormalities in a variety of neurologic disorders associated with motor speech disorders. Our classification system is based on that used by Ropper and Brown (2005). Admittedly, this list is not exhaustive but is suitable for an overview.

Cerebrovascular Disease

Stroke occurs when blood supply to the nervous system is disrupted by the rupturing of a vessel or its blockage by a clot. The signs of a stroke depend on what part of the nervous system is robbed of its blood supply. As discussed in an earlier section, multiple areas of the nervous system from cortex to individual cranial nerves coursing to the face, tongue, velopharynx, larynx, and pharynx comprise a network in support of swallowing. Therefore, dysphagia occurs commonly after stroke, with some series reporting dysphagia in up to 81% (Meng, Wang, & Lien, 2000) to 90% (Kidd, Lawson, Nesbitt, & MacMahon, 1993) of patients in the acute poststroke stage (the period of a few days after a stroke occurs). Approximately 10% of patients remain dysphagic when evaluated six months after stroke (O'Neill, 2000). The incidence is highest and the dysphagia is most likely to persist if the stroke involves the brainstem and in persons who suffer more than one stroke, especially if damage includes bilateral cortical and subcortical areas (Daniels & Foundas, 1999). However, dysphagia can occur even after a single left- or right-hemisphere stroke (Robbins, Levine, Maser, Rosenbek, & Kempster, 1993), although the dysphagia tends to be less severe and to resolve relatively rapidly in most persons. The relationship of the signs of dysphagia to the location of the lesion is seldom very strong—with one notable exception. A stroke involving the medulla of the brainstem is likely to produce a fairly predictable and severe dysphagia (Martino, Terrault, Ezerzer, Mikulis, & Diamant, 2001; Robbins & Levine, 1993). Patients with what is often called *Wallenberg's syndrome* have two main impairments: difficulty tightly closing the larynx and opening the upper esophageal sphincter during the swallow. In the most severe form of this dysphagia, they may be unable to swallow at all and are forced to spit even their saliva into a cup. Such persons are forced to take their nourishment from a feeding tube unless rehabilitation can restore their swallowing.

Bilateral strokes, especially if they involve critical motor areas of the left and right hemispheres or subcortical structures such as the basal ganglia, often cause both oral and pharyngeal stage abnormalities (Horner, Massey, & Brazer, 1990). Oral stage signs can include slow inadequate chewing, difficulty with bolus formation and movement, and slowed initiation of the swallow. Pharyngeal abnormalities may include postswallow pharyngeal residue and aspiration. In contrast, unilateral strokes are more likely to produce oral stage abnormalities, such as difficulty with bolus preparation and movement, than they are to produce pharyngeal stage abnormalities (Aydogdu, Ertekin, Tarlaci, Turman, Kiylioglu, & Secil, 2001; Han, Chang, Lu, & Wang, 2005). Robbins and colleagues (1993), however, have reported that aspiration is more likely after a stroke involving the right hemisphere than the left and, conversely, that oral stage abnormalities are more likely after a stroke in the left hemisphere than in the right. Finally, it also appears that anterior cortical lesions in either hemisphere are more likely than posterior ones to produce a clinically significant dysphagia (Daniels & Foundas, 1999).

Weakness, abnormal tone, abnormal motor programming, and discoordination all have been hypothesized to explain the signs of abnormal swallowing in various groups of dysphagic stroke patients. These explanations need to be tested experimentally, just as in dysarthria. However, one explanation for dysphagia following unilateral hemispheric stroke is supported by data. Hamdy and colleagues (1998) posit that each of us has a swallowing dominant hemisphere. In some of us the right hemisphere is dominant and in some it is the left. A stroke in the dominant hemisphere results in dysphagia involving both oral and pharyngeal stages, which may improve with cortical reorganization in the unaffected hemisphere. For students, the point to remember is that dysphagia commonly occurs after stroke, particularly in the acute period of recovery, regardless of the exact pathophysiology.

Degenerative Diseases of the Nervous System

Diseases Characterized by Abnormalities of Movement and Posture

Parkinson's disease (PD) is a relatively common progressive neurodegenerative disease associated primarily with basal ganglia pathology. Hallmark symptoms of PD include a resting tremor, bradykinesia, rigidity, akinesia, and loss of postural reflexes. Speech disorders also occur frequently in PD and the dysarthria of PD is, in fact, the prototypical example of hypokinetic dysarthria. Hypokinetic dysathria occurs in up to 90% of individuals with PD at some point during the progression of the disease (Logemann, Fisher, Boshes, & Blonsky, 1978; Müller et al., 2001). Swallowing impairments also occur frequently in PD, with some reports indicating 75% or more of patients with PD have oropharyngeal dysphagia (Leopold & Kagel, 1996, 1997b, 1997c; Nilsson, Ekberg, Olsson, & Hindfelt, 1996; Robbins, Logemann, & Kirshner, 1986). It has been suggested that dysphagia severity is correlated to the severity of PD (Leopold & Kagel, 1997b), but other data do not support this notion (Nilsson, Ekberg, Olsson, & Hindfelt, 1996).

Oral, pharyngeal, and esophageal phases of swallowing can be impaired in patients with PD. Oral stage deficits probably occur most frequently (Volonté, Porta, & Comi, 2002). Patients with PD often exhibit a characteristic "rocking" motion of the tongue in which the posterior tongue remains elevated, preventing material from exiting the oral cavity (Ertekin et al., 2002; Logemann, 1998; Yorkston, Miller, & Strand, 1995). Other oral state deficits in patients with PD may include drooling, increased oral transit time, lingual tremor, impaired initiation of lingual movement, and premature spillage of the bolus into the pharynx (Yorkston, Miller, & Strand, 1995). Pharyngeal stage dysphagia often occurs with disease progression after an initial presentation of primarily oral stage deficits (Logemann, 1998). Pharyngeal stage impairments may include a pharyngeal swallow delay, impaired pharyngeal clearance, decreased laryngeal elevation and closure, and laryngeal penetration and aspiration (Leopold & Kagel, 1997b, 1997c; Leopold & Kagel, 1996; Yorkston, Miller, & Strand, 1995). Esophageal dysphagia has also been described, including cricopharyngeal dysfunction, esophageal dysmotility (Castell, Johnston, Colcher, Li, Gideon, & Castell, 2001; Yorkston, Miller, & Strand, 1995), tertiary contractions, abnormalities of the LES, and gastroesophageal reflux (Leopold & Kagel, 1997c).

Dysphagia may at times be the presenting symptom of neurodegenerative disease in PD. Logemann (1998) suggests that the aforementioned "rocking" motion of the tongue in patients with PD is "a particularly pathognomonic sign of this disease" (p. 335). Patients with PD often have poor insight into their dysphagia (Volonté, Porta, & Comi, 2002). They may not complain of swallowing difficulty, even in the setting of weight loss, dehydration, and pneumonia. When they do report dysphagia, patients with PD often describe oral stage deficits, a sticking sensation in the throat, and coughing or choking during meals. Esophageal stage deficits usually go unnoticed by patients (Yorkston, Miller, & Strand, 1995).

Multiple system atrophy (MSA) is a *parkinson-plus syndrome* (PPS). The term PPS is used to refer to a number of conditions in which parkinsonian symptoms are present with additional symptoms suggestive of more widespread neural degeneration than is encountered in PD. In contrast to patients with PD, patients with PPS are often younger at diagnosis, have a more aggressive progression of symptoms, and progress more rapidly to death. Parkinsonian symptoms in patients with PPS often do not respond or have limited response to treatments for PD, such as the use of levodopa (Wszolek, Markopoulou, & Chase, 2004).

MSA is a PPS characterized by the gradual onset of parkinsonism, cerebellar dysfunction, and autonomic failure (Shulman, Minagar, & Weiner, 2004). The use of the terminology MSA is complicated and involves three related neurodegenerative diseases—*olivopontocerebellar atrophy (OPCA)*, *Shy-Drager syndrome (SDS)*, and *striatonigral degeneration (SND)*. Shulman, Minagar, and Weiner (2004) describe the history of the use of these terms:

Dejerine and Thomas first coined the term OPCA in 1900 to describe two sporadic cases of progressive cerebellar degeneration with parkinsonism. Sixty years later, Shy and Drager published the first clinicopathological study of a patient with idiopathic orthostatic hypotension . . . Also in 1960, van der Eecken et al. described a unique pathological subgroup among a large number of patients with paralysis agitans. Striatopallidonigral degeneration was identified . . . in a few patients with extrapyramidal rigidity but minimal tremor (p. 359).

Whereas OPCA is associated with cerebellar dysfunction, SDS with autonomic failure, and SND with extrapyramidal signs (i.e., parkinsonism), "emergence of the other two syndromes can be predicted (if) the patient survives long enough" (Shulman, Minagar, & Weiner, 2004, p. 360). Graham and Oppenheimer first suggested the term MSA in 1969 to cover all three of these overlapping syndromes. Plate 13 details the relationship between these conditions.

More recently, a consensus statement on the diagnosis of MSA recommended discontinuing the use of terms SND, SDS, and OPCA, instead suggesting that patients be designated "as having *MSA-P* if parkinsonian features predominate or *MSA-C* if cerebellar features predominate" (Gilman et al., 1999, p. 97). Although this notion appears to be gathering support, any of the aforementioned terms can still be encountered and the classification of this disorder will likely remain somewhat confusing. We primarily use the term MSA in the following discussion.

Dysarthria is a common symptom of MSA and a mixed dysarthria with features of hypokinetic, ataxic, and spastic dysarthria types is described most frequently (Duffy, 2005). Dysphagia is also a well-known symptom of MSA, though the nature of the swallowing impairment in these patients has not been well studied. Higo and colleagues (2003, 2005) have performed the most extensive research on the swallowing function in patients with

MSA using VFSE. Higo et al. (2003) first reported on 29 patients with MSA who participated in VFSE and manometry. Their results indicated significant oral stage dysphagia, including difficulty with holding and transporting the bolus. Pharyngeal stage function was also found to be impaired, but much less so than the oral stage. Manometry revealed decreased oropharyngeal and hypopharyngeal swallowing pressures, as well as incomplete relaxation of the UES in 60% of patients who had MSA for at least five years.

Higo et al. (2005) next used VFSE to investigate oropharyngeal swallowing function in 21 patients diagnosed with MSA-C. Subjects were divided into three groups depending on length of disease duration. Individuals in the early stage of MSA were those with 1 to 3 years since onset, middle stage patients were those 4 to 6 years after onset, and late stage patients had had the onset of symptoms more than seven years before the study. Results suggested that oral stage dysphagia was often involved even in the early stage of the disease and this increased over the duration of the disease until it was "remarkably disturbed" in patients in the late stages of the disease (p. 646). Pharyngeal stage involvement was less common than oral deficits in the early stage, although increasing pharyngeal dysphagia, including reduced pharyngeal clearance and impaired laryngeal elevation, was noted in patients in the middle and late stage of the disease.

Dysphagia is also reported to occur frequently in the literature, which uses the terminology SND, SDS, and OPCA, although it has received little systematic attention. For example, Berciano (1982) reviewed 117 cases of familial and sporadic OPCA and found that dysphagia was a "neurological finding" in 24 to 33% of cases and that dysphagia was the initial symptom in one case (p. 260). Other authors have also reported the presence of pharyngeal and esophageal dysphagia in patients with OPCA (Kurihara, Kita, Hirayama, Hara, & Toyama, 1990). Gouider-Khouja and colleagues (1995) described the presence of dysphagia in 44% of the 18 patients with SND they investigated and reported dysphagia as the initial patient complaint in one case. Dysphagia in SDS has received little attention and it can be hypothesized that oropharyngeal dysphagia may be relatively uncommon in "pure" autonomic failure. Of course, with disease progression and the additional involvement of the extrapyramidal and cerebellar systems, oropharyngeal dysphagia becomes increasingly likely.

Progressive supranuclear palsy (PSP) (sometimes known as *Steele-Richardson-Olszewski syndrome*) is a PPS of insidious onset characterized by parkinsonism that is poorly responsive to levodopa, vertical gaze palsy, poor balance, frequent falls, dysarthria, and personality changes (Adams & Victor, 1991; Ropper & Brown, 2005). PSP is associated with pathologic changes in the basal ganglia, brainstem, and cerebellum.

Dysarthria and dysphagia are frequently associated with PSP and each may be the presenting sign of neurologic disease (Diroma et al., 2003). Individuals with PSP most commonly present with a mixed dysarthria with features of hypokinetic, spastic, and ataxic dysarthria types (Duffy, 2005). Videofluoroscopy has been used to assess oropharyngeal swallow function in patients with PSP and results indicate swallowing deficits similar to those encountered in patients with PD. Reported deficits include impaired bolus preparation and lingual movements, premature spillage, delayed swallowing initiation, impaired laryngeal movement, and postswallow pharyngeal residue (Leopold & Kagel, 1997a). In contrast to patients with PD, Leopold

and Kagel (1997a) describe increased velar incompetency in patients with PSP. Patients with PSP and dysphagia are also often aware of their difficulty swallowing, even when they present with cognitive impairments (Müller et al., 2001).

Corticobasal degeneration (CBD), also known as *corticobasal-ganglionic degeneration*, is a PPS of insidious, asymmetric onset characterized by motor deficits, deficits in higher cortical function, and neuropsychiatric abnormalities. Limb clumsiness with or without rigidity is often the first symptom. An asymmetric akinetic-rigid parkinsonism, with or without temor, is also common. Other symptoms of motor dysfunction may include tremor, myoclonus, limb or upper face dystonia, abnormalities in eye movements, and speech and swallowing problems. Deficits in what Stover and colleagues (2004) describe as higher cortical function may include limb apraxia, apraxia of speech, aphasia, and alien limb phenomenon. Neuropsychiatric abnormalities in patients with CBD include depression, apathy, anxiety, agitation, and disinhibition. Much like other PPS, CBD is not typically levodopa responsive (Stover, Wainer, & Watts, 2004).

Speech and swallowing disorders occur commonly in CBD. Hypokinetic, spastic, and ataxic dysarthria types, either in isolation or presenting as a mixed dysarthria, occur most frequently (Duffy, 2005; Ozsancak, Auzou, Jan, Defebvre, Derambure, & Destee, 2006), often with hypokinetic features predominating (Frattali & Sonies, 2000). A variety of oral, pharyngeal, and esophageal stage abnormalities may be encountered in patients with CBD. Oral stage deficits may include piecemeal deglutition, excessive lingual movements, oral dysmotility, premature spillage, and nasal regurgitation. Pharyngeal stage deficits may be characterized by a pharyngeal swallow delay, postswallow pharyngeal residue, penetration, and aspiration. Esophageal dysmotility and gastroesophageal reflux may also occur (Frattali & Sonies, 2000).

Dystonia is a movement disorder characterized by involuntary sustained muscle contractions that result in repetitive twisting movements or abnormalities in posture. Dystonia can be classified by etiology (i.e., primary or secondary), age of onset (early or late onset), or distribution (i.e., focal, segmental, or generalized) (Albanese et al., 2006). For simplification, the present discussion classifies dystonic syndromes by their distribution. For example, in generalized dystonia multiple body areas are involved, such as the legs, trunk, and at least one other body region. Segmental dystonia involves at least two contiguous areas of the body. Examples include the cranial muscles (i.e., face, jaw, tongue, and/or vocal folds) or axial muscles (i.e., trunk and neck). Focal dystonia is restricted to a single body area, such as the upper or lower face muscles, larynx, or neck (Tagliati, Golden, & Bressman, 2004).

When the distribution of dystonia targets any of the components of the swallowing mechanism, dysphagia may occur. In patients with generalized dystonia involving the trunk and, therefore, the respiratory mechanism, difficulty coordinating swallowing with respiration may be exhibited. A number of segmental or focal dystonias that involve the structures involved in swallowing are also associated with swallowing abnormalities. Neck dystonia, often known as *cervical dystonia* or *spasmodic torticollis*, has been reported to be associated with dysphagia in approximately 50% of unselected patients is some series. Most frequent swallowing abnormalities include a delay in swallow initiation and vallecular residue (Riski, Horner, & Nashold, 1990). Mouth and face dysto-

nia or *oromandibular dystonia (OMD)* involves the masticatory, lower facial, and tongue muscles in a variety of combinations. When coupled with upper facial dystonia (also known as *blepharospasm*) this condition is often known as *Meige syndrome* or *Brueghel's syndrome*. All forms of OMD can have a negative influence on swallow function. In a series of unselected patients with Meige syndrome, 90% presented with swallowing abnormalities which included premature spillage of the bolus and vallecular residue (Cersosimo, Juri, Suarez de Chandler, Clerici, & Micheli, 2005). Not surprisingly, other swallowing abnormalities in OMD may include chewing difficulties and other deficits in oral preparation of the bolus (Mascia, Valls-Sole, Marti, & Sanz, 2005). Jaw dystonia can result in either *jaw-opening* or *jaw-closing OMD*. This may often result in a variety of oral and pharyngeal stage deficits, which can be severe in some cases. Lingual dystonia also often results in dysphagia. For example, in patients with tongue protrusion, lingual dystonia with or without OMD, biting of the tongue, and pushing food out of the oral cavity with the tongue has been described (Charles, Davis, Shannon, Hook, & Warner, 1997). Finally, laryngeal dystonia or *spasmodic dysphonia (adductor, abductor,* or *mixed* types) may result in complaints of dysphagia, but swallowing is usually relatively preserved in comparison to speech deficits.

Extrapyramidal Syndromes with Hereditary Metabolic Disease

Wilson's disease (WD) is a rare autosomal recessive genetic disease associated with copper accumulation in the liver, brain, and eyes due to an impairment of gastrointestinal elimination of this material. Hepatic (or liver) manifestations of WD include spleen and liver enlargement, acute and/or chronic hepatitis, and progressive cirrhosis. Neurologic symptoms most frequently include tremor, dysarthria, cerebellar dysfunction, dystonia, and abnormalities in gait. Psychiatric symptoms such as personality changes and mood disturbances may also be present. Ophthalmologic symptoms of WD include the presence of pigmented corneal rings known as *Kayser-Fleisher rings*, which are considered a pathognomic sign of WD (Pfeiffer, 2004).

Dysarthria occurs frequently in WD and is reported in over 90% of unselected patients with neurologic manifestations of WD in some studies (Oder, Grimm, Kollegger, Ferenci, Schneider, & Deecke, 1991; Wang et al., 2005). WD is most commonly associated with a mixed dysarthria with features of hypokinetic, spastic, and ataxic dysarthria types (Duffy, 2005). Dysphagia in WD has received little attention and is apparently a much less frequent neurologic manifestation of the disease. However, both pharyngeal and esophageal dysmotility has been described in select cases (Gulyas & Salazar-Grueso, 1988; Haggstrom & Hirschowitz, 1980). *Sialorrhea*, or an excessive secretion of saliva, has also been described (Wang et al., 2005). This problem is likely related to oropharyngeal dysphagia and decreased frequency of swallowing rather than a true excess in the production of saliva.

Diseases Characterized Primarily by Progressive Dementia

Alzheimer's disease (AD), named for Alois Alzheimer who described the case of a rapidly dementing 51-year-old woman in 1907, is the most common form of dementia. When intellectual functions such as memory, attention, and interest begin to fail, a person is said to have dementia. AD occurs in about 50% of those adults with intellectual decline and dementia (Ropper & Brown, 2005). In AD, abnormalities such as senile plaques occur in diffuse areas of the brain. AD usually begins with forgetfulness and can advance over several years to result in a person's being bedridden, nonresponsive, and dependent on others for even the simplest of self-care activities.

Swallowing problems in AD take up most of this discussion, but it is important to recognize that other dementia syndromes can occur and the notions about swallowing in AD may have to be revised when evaluating and treating persons with non-AD dementia. After AD, the next most frequent dementia type is *multi-infarct dementia*. In this condition, intellectual decline results from a series of strokes often distributed within the cortex and subcortex. Additionally, what Ropper and Brown (2005) call circumscribed cerebral atrophies can occur, in which the abnormalities are much more focal or localized. Included in this group are *Pick disease, frontotemporal dementia (FTD)*, and *primary progressive aphasia*. Swallowing problems in these conditions, with the possible exception of cases of multi-infarct dementia associated with lesions in the neural network supporting swallowing, are less frequent than in AD until a full-blown dementia occurs, as it inevitably does. Dementia also can occur as part of a number of other neurologic diseases such as PD and ALS. In these instances, discussion of the dysphagia in relation to those disorders will be relevant, as is the following discussion of swallowing in AD.

In addition to broad intellectual decline, AD often results in both speech and swallowing disorders. The motor speech disorders associated with AD may include hypokinetic dysarthria and apraxia of speech (Duffy, 2005). Clinically significant dysphagia is most likely during the latter stages of dementia when many such persons have been institutionalized (Feinberg, Ekberg, Segall, & Tully, 1992; Ikeda, Brown, Holland, Fukuhara, & Hodges, 2002; Kalia, 2003). Feinberg and colleagues (1992) studied the swallow function of 131 institutionalized demented patients using VFSE. Seventy-four had AD, 27 had multi-infarct dementia, and 30 had dementia as part of PD. Because these patients were all suffering from advanced dementia, the medical diagnosis is mentioned only once in the discussion of results. Those patients with PD had the highest proportion of oral stage abnormalities, although 71% of the total group of 131 had some oral stage abnormality. Oral stage abnormalities included premature spillage in which material leaked from the mouth into the pharynx. Pharyngeal stage deficits occurred in 43% of all subjects and included postswallow pharyngeal residue and aspiration. Forty-two percent of subjects presented with both oral and pharyngeal stage abnormalities. Only 7% of these persons had normal swallow function. Aspiration and pneumonia are reported by some to be the most serious medical problems of those with advanced AD (Kalia, 2003).

Swallowing deficits can sometimes occur earlier in dementing illness. This is especially true when dementia is part of a disease process such as ALS or PD. Priefer and Robbins (1997) report early onset of dyphagia even in some patients with AD. These abnormalities take the form of slowed oral and pharyngeal stages. Diagnosing dysphagia in early AD requires the clinical scientist to understand how nor-mal swallowing changes with aging. Swallowing slows with aging, but critical components such as laryngeal closure remain functional. Therefore, it is important that slowing be greater than normal for a confident diagnosis of dysphagia in dementia, and the most confident diagnosis can be made if other bolus flow problems such as pharyngeal residue or aspiration are also present. Early identification of swallowing abnormalities may be important because aspiration in the early stage of AD predicts long-term outcome with death being more likely in the severely demented and in those with early stage dementia who aspirate and have weight loss (Kalia, 2003).

Normal eating and drinking require more than simply an intact swallow, however. One must remain interested in eating, have sufficient coordination to move food and drink into the mouth, and have adequate attention to accomplish chewing and the other more cognitive aspects of swallowing. These abilities also decline in demented patients. Ikeda and colleagues (2002) report the results of a caregiver questionnaire in which the caregivers of those with FTD and AD were compared. Changes in food preferences and eating habits were more frequent early signs of changes in those with FTD than in those with AD. Specific swallowing difficulties occurred earlier than changes in food preferences and eating habits in AD as compared to FTD. Nonetheless, in all dementing illnesses, aspects of eating, drinking, and swallowing usually decline so that persons are totally dependent on caregivers or tube feedings.

The pathophysiology of dysphagia in dementing illness has been inadequately studied, but several hypotheses have been formulated. Chouinard (2000) posits a pseudobulbar state leading to dysphagia in dementia. It may well be that the spasticity and weakness that define so-called pseudobulbar palsy contribute to end-stage swallowing difficulty. Other factors are probably at work as well. Intention to swallow and the programming and planning of swallowing that depend on an elaborate cortical and subcortical network probably also decline (Horner, Alberts, Dawson, & Cook, 1994). For example, Horner and her colleagues (1994) identified oral apraxia as a predictor of swallowing difficulty in demented persons. These conditions can lead to a situation in which a caregiver places food in the demented person's mouth and then has to urge that person to swallow, an effort that often, but not inevitably, fails. Perhaps a greater influence than pseudobulbar palsy is *sarcopenia* or muscle wasting. It is frequent in aging when muscles for walking, turning, lifting, and swallowing are used with less frequency. Dependence leads nearly inexorably to reduced use and to sarcopenia. The result is loss of muscle bulk and strength which, when they occur in swallowing musculature, lead to increasingly severe dysphagia. One final complicating factor is medication. Most demented persons are on multiple medications that may negatively influence swallowing function.

Despite only a modest treatment literature, there does seem to be agreement that clinical attention to the abnormal swallow is important. Neither the goals nor the methods, however, are agreed upon, especially by those with the most experience in managing men and women with dementia. It has been common clinical wisdom to argue that dysphagia management reduces chances of aspiration pneumonia in the demented. The evidence in support of this wisdom is not abundant, but the assumption of influence is not harmful unless inappropriately high expectations or inappropriate management decisions are the result. Chouinard's (2000) guidelines for management are adequate given the present state of knowledge. He suggests that managing dysphagia, optimizing function generally, and doing what is possible to guarantee adequate nutrition and hydration, are the cornerstones of management for demented persons. Dysphagia management seldom involves exercises as cognitive impairment makes following directions difficult or impossible and independent practice unlikely. However, selecting the best food and liquid preparation and consistency may be useful so long as what is provided is of interest and acceptable to the patient. Special positioning so that the person is supported in the best possible sitting posture may also be important. It is over the issue of how to provide adequate nutrition that the greatest controversy arises. Tube feedings were increasingly popular in the 1980s and 1990s, but evidence they prolong life or increase quality of life when compared to having knowledgeable persons feed patients is weak at best. Indeed, the contemporary approach in many centers is to employ feeding programs conducted by skilled nurses and others (Chouinard, 2000). These feeding programs, combined with best possible oral hygiene, general care, and attention to medications, appear to have the best chance of preserving each patient's health and dignity to the degree possible.

Diseases in Which Dementia Is a Prominent Feature With Other Neurologic Abnormalities

Huntington's disease (HD) is an inherited autosomal dominant neurodegenerative disease. It occurs most frequently in midadult life with a relentless course to death in 12 to 15 years. The primary symptoms of HD include movement disorders, such as chorea, rigidity, and dystonia, and neuropsychological changes such as changes in personality and emotion, behavior disorders, intellectual decline, and dementia (Ropper & Brown, 2005; Yorkston, Miller, & Strand, 1995).

Both dysarthria and dysphagia are common, but not inevitable, in patients with HD. HD is typically associated with hyperkinetic dysarthria (Duffy, 2005). Kagel and Leopold (1992; see also Leopold & Kagel, 1985) have been pioneers in the use of VFSE to evaluate oropharyngeal swallow function in patients with HD. In patients with HD and prominent chorea, swallowing difficulties may include uncontrolled *tachyphagia* (rapid uncontrolled swallowing), lingual abnormalities due to chorea, uninhibited swallow initiation, impaired inhibition of respiration during swallowing, and postswallow pharyngeal residue. Tachyphagia is a particularly prominent symptom of dysphagia in these patients. Although death secondary to respiratory complications associated with dysphagia in HD has been reported, penetration and aspiration have not been frequently observed during VFSE (Hamakawa et al., 2004; Kagel & Leopold, 1992; Leopold & Kagel, 1985). Although less common, some patients with HD exhibit prominent rigidity and bradykinesia rather than chorea. Patients with this symptomatology may exhibit mandibular rigidity, inefficient mastication, and slow oral transit in a pattern of dysphagia more typical of patients with PD. Postswallow pharyngeal residue and laryngeal penetration and aspiration occur more frequently in patients with this presentation. Finally, esophageal dysphagia has been reported to occur relatively infrequently in patients

with HD, though *eructation* (excessive belching), *aerophagia* (swallowing air), vomiting, and esophageal dysmotility have been described in some patients (Leopold & Kagel, 1985; Kagel & Leopold, 1992).

Due to the frequent presence of swallowing difficulties in individuals with HD, dysphagia assessment and treatment is critical in this population. General management approaches often used in patients with HD include postural and position changes, assistive devices, supervision with meals to control rate of consumption and bolus size, dietary changes, and alternative feeding (Yorkston, Miller, & Strand, 1995). Successful implementation of many, if not all, of these techniques requires a great deal of caregiver assistance due to the cognitive deficits in patients with HD, but they have been reported to have considerable and persistent benefit (Leopold & Kagel, 1985). Patients with HD are also at nutritional risk due to a multitude of factors that include dysphagia, difficulty with food preparation due to chorea and cognitive deficits, impaired self-feeding skills, and increased calorie consumption due to chorea. Dietary supplements and consultations with dieticians may be beneficial in patients with HD (Trejo, Tarrats, Alonso, Boll, Ochoa, & Velásquez, 2004)

Syndromes of Progressive Ataxia

A number of chronic, progressive neurologic diseases characterized primarily by *ataxia* or incoordination of volitional movement are associated with cerebellar disease. In addition to ataxia, cerebellar lesions frequently result in the loss of muscle tone, as well as gait and equilibrium disturbances (Adams & Victor, 1991). Classification of the diseases that result in progressive ataxia is notoriously challenging, but can be thought of as comprising three broad groups— the *spinocerebellar ataxias* with involvement of the cerebellum and spinal cord, *"pure" cerebellar ataxias* without other involvement of other neurologic structures, and the *complicated cerebellar ataxias* involving multiple other structures (Ropper & Brown, 2005).

Friedreich's ataxia (FRDA) is an example of one of the spinocerebellar ataxias and is probably the most frequently occurring of the forms of hereditary ataxia (Wilmot & Subramony, 2004). Onset is almost always before the 25th year of life and ataxia of gait is typically the initial symptom of neurologic disease. With disease progression, symptoms include progressive ataxia of the limbs and trunk, dysarthria (usually within five years of onset), lower limb areflexia, and sensory changes, such as loss of joint position and vibratory sense (Harding, 1981; Wilmont & Subramony, 2004). A number of other hereditary spinocerebellar ataxias have been identified.

"Pure" cerebellar ataxias without associated neurologic disease may also be encountered. *Holmes-type ataxia* is the prototype of pure cerebellar degeneration and both hereditary and sporadic cases have been described. Clinical features include an insidious onset in the fourth or fifth decade with a slow progression of symptoms, an ataxic gait, trunk instability, a hand and head tremor, and dysarthria (Ropper & Brown, 2005).

Complicated cerebellar ataxias combining cerebellar atrophy with changes in other structures have also been described, such as in OPCA (see the section on MSA). Other examples of complicated cerebellar ataxias combine cerebellar atrophy with involvement of the basal ganglia, such as encountered in *Machado-Joseph-Azorean disease* and MSA-C (Ropper & Brown, 2005).

Dysarthria occurs frequently in the forms of progressive ataxias and, not surprisingly, ataxic dysarthria is the dysarthria type most frequently described in these patients. Mixed dysarthria may also be encountered when neurologic involvement is not restricted to the cerebellum (Duffy, 2005). Dysphagia in patients with ataxia has received surprisingly little systematic attention, although dysphagia has been reported with a variety of the progressive ataxias (Arpa, Cuesta, Cruz-Martinez, Santiago, Sarria, & Palau, 1999; Baba, Uitti, Farrer, & Wszolek, 2005; Jardim et al., 2001; Rub et al., 2003). Although dysphagia appears to occur less often than dysarthria with progressive ataxia, oropharyngeal dysphagia has been described including premature spillage of the bolus, piecemeal deglutition, pharyngeal residue, and aspiration (Nagaya, Kachi, Yamada, & Sumi, 2004). A likely explanation for dysphagic signs in syndromes of progressive ataxia is discoordination of oral, pharyngeal, and respiratory movements

Syndromes of Muscular Weakness and Wasting Without Sensory Changes

Motor neuron disease (MND)/amyotrophic lateral sclerosis (ALS) is a progressive degenerative disorder of motor neurons in the spinal cord, brainstem, and cortex (Ropper & Brown, 2005). Understanding that the disease can begin by involving only the spinal (arms, legs, trunk, including respiratory muscles) or bulbar (jaw, face, tongue, palate, pharynx, larynx) musculature is critical to understanding why patients can differ from one another. They also differ according to whether the site of involvement is to upper motor neurons (neurons that are above the brainstem or spinal cord) or lower motor neuron (neurons of the brainstem or spine). Some reserve the term ALS for the condition in which there is upper and lower motor neuron involvement affecting both spinal and bulbar musculature. These experts would argue that MND should be the generic name for these various combinations. Additional subtypes include *primary lateral sclerosis* in which involvement is restricted primarily to upper motor neurons and *spinal musculature atrophy* in which the involvement is primarily of the lower motor neurons, especially of the spinal system. In this system of nomenclature, both upper and lower motor neuron involvement of the bulbar system is called *progressive bulbar palsy*. For the introductory reader, the most important consideration when considering swallowing disorders in MND is that persons may be seen at the time they have either primarily or exclusively spinal or bulbar involvement. In addition, a portion of such persons may have an accompanying dementia that potentially complicates both diagnosis and treatment.

Disordered swallowing is a major complication in MND for the vast majority of patients and tube feeding is necessary if safe and adequate nutrition and hydration are to be maintained. Even for tube-fed patients, however, aspiration and its consequences are a major cause of death, and tube feeding has been found to be associated with a median survival rate of 185 days (Chio, Finocchiaro, Meineri, Bottacchi, & Schiffer, 1999). The signs of dysphagia have been reported by multiple authors (Briani et al., 1998; Kawai et al., 2003; Robbins, 1987). However, the majority of such studies provide only one examination of swallowing so that the pattern of decline in swallowing must be pieced together from this literature, from clinical experience, and from a small number of studies in which patients were followed over time. Nonetheless, certain central tendencies emerge from the literature. First, substantial differences in onset and course of signs exist among patients. Dysphagia can occur early or somewhat later and can progress rapidly or slowly. Second, swallow decline mirrors speech decline in the majority of patients (Strand, Miller, Yorkston, & Hillel, 1996; Yorkston, Miller, & Strand, 1995). Third, dysphagia appears to occur earlier and increase more rapidly in females than males. Fourth, signs of oral stage involvement such as escape of food or liquid from the mouth, difficulty chewing, and decreased ability to move a bolus posteriorly to initiate the pharyngeal stage of swallowing, often occur earlier than do pharyngeal signs. Indeed, Robbins (1987) posits that oral stage abnormalities may lead to the appearance of pharyngeal abnormality early in the disease. She reasons that abnormal propulsion of material from the mouth into the pharynx may result in postswallow pharyngeal residue that can subsequently be aspirated. Fifth, pharyngeal signs including pharyngeal residue remaining after the swallow and penetration and aspiration inevitably occur in the course of the disease. However, it may be that not all pharyngeal signs appear simultaneously. Ertekin and colleagues suggest that elevation of the hyolaryngeal complex and opening of the UES may be relatively well preserved until later in the disease's course despite the appearance of other pharyngeal signs such as residue (Ertekin, Aydogdu, Yuceyar, et al., 2000). Sixth, the early onset of speech and swallowing abnormalities, especially if the person is also older and suffering from breathing difficulties because of weak respiratory muscles, is a negative prognostic sign. In other words, such patients are likely to live less long than persons without this cluster of abnormalities. Seventh, respiratory status is very often compromised in this group and this compromise is as important as the decline in bulbar swallowing structures. Safe swallowing requires an apneic or breath-holding period while material is being swallowed. A person with inadequate respiration may not be able to stop breathing long enough to swallow safely or may have difficulty coordinating respiration and swallowing movements. Either condition can put a person at risk for aspiration. Therefore, when evaluating and treating dysphagia in MND/ALS, clinicians must be very attentive to the person's breathing.

It is traditional to expect that the speech of a person with MND will be a mixed dysarthria with spastic (increased tone) and flaccid (decreased tone) components. That expectation is not present in dysphagia. Rather the assumption is usually that the dysphagia results from weakness. This assumption is in need of testing. We are not aware of any attempt to differentiate swallowing patterns in the various subtypes of MND. One might hypothesize that patterns would differ in those whose bulbar muscles are primarily or exclusively weak and hypotonic when compared to those who are primarily or exclusively weak and hypertonic.

No medical treatment of known efficacy is available for MND. Similarly no data confirm the efficacy of medical, surgical, or behavioral treatments for dysphagia in MND and most efforts are directed toward palliation or helping the person make the best use of whatever ability remains. A common reason for suggesting a feeding tube is respiratory system decline. Yorkston, Miller, and Strand (1995) recommend that respiratory status be monitored closely when decisions about tube feeding are being considered due to increased surgical risk in patients with poor respiratory sup-

port. These authors suggest that patients with patients with a vital capacity between 1.0 and 1.5 liters are "marginal" candidates for surgical procedures, whereas those with a vital capacity of less than 1.0 liter are generally considered "poor" surgical candidates. Yorkston et al. (1995) further suggest that placement of a feeding tube may be recommended "prior to the time when it is mandatory in terms of swallowing function (because) such surgery needs to be carried out before poor respiratory status makes the surgical risks too high" (p. 59). SLPs often recommend soft and even pureed foods and thickened liquids to keep individuals with MND/ALS eating at least something by mouth for as long as possible. Exercises are usually discouraged in MND and instead conserving strength for critical eating and swallowing activities is recommended.

Craniocerebral Trauma

Traumatic brain injury (TBI) is a frequent cause of neurologic deficits, especially in the young. Severity of injury varies from patient to patient, as do the signs and symptoms. Dysphagia occurs in as many as one-third overall and in a higher percentage of those with moderate or severe trauma, especially when first admitted into a trauma care unit. In these cases, coma is common and may last from hours to weeks. During this period, patients may also often have a tracheostomy, a surgically prepared hole in the neck into which is inserted a breathing tube connected to a ventilator for respiratory support. During this time, feeding is via a tube, usually inserted into the patient's stomach. Such patients may or may not be able to swallow their saliva during this period. Swallowing, however, is not the care team's paramount concern during this period, but identifying the presence of dysphagia can be critical to long-term planning (Mackay, Morgan, & Bernstein, 1999). Establishing swallowing integrity is especially critical when patients emerge from coma and begin breathing independently (not that these two things occur simultaneously, however). A major reason for this interest, of course, is to establish the person's ability to swallow so that oral nutrition or swallowing treatment can begin. Another reason is prognostic. Dysphagia is associated with how long a person is likely to be hospitalized (Morgan, Ward, Murdoch, Kennedy, & Murison, 2003) and with time to begin oral nutrition (Mackay, Morgan, & Bernstein, 1999). It has also been demonstrated that dysphagia is predictive of the need for assistance with eating (Duong, Englander, Wright, Cifu, Greenwald, & Brown, 2004) and of long-term functional ability (Halper, Cherney, Cichowski, & Zhang, 1999). Finally, it is important to remember that dysphagia often occurs in the context of other, sometimes severe, physical and cognitive impairments, and that substantial differences can characterize individuals with TBI.

A number of studies report the major signs of dysphagia in TBI in children and adults. Morgan, Ward, Murdoch, and Bilbie (2002) studied 18 children. The signs they identified included poor bolus formation and movement, delayed initiation of the swallow, aspiration, and reduced movement of the bolus through the pharynx resulting in substantial residuals after the swallow was completed. Subsequently data from the same laboratory (Morgan, Ward, Murdoch, Kennedy, & Murison, 2003) on 1,145 children with TBI provided a profile of swallowing incidence, severity, and signs. Only 5.3% of these children had dysphagia but the incidence was 68% for those with severe head injury. Again, signs of dysphagia were similar to those

reported in the earlier study. This study had the additional benefit of providing data on which children are likely to have difficulty swallowing. Predictors include score on the Glasgow Coma Scale (GCS) at time of admission. The GCS measures individuals' best eye response, best verbal response, and motor response. Not surprisingly, a low score suggestive of a greater severity of damage is related to presence and severity of swallowing impairment. Signs are similar for adults. Mackay, Morgan, and Bernstein (1999) report that what they call loss of bolus control and reduced lingual control were the most frequent signs, followed by decreased tongue base retraction, a delay in the initiation of the pharyngeal swallow, and reduced laryngeal closure leading to aspiration. Lazarus and Logemann (1987) report similar signs. In their study, delayed initiation of the swallow was the most frequent sign, followed by poor bolus control.

Dysphagia occurs in patients with TBI for a multitude of reasons. A somewhat older study (Winstein, 1983) identified cognitive changes as a major contributor, and the importance of impaired cognition has been confirmed more recently by other researchers (Halper et al., 1999). Cognitive impairment can explain the oral stage abnormalities in this population because the oral stage is the most volitional of all the swallowing stages. Another contributor to oral stage abnormalities in some persons is damage to facial structures that may occur in an accident. Mackay, Morgan, and Bernstein (1999) also implicate sensory, strength, and tone deficits as explanations for oral and pharyngeal deficits. Perhaps the most complete list of the variables that may explain dysphagia is provided by Morgan, Ward, and Murdoch (2004). They cite cognitive impairment, behavioral abnormalities, tone and posture deficits, and "oral sensitivity issues." A final influence on some patients is the presence of a tracheostomy. The alterations in sensation and swallowing pressures that result may also influence swallowing, although this remains a controversial subject.

Treatment for dysphagia in TBI usually involves a team. In the period right after injury, depending on a person's level of consciousness, the emphasis will likely be on tube feeding. During this period, the emphasis is also on preventing or controlling pulmonary infections to which intubated and ventilator-dependent persons are prone. As soon as the medical team deems it appropriate, a swallowing evaluation to determine the presence, severity, and signs of dysphagia is warranted, along with ongoing assessments of cognitive and general functional status. If an individual has no or only a minor dysphagia, the emphasis may well be on providing the opportunity for the person to begin switching from tube to oral nutrition. Behavioral problems secondary to impaired memory and attention and agitation may well complicate this effort. The dysphagic person will require a focused rehabilitative effort from the SLP. Special food and liquid preparations such as pureed food and thickened liquids may be recommended after the swallowing evaluation. In addition, recommendations about bolus size, rate of feeding, and special positioning such as a chin tuck may be made. As a person has the ability to attend and cooperate, more direct rehabilitative approaches, such as muscle strengthening, may be introduced. All such procedures occur in the context of aggressive pulmonary, occupational, and physical therapy, cognitive rehabilitation, and nursing care to maximize rehabilitation.

Intracranial Neoplasms

Intracranial neoplasms are masses or tumors that can invade or grow in any part of the body, including the nervous system. They can be benign which means they are self-contained and do not spread into other areas (metastasize), or they can be cancerous in which case they may not only grow but also spread into other areas of the body. A cancerous tumor in the lung, for example, may metastasize to the central nervous system. Like strokes, tumors produce dysphagia if they are located in those parts of the nervous system important to swallowing. The dysphagia following stroke is usually most severe in the immediate poststroke period and then either stabilizes or more likely improves. The effects of tumors are different. First, if a tumor occurs in a part of the nervous system important to swallowing, dysphagia may be the first sign of illness and the signs of dysphagia will often worsen until the tumor is identified and treated. Surgery and/or radiation treatments are the treatments of choice. Even if these treatments are successful in removing the tumor, however, they may fail to restore the nervous system to normal and may even cause additional damage to critical tissues. In these cases, dysphagia may persist or worsen.

The signs of dysphagia resulting from tumors depend, in part, on where the tumor is located. Overall, cognitive deficits in such abilities as memory and attention are the most frequent results of nervous system tumor, especially in adults. Swallowing disorders can occur, however (Mukand, Blackinton, Crincoli, Lee, & Santos, 2001). In children, brainstem and cerebellar masses are more frequent locations for tumor than in adults (Siffert et al., 2000) and dysphagia is a frequent sign.

More specifically, as in brainstem stroke, brainstem tumors may result in Wallenberg's syndrome, including dysphagia in which laryngeal valving to protect the airway is reduced as is opening of the upper esophageal sphincter. This syndrome may be present prior to the diagnosis and persist after surgical treatment. This possibility prompted Wesling and colleagues (2003) to recommend that aggressive swallowing rehabilitation be initiated just as it is in stroke. Cerebellar tumors and their surgical management often produce a specific syndrome of mutism or inability to speak. This syndrome may (Siffert et al., 2000) or may not be accompanied by dysphagia (al-Jarallah, Cook, Gascon, Kanaan, & Sigueira, 1994). Breathing can be a special problem for such children, further complicating the swallowing difficulty (Chen et al., 2005). The resulting swallowing problems can involve both the oral and pharyngeal stages of swallowing (Cornwell, Murdoch, Ward, & Morgan, 2003) and both presurgical counseling of children and their parents and postsurgery treatment are recommended (Kirk, Howard, & Scott, 1995). One especially interesting observation about dysphagia in brain tumor patients is that they may have much more severe swallowing disorders than one would expect from their self-reports, making formal swallowing examination especially critical (Newton, Newton, Pearl, & Davidson, 1994). Finally, dysphagia following tumors involving the brainstem and cerebellum are often very severe (Prosiegel, Holing, Heintze, Wagner-Sonntag, & Wiseman, 2005a, 2005b) and may be more severe than in stroke, perhaps because involvement is more likely to be bilateral in cases of tumor. As in stroke, the presumed reasons for the dysphagia are weakness, abnormal tone, and discoordination.

Demyelinating Disorders

Multiple sclerosis (MS) is a progressive disease characterized by demyelination of nerve fibers in the brain and spinal cord that results in neurologic deficits. MS is most frequently diagnosed in young to middle-aged adults and often has a remitting and relapsing course (Yorkston, Miller, & Strand, 1995). Dysarthria occurs in 40 to 50% of individuals with MS. Dysarthria types associated most frequently with MS include ataxic and spastic dysarthria, often in combination to form a mixed dysarthria (Duffy, 2005; Yorkston, Miller, & Strand, 1995).

Dysphagia in people with MS appears to occur in at least one-third of cases, though patients often do not complain about difficulty swallowing (Calcagno, Ruoppolo, Grasso, De Vincentiis, & Paolucci, 2002; Prosiegel, Schelling, & Wagner-Sonntag, 2004; Thomas & Wiles, 1999). Pharyngeal stage deficits occur much more frequently than oral stage deficits (Calcagno et al., 2002). Patients with brainstem involvement show an increased risk of dysphagia (Calcagno et al., 2002; Thomas & Wiles, 1999) and patients who are nonambulatory may have an increased risk for dysphagia in comparison to ambulatory patients (Calcagno et al., 2002).

Although dysphagia may be under reported by patients, the high frequency of dysphagia suggests the value of a comprehensive evaluation of swallowing in patients with MS. Furthermore, Calcagno and colleagues (2002) reported that compensatory swallowing strategies as determined with FEES, such as postural changes or diet modifications, were sufficient to improve swallowing function in most of their patients. Weisner et al. (2002) suggested dysphagia should be regarded as a serious problem even in the early stages of MS and recommend the use of video-fluoroscopy for provision of specific swallowing recommendations (Weisner et al., 2002).

Disorders of the Neuromuscular Junction

Myasthenia gravis (MG) is an autoimmune disease of the neuromuscular junction. The main symptom of MG is a fluctuating muscular weakness, particularly of the bulbar and ocular muscles. Eye and facial movements, swallowing, and speech are involved in up to 80% of cases (Ropper & Brown, 2005). Between 6 to 24% of patients with MG may have oropharyngeal dysphagia as their presenting symptom due to bulbar weakness (Emilia-Romagna Study Group, 1998; Grob, Arsura, Brunner, & Namba, 1987) and dysphagia may also be the only symptom of MG (Llabrés, Molina-Martinez, & Miralles, 2005). Speech is also frequently affected in MG and the dysarthria type associated with MG is flaccid dysarthria due to lower motor neuron involvement (Duffy, 2005).

Colton-Hudson and colleagues (2002; Koopman et al., 2004) investigated oropharyngeal swallow function in 20 patients with MG and dysphagia. Oral phase dysphagia was relatively mild, whereas pharyngeal dysphagia was more severely involved in this group. All 20 patients were found to have a delay in the initiation of the pharyngeal swallow. Aspiration was seen in seven patients and it usually occurred without a cough reflex from the patient. Penetration reportedly occurred much more frequently (Colton-Hudson et al., 2002; Koopman et al., 2004). Kluin and colleagues (1996) also reported on eight men with MG and prominent pharyngeal dysphagia, including reduced pharyngeal motility, penetration, and silent aspiration. Esophageal dysphagia has also been reported in patients with MG (Huang, King, & Chien, 1998; Linke, Witt, & Tatsch, 2003).

Dysphagia evaluation may be particularly critical for patients with MG due to the role of dysphagia in myasthenic crises. A myasthenic crisis can occur in a matter of hours and can result in respiratory failure and quadriparesis. Oropharyngeal dysphagia and aspiration pneumonia are often implicated in a myasthenic crisis (Ropper & Brown, 2005; Thomas et al., 1997). Clearly, the need for the careful assessment and management of swallowing can be critical in patients with MG.

Diseases of Peripheral Nerves

Guillain-Barré syndrome (GBS) is progressive disease of acute onset that is one of the most common causes of acute or subacute paralysis. The first symptoms are often paresthesias and numbness in the toes and fingers. A primary symptom of progressive muscular weakness due to demyelization develops over days and weeks. Weakness evolves to include the muscles of the proximal and distal legs and arms, the trunk, neck, and cranial nerves (Ropper & Brown, 2005). In a few cases, muscle weakness results in total paralysis with respiratory failure. Recovery is sporadic and can occur over weeks and months. Some residual weakness may persist.

With cranial nerve involvement in patients with GBS, dysarthria and dysphagia often occur. Involvement of the facial and oropharyngeal muscles with consequent dysarthria and dysphagia may occur in 50% of cases. The dysarthria associated with GBS is a flaccid type (Duffy, 2005).

The pattern of swallowing abnormalities encountered in GBS has not been well described. Chen and colleagues (1996) report both oral and pharyngeal stage dysphagia, with greater severity for pharyngeal involvement. Dysphagia often improves during the recovery period, but dysphagia may persist, particularly in severe cases. Follow-up assessment of swallowing during the recovery period approximately four to eight weeks after the onset of symptoms has been recommended (Chen, Donofrio, Frederick, Ott, & Pikna, 1996).

Inflammatory Myopathies

Polymyositis (PM) and *dermatomyositis (DM)* are idiopathic inflammatory muscle diseases. PM is characterized principally by proximal limb and trunk weakness. DM presents with a similar pattern of muscle weakness with the addition of a rash (Ropper & Brown, 2005; Scola, Werneck, Prevedello, Toderke, & Iwamoto, 2000). The muscles of the trunk, shoulders, hips, upper arms, and thighs are often involved initially. Pharyngeal, striated esophageal, and laryngeal muscles may also be involved, and, less often, the jaw, tongue, and facial muscles may be affected (Ropper & Brown, 2005). Not surprisingly, PM and DM are often associated with a flaccid dysarthria and, more frequently, dysphagia (Chwalinska-Sadowska & Maldykowa,1990; Ertekin, Secil, Yuceyar, & Aydogdu, 2004). The prevalence of dysphagia in these groups has been found to be over 50% (Chwalinska-Sadowska & Maldykowa, 1990; Wang, Lin, Hsu, Kao, Chang, & Lau, 1993) and swallowing difficulty occurs more often frequently in patients with DM than in patients with PM (Chwalinska-Sadowska & Maldykowa, 1990; Scola et al., 2000).

The oropharyngeal swallowing difficulties seen in PM/DM have not been well described, but appear to be primarily due to weakness of the striated muscles of the pharynx (Ertekin, Secil, Yuceyar, & Aydogdu, 2004). Sonies (1997) reported that tongue weakness and are often the first signs of dysphagia. *Xerostomia* (decreased salivation) is another frequent complaint (Willig, Paulus, Lacau Saint Guily, Béon, & Navarro, 1994). Esophageal dysphagia also occurs frequently in PM/DM and cricopharyngeal muscle obstruction with esophageal dysmotility has been described as the most frequent cause of dysphagia in these patients. Corticosteroids are often used to treat PM/DM (Ropper & Brown, 2005) and these medications have been described as having a beneficial effect on pharyngeal and esophageal functioning. Cricopharyngeal myotomy has also been reported to be a beneficial surgical technique in some individuals with PM/DM (Sonies, 1997).

Inclusion-body myositis (IBM) is the third major type of inflammatory myopathy (Ropper & Brown, 2005). In contrast to PM/DM, IBM is associated with primarily distal muscle weakness, most frequently of the quadriceps, wrist or finger flexors, and/or pharyngeal muscles (Badrising et al., 2005; Christopher-Stine & Plotz, 2004; Ropper & Brown, 2005). Other distinguishing characteristics of IBM versus PM/DM are the frequent occurrence of facial weakness (Badrising et al., 2005; Christopher-Stine & Plotz, 2004) and lack of response to corticosteroids in patients with IBM (Ropper & Brown, 2005).

Dysphagia occurs frequently in IBM, with patients subjectively reporting dysphagia in up to 66 to 80% of cases (Badrising et al., 2005; Houser, Calabrese, & Strome, 1998) Dysphagia may also be the presenting symptom of neurologic disease (Badrising et al., 2005). The nature of swallowing difficulties in IBM has not been studied systematically but has been hypothesized to be primarily pharyngeal in nature (Houser, Calabrese, & Strome, 1998).

Developmental Disorders of the Nervous System

Cerebral palsy (CP) is the name given to a variety of neurologically based sensorimotor disorders present at birth. Considerable heterogeneity exists within the population of children diagnosed with CP. In part the heterogeneity is accounted for by the primary neurologic deficit, whether it is spasticity, flaccidity, *athetosis* (slow, writhing movements), or some combination. These children also differ in their other abnormalities. Some may have mental retardation, some not; some may have learning disabilities, some not; some may be severe, others may have only mild or moderate motor problems; some may have speech problems, some may not.

The proportion of CP infants and children with swallowing problems is difficult to know with surety. Reilly, Skuse, and Poblete (1996) identified what they called clinically significant oral motor, including eating problems, in 49 children with CP, 12 to 72 months of age. Rogers and colleagues (1994) completed VFSE with 90 children with CP and identified the full range of oral and pharyngeal stage abnormalities in nearly all the participants; 80% had to be fed by another person. One especially alarming statistic was that when these children aspirated, 97% of them did so silently. In other words, they did not cough or otherwise show signs of having aspirated. It is important to note that these were children already identified as probably having swallowing difficulty. This raises the issue of how such individuals can be identified early. Interestingly, how

well an infant sucks may not be a predictor of later swallowing problems (Selley et al., 2001). Drooling (Senner, Logemann, Zecker, & Gaebler-Spira, 2004) and poor oral motor skills with activities such as eating from a spoon and chewing may be a predictor of dysphagia (Gisel, Applegate-Ferrante, Benson, & Bosma, 1996). Both impaired oral motor ability (Gisel et al., 1996) and reduced pharyngeal coordination may predict aspiration specifically. The search for easily observable signs of dysphagia and predictors of aspiration is especially critical in infants and children because VFSE and the attendant radiation exposure are of special concern for children with years of life ahead of them (Cockerill & Carroll-Few, 2001).

Children with CP present special challenges for the speech pathologist. First, a very high proportion of CP children have what is known as gastroesophageal reflex disease (GERD) (Chong, 2001; Del Giudice et al., 1999) in which food and liquid do not pass into the esophagus and stomach and stay there but instead return up the esophagus and into the pharynx and sometimes into the mouth. Although GERD is also encountered frequently in adults, the results can be more tragic for children, including as they do reluctance or refusal to eat. In addition, many children with CP, unlike adults who acquire a neurologic disease later in life, do not develop normal eating. Therefore, the swallowing problem in a child is often an eating/swallowing problem and management is of necessity a matter of influencing both eating and swallowing. Furthermore, because infant development depends so heavily on adequate nutrition, decisions about tube feeding (Brant, Stanich, & Ferrari, 1999) are especially critical and a dysphagia team is more likely to recommend a period of tube feeding in a child with

CP than in an adult with one of a variety of acquired neurologic disorders. Such a recommendation often requires special counseling about the health benefits and potential that the tube will not be necessary for a lifetime (Craig, Scambler, & Spitz, 2003). The treatment of dysphagic CP children is often even more interdisciplinary and directed at a wider variety of targets than is rehabilitation with adults. Feeding and not merely swallowing is an emphasis (Parrott et al., 1992) and because posture is so often abnormal in CP children, postural adjustment and training is often a first treatment step (Redstone & West, 2004). Mechanisms of dysphagia are not yet specified in CP. What is known is that successful evaluation and treatment require attention to motor, cognitive, developmental, and behavioral strengths and weaknesses. A lone SLP has little chance of success.

Treatment of Oropharyngeal Dysphagia

Dysphagia treatment developed nearly independently of medical diagnosis. Instead, the emphasis has been and continues to be on identifying the signs and the underlying abnormal physiology as guides for treatment. This approach is best understood by example. In typical practice, if aspiration is observed on VFSE, the clinician first notes whether it occurred before, during, or after the swallow. Next, a biomechanical explanation to the dysphagia is created based on the movements of the bolus and the swallowing structures during the aspiration episode. Delayed initiation of the swallow is often identified as the reason for aspiration before the swallow. Similarly, inadequate laryngeal closure

is often hypothesized to be the reason for aspiration during the swallow. Residual material remaining in the pharynx after the swallow is often identified as the reason for postswallow aspiration. As in dysarthria, many clinicians also speculate about the contribution of assumed weakness, abnormal tone, or discoordination to the observed pattern, but such speculations have never been verified experimentally. The clinician next selects a method to treat a swallow delay, poor laryngeal closure, or large residuals and sometimes the selection is motivated by the clinician's hypothesis about strength, tone, and coordination and sometimes it is not. In most clinical practice, these methods are the same regardless of whether the patient has PD, stroke, or some other neurologic disease.

A relatively recent development is the attempt to identify the influence of particular therapeutic approaches on the swallowing of certain populations. Perhaps the best examples are the use of expiratory muscle strength training (EMST) (Kim & Sapienza, 2005) and the Lee Silverman Voice Treatment (LSVT) (Sharkawi et al., 2002) as management approaches for the dysphagia of PD. Early results are promising. However, there is no expectation that dysphagia in PD will be the only pattern of dysphagia modifiable by these methods, just as LSVT, for example, is not limited to use with hypokinetic dysarthria. Indeed, the present trend of drawing from a large array of treatments regardless of the neurologic disease will doubtless continue.

Future Directions

A large-scale research effort patterned after the work of Darley, Aronson, and Brown (1969a, 1969b, 1975) will be required if specific dysphagia syndromes are to be identified. The contributions and future of the Darley, Aronson, and Brown classification system of speech disorders was reviewed by Kent and colleagues (Kent, Kent, Duffy, & Weismer, 1998). Similarly, there will be benefits to such an effort in dysphagia, one of which would be to increase the power of swallowing evaluations to aid differential diagnosis. A second benefit would be that such a system could guide sophisticated kinematic or movement analysis as a basis for enhanced understanding of why certain patterns of abnormality occur. A third benefit would be that such a system and the science it engenders could provide a basis for more specific evaluation and treatment planning. In the absence of such a monumental effort, the literature in neurogenic dysphagia will continue to develop steadily but haphazardly. But even if such a study is undertaken, students will still be required to do what Ray Kent has done for decades: they will need to read widely and carefully, they will need to think creatively, and they will need to remain humble. Dysphagia, like dysarthria, represents the involvement of one of humankind's most complex and important abilities. Neither readily gives up its secrets. Kent has spent a career in search of those secrets. Among many other things, this volume is a testament to his successes.

Acknowledgments. The authors would like to thank the many individuals who helped make this chapter possible. Thank you to Nan Musson (Malcolm Randall VAMC) and Joe Murray (Ann Arbor VAMC) for sharing many of the illustrations from their CD titled "Understanding Dysphagia" (1.0). This CD is available by contacting the North Florida Foundation for Research and Education, Inc., c/o Joy Mitchell, CCRC, CCRA, Executive Director, North Florida/ South Georgia Veterans Health System, 1601 SW Archer Rd. (151), Gainesville, FL 32608, Telephone (352) 376-1611, extension 5832, Fax (352) 379-4102. Greg Westlye and John Richardson of the Medical Media Department and Neal Musson of the VA Brain Rehabilitation Research Center (BRRC) at the Malcolm Randall VAMC were all instrumental in preparing the illustrations and images in this chapter for publication and we are grateful for their assistance. Many thanks also to Marilyn Gresser and the staff at the Malcolm Randall VAMC Medical Library for their research assistance. We are also grateful to Christine Joyner of the University of Florida's Department of Communicative Disorders for her administrative assistance. Finally, both authors would like to thank the BRRC at the Malcolm Randall VAMC in Gainesville, FL and the Department of Communication Disorders at the University of Florida for their support. Mr. Jones was supported in part by a Speech Pathology Pre-Doctoral Traineeship at the BRRC, Malcolm Randall VAMC.

References

Adams, R. D., & Victor, M. (1991). *Principles of neurology companion handbook* (4th ed.). New York: McGraw-Hill.

Albanese, A., Barnes, M. B., Bhatia, K. P., Fernandez-Albareze, E., Filippini, G., Gasser, T., et al. (2006). A systematic review on the diagnosis and treatment of primary (idiopathic) dystonia and dystonia plus syndromes: Reports an ESNS/MDS-ES task force. *European Journal of Neurology, 13*, 433–444.

al-Jarallah, A., Cook, J. D., Gascon, G., Kanaan, I., & Sigueira, E. (1994). Transient mutism following posterior fossa surgery in children. *Journal of Surgical Oncology, 55*, 126–131.

Arpa, J., Cuesta, A., Cruz-Martinez, A. Santiago, S., Sarria, J., & Palau, F. (1999). Clinical features in genetic analysis of a Spanish family with spinal cerebellar ataxia 6. *Acta Neurologica Scandinavica, 99*, 43-47.

Aviv, J. E., Kim, T., Sacco, R. L., Kaplin, S., Goodhart, K., Diamond, B., et al. (1998). FEESST: A new bedside endoscopic test of the motor and sensory components of swallowing. *Annals of Otology, Rhinology, and Laryngology, 107*, 378-387.

Aviv, J. E., Murry, T., Zschommler, A., Cohen, M., & Gartner, C. (2005). Flexible endoscopic evaluation of swallowing with sensory testing: Patient characteristics and analysis of safety in 1,340 consecutive examinations. *Annals of Otology, Rhinology, and Laryngology, 114*, 173-176.

Aydogdu, I., Ertekin, C., Tarlaci, S., Turman, B., Kiyliouglu, N., & Secil, Y. (2001). Dysphagia in lateral medullary infarction (Wallenberg's syndrome): An acute disconnection syndrome in premotor neurons related to swallowing activity. *Stroke, 32*, 2081-2087.

Baba, Y., Uitti, R. J., Farrer, M. J., & Wszolek, Z. K. (2005). Sporadic SCA 8 mutation resembling corticobasal degeneration. *Parkinsonism and Related Disorders, 11*, 147-150.

Badrising, U. A., Maat-Schieman, M. L. C., van Houwelingen, J. C., van Doorn, P. A., van Duinen, S. G., van Engelen, B. G. M., et al. (2005). Inclusion body myositis: Clinical features and clinical course of the disease in 64 patients. *Journal of Neurology, 252*, 1448-1454.

Berciano, J. (1982). Olivopontocerebellar atrophy: A review of 117 cases. *Journal of the Neurological Sciences, 53*, 253-272.

Brant, C. Q., Stanich, P., & Ferrari, A. P. Jr. (1999). Improvement of children's nutritional status after enteral feeding by PEG: An interim report. *Gastrointestinal Endoscopy, 50*, 183-188.

Briani, C., Marcon, N., Ermani, M., Costantini, M., Bottin, R., Iurilli, V., et al. (1998). Radiological evidence of subclinical dysphagia in motor neuron disease. *Journal of Neurology, 245*, 211-216.

Calcagno, P., Ruoppolo, G., Grasso, M. G., De Vincentiis, M., & Paolucci, S. (2002). Dysphagia in multiple sclerosis—Prevalence and prognostic factors. *Acta Neurologica Scandinavica, 105*, 40-43.

Castell, J. A., Johnston, B. T., Colcher, A., Li, Q., Gideon, R. M., & Castell, D. L. (2001). Manometric abnormalities of the esophagus in patients with Parkinson's disease. *Neurogastroenterology and Motility, 13*, 361-364.

Cersosimo, M. G., Juri, S., Suarez de Chandler, S., Clerici, R., & Micheli, S. E. (2005). Swallowing disorders in patients with blepharospasm. *Medicina, 65*, 117-120.

Charles, P. D., Davis, T. L., Shannon, K. M., Hook, M. A., & Warner, J. S. (1997). Tongue protrusion dystonia: Treatment with Botulinum toxin. *Southern Medical Journal, 90*, 522-526.

Chen, M. Y. M., Donofrio, T. V., Frederick, M. G., Ott, D. J., & Pikna, L. A. (1996). Videofluoroscopic evaluation of patients with Guillain-Barré syndrome. *Dysphagia, 11*, 11-13.

Chen, M. L., Witmans, M. B., Tablizo, M. A., Jubran, R. F., Turkel, S. B., Tavare, C. J., et al. (2005). Disordered respiratory control in children with partial cerebellar resections. *Pediatric Pulmonology, 40*, 88-91.

Chio, A., Finocchiaro, E., Meineri, P., Bottacchi, E., & Schiffer, D. (1999). Safety and factors related to survival percutaneous endoscopic gastrostomy and ALS. *Neurology, 53*, 1123-1125.

Chong, S. K. (2001). Gastrointestinal problems in the handicapped child. *Current Opinion in Pediatrics, 13*, 441-446.

Chouinard, J. (2000). Dysphagia in Alzheimer disease: A review. *Journal of Nutrition, Health and Aging, 4*, 214-217.

Christopher-Stine, L., & Plotz, P. H. (2004). Adult inflammatory myopathies. *Best Practice and Research Clinical Rheumatology, 18*, 331-344.

Chwalinska-Sadowska, H., & Maldykowa, H. (1990). Polymyositis-dermatomyositis—a 25-year follow-up of 50 patients (analysis of clinical symptoms and signs and results of laboratory test). *Materia Medica Polona*, *22*, 205-212.

Cockerill, H., & Carroll-Few, L. (2001). Non-invasive technique for assessment and management planning of oral-pharyngeal dysphagia in children with cerebral palsy. *Developmental Medicine and Child Neurology*, *42*, 429-430.

Colodny, N. (2002). Interjudge and intrajudge reliabilities in fiberoptic endoscopic evaluation of swallowing (FEES) using the penetration-aspiration scale: A replication study. *Dysphagia*, *17*, 308-315.

Colton-Hudson, A., Koopman, W. J., Moosa, T., Smith, D., Bach, D., & Nicolle, M. (2002). A prospective assessment of the characteristics of dysphagia in myasthenia gravis. *Dysphagia*, *17*, 147-151.

Corbin-Lewis, J. M., Liss, J. M., & Sciortino, K. L. (2004). *Clinical anatomy and physiology of the swallowing mechanism*. Clifton Park, NY: Thomson Delmar Learning.

Cornwell, P. L., Murdoch, B. E., Ward, E. C., & Morgan, A. (2003). Dysarthria and dysphagia as long-term sequelae in a child treated for posterior fossa tumour. *Pediatric Rehabilitation*, *6*, 67-75.

Craig, G. M., Scambler, G., & Spitz, L. (2003). Why parents of children with neurodevelopmental disabilities requiring gastrostomy feeding need more support. *Developmental Medicine and Child Neurology*, *45*, 183-188.

Daniels S. K., & Foundas, A. L. (1999). Lesion localization in acute stroke patients with risk of aspiration. *Journal of Neuroimaging*, *9*, 91-98.

Darley, F. L., Aronson, A. E., & Brown, J. R. (1969a). Cluster of deviant speech dimensions in the dysarthrias. *Journal of Speech and Hearing Research*, *12*, 462-496.

Darley, F. L., Aronson, A. E., & Brown, J. R. (1969b). Differential diagnostic patterns of dysarthria. *Journal of Speech and Hearing Research*, *12*, 249-269.

Darley, S. L., Aronson, A. E., & Brown, J. R. (1975). *Motor speech disorders*. Philadelphia: W. B. Saunders.

Del Giudice, E., Staiano, A., Capano, G., Romano, A., Florimonte, L., Miele, E., et al. (1999). Gastrointestinal manifestations in children with cerebral palsy. *Brain Development*, *21*, 307-311.

Diroma, C., Del'Aquila, C., Fraddosci, A., Lamberti, S., Masternardi, R., Russo, I., et al. (2003). Natural history and clinical features of progressive supranuclear palsy: A clinical study. *Neurological Sciences*, *24*, 176-177.

Duffy, J. R. (2005). *Motor speech disorders: Substrates, differential diagnosis, and management* (2nd ed.). St. Louis, MO: Elsevier-Mosby.

Duong, T., T., Englander, J., Wright, J., Cifu, D. X., Greenwald, B. A., & Brown, A. W. (2004). Relationship between strength, balance, and swallowing deficits and outcome after traumatic brain injury: A multicenter analysis. *Archives of Physical Medicine and Rehabilitation*, *85*, 1291-1297.

Emilia-Romagna study group on clinical and epidemiological problems in neurology. (1998). Incidence of myasthenia gravis in the Emilia-Romagna region: A prospective multi-center study. *Neurology*, *51*, 255-258.

Ertekin, C., & Aydogdu, I. (2003). Neurophysiology of swallowing. *Clinical Neurophysiology*, *114*, 2226-2244.

Ertekin, C., Aydogdu, I., Yuceyar, N., Kiylioglu, N., Tarlaci, S., & Uludag, B. (2000). Pathological mechanisms of oropharyngeal dysphagia in amyotrophic lateral sclerosis. *Brain*, *123*, 125-140.

Ertekin, C., Secil, Y., Yuceyar, N., & Aydogdu, I. (2004). Oropharyngeal dysphagia in polymyositis/dermatomyositis. *Clinical Neurology and Neurosurgery*, *107*, 32-37.

Ertekin, C., Tarlaci, S., Aydogdu, I., Kiylioglu, N., Yuceyar, N., Turman, A. B., et al. (2002). Electrophysiological evaluation of pharyngeal phase of swallowing in patients with Parkinson's disease. *Movement Disorders*, *17*, 942-949.

Feinberg, M. J., Ekberg, O., Segall, L., & Tully, J. (1992). Deglutition in elderly patients with dementia: Findings of videofluorographic evaluation and impact on staging and management. *Radiology*, *183*, 811-814.

Frattali, C. M., & Sonies, B. C. (2000). Speech and swallowing disturbances in cortical basal degeneration. *Advances in Neurology, 82,* 163-160.

Gilman, S., Low, P. A., Quinn, N., Albanese, A., Ben-Schlomo, Y., Fowler, C. J. et al. (1999). Consensus statement on the diagnosis of multiple system atrophy. *Journal of the Neurological Sciences, 163,* 94-98.

Gisel, E. G., Applegate-Ferrante, T., Benson, J., & Bosma, J. F. (1996). Oral-motor skills following sensorimotor therapy in two groups of moderately dysphagic children with cerebral palsy: Aspiration vs. nonaspiration. *Dysphagia, 11,* 59-71.

Gouider-Khouja, N., Bidailhet, M., Bonnet, A.-M., Pischon, J., & Agid, Y. (1995). "Pure" striatonigral degeneration and Parkinson's disease: A comparative clinical study. *Movement Disorders, 10,* 288-294.

Graham, J. G., & Oppenheimer, D. R. (1969). Orthostatic hypotension and nicotine sensitivity in a case of multiple system atrophy. *Journal of Neurology, Neurosurgery, and Psychiatry, 32,* 28-34.

Grob, D., Arsura, L., Brunner, N. G., & Namba, T. (1987). The course of myasthenia gravis and therapies affecting outcome. *Annals of the New York Academy of Sciences, 505,* 472-499.

Gulyas, A. E., & Salazar-Grueso, E. F. (1988). Pharyngeal dysmotility in patient with Wilson's disease. *Dysphagia, 2,* 230-234.

Haggstrom, G., & Hirschowitz, B. I. (1980). Disorder esophageal motility in Wilson's disease. *Journal of Clinical Gastroenterology, 2,* 273-275.

Halper, A. S., Cherney, L. R., Cichowski, K., & Zhang, M. (1999). Dysphagia after head trauma: The effect of cognitive-communicative impairments on functional outcomes. *Journal of Head Trauma Rehabilitation, 14,* 486-496.

Hamdy, S., Aziz, Q., Rothwell, J. C., Power, M., Singh, K. D., Nicholson, D. A., et al. (1998). Recovery of swallowing after dysphagic stroke relates to functional reorganization in the intact motor cortex. *Gastroenterology, 115,* 1104-1112.

Hamdy, S., Aziz, Q., Rothwell, J. C., Singh, K. D., Barlow, J., Hughes, D. G., et al. (1996). The cortical topography of human swallowing musculature in health and disease. *Nature Medicine, 2,* 1217-1224.

Hamkawa, S., Koda, C., Umeno, H., Yshida, Y., Nakashima, T., Asaoka, K., et al. (2004). Oral-pharyngeal dysphagia in the case of Huntington's disease. *Auris Nasus Larynx, 31,* 171-176.

Han, D. S., Chang Y. C., Lu, C. H., & Wang, T. G. (2005). Comparison of disordered swallowing patterns in patients with recurrent cortical /subcortical stroke and first-time brainstem stroke. *Journal of Rehabilitation Medicine, 37,* 189-191.

Harding, A. E. (1981). Friedreich's ataxia: A clinical and genetic study of 90 families with an analysis of early diagnostic criteria intrafamilial clustering of clinical features. *Brain, 104,* 589-620.

Higo, R., Nito, T., & Tayama, N. (2005). Swallowing function in patients with multiple-system atrophy with a clinical predominance of cerebellar symptoms (MSA-C). *European Archives of Oto-Rhino-Laryngology, 262,* 646-650.

Higo, R., Tayama, N., Watanabe, T., Nitou, T., & Ugaway. (2003). Videofluoroscopic and manometric evaluation of swallowing function in patients with multiple system atrophy. *Annals of Otology, Rhinology, and Laryngology, 112,* 630-636.

Horner, J., Alberts, M. J., Dawson, D., V., & Cook, G. M. (1994). Swallowing in Alzheimer's disease. *Alzheimer Disease and Associated Disorders, 8,* 177-189.

Horner, J., Massey, E. W., & Brazer, S. R. (1990). Aspiration in bilateral stroke patients. *Neurology, 40,* 1686-1688.

Houser, S. M., Calabrese, L. H., & Strome, M. (1998). Dysphagia in patients with inclusion body myositis. *Laryngoscope, 108,* 1001-1005.

Huang, M.-H., King, K.-L., & Chien, K.-U. (1988). Esophageal manometric in patients with myasthenia gravis. *Journal of Thoracic Cardiovascular Surgery*, *95*, 281-285.

Huckabee, M. L., & Pelletier, C. A. (1998). *Management of adult neurogenic dysphagia*. San Diego, CA: Singular Publishing Group.

Ikeda, M., Brown, J., Holland, A. J., Fukuhara, R. & Hodges, J. R. (2002). Changes in appetite, food preference, and eating habits in frontotemporal dementia and Alzheimer's disease. *Journal of Neurology, Neurosurgery, and Psychiatry*, *73*, 371-376.

Jardim, L. B., Pereira, M. L., Silveira, I., Ferro, A., Sequeiros, J., & Giugliani, R. (2001). Neurologic findings in Machado-Joseph disease: Relation with disease duration, subtypes, and (CAG)n. *Archives of Neurology*, *58*, 899-904.

Kagel, M. C., & Leopold, N. A. (1992). Dysphagia in Huntington's disease: A 16-year retrospective. *Dysphagia*, *7*, 106-114.

Kalia, M. (2003). Dysphagia and aspiration pneumonia in patients with Alzheimer's disease. *Metabolism*, *52*, 36-38.

Kawai, S., Tsukuda, M., Mochimatsu, I., Enomoto, H., Kagesato, Y., Hirose, H., et al. (2003). A study of the early stage of dysphagia and amiotrophic lateral sclerosis. *Dysphagia*, *18*, 1-8.

Kennedy III, J. D., & Kent, R. (1985). Anatomy and physiology of deglutition and related functions. *Seminars in Speech and Language*, *6*, 1-12.

Kennedy III, J. G., & Kent, R. D. (1988). Physiological substrates of normal deglutition. *Dysphagia*, *3*, 24-37.

Kent, R. D., Kent, J. F., Duffy, J., & Weiser, G. (1998). Dysarthrias: Speech-voice profiles, related dysfunctions, and neuropathology. *Journal of Medical Speech-Language Pathology*, *6*, 165-211.

Kidd, D., Lawson, J., Nesbitt, R., & McMahon, J. (1993). Aspiration in acute stroke: A clinical study with videofluoroscopy. *Quarterly Journal of Medicine*, *86*, 825-829.

Kim, J., & Sapienza, C. M. (2005). Implications of expiratory muscle strength training for rehabilitation of the elderly: A tutorial. *Journal of Rehabilitation Research and Development*, *42*, 211-224.

Kirk, E. A, Howard, V. C., & Scott, C. A. (1995). Description of posterior fossa syndrome in children after posterior fossa brain tumor surgery. *Journal of Pediatric Oncology Nursing*, *12*, 181-187.

Kluin, K. J., Bromberg, M. B., Feldman, E. L., & Simmons, Z. (1996). Dysphagia in elderly men with myasthenia gravis. *Journal of the Neurological Sciences*, *138*, 49-52.

Koopman, W. J., Wiebe, S., Colton-Hudson, A., Moosa, T., Smith, D., Bach, D., et al. (2004). Prediction of aspiration in myasthenia gravis. *Muscle and Nerve*, *29*, 256-260.

Kurihara, K., Kita, K., Hirayama, K., Hara, T., & Toyama, M. (1990). Dysphagia and olibopontocerebellar atrophy [Abstract]. *Rinsho Shinkeigaku*, *30*, 146-150.

Langmore, S. E., Schatz, K., & Olsen, N. (1988). Fiberoptic endoscopic examination of swallowing safety: A new procedure. *Dysphagia*, *2*, 216-219.

Lazarus, C., & Logeman, J. A. (1987). Swallowing disorders in closed head trauma patients. *Archives of Physical Medicine and Rehabilitation*, *68*, 79-84.

Leopold, N. A., & Kagel, M. C. (1985). Dysphagia in Huntington's disease. *Archives of Neurology*, *42*, 57-60.

Leopold, N. A., & Kagel, M. C., (1996). Prepharyngeal dysphagia in Parkinson's disease. *Dysphagia*, *11*, 14-22.

Leopold, N. A., & Kagel, M. C. (1997a). Dysphagia in progressive supranuclear palsy: Radiologic features. *Dysphagia*, *12*, 140-143.

Leopold, N. A., & Kagel, M. C. (1997b). Laryngeal deglutition movement in Parkinson's disease. *Neurology*, *48*, 373-376.

Leopold, N. A., & Kagel, M. C. (1997c). Pharyngoesophageal dysphagia in Parkinson's disease. *Dysphagia*, *12*, 11-18.

Linke, R., Witt, T. N., & Tatsch, A. (2003). Assessment of esophageal function in patients with myasthenia gravis. *Journal of Neurology*, *250*, 601-606.

Llabrés, M., Molina-Martinez, F. J., & Miralles, S. (2005). Dysphagia as the sole manifestation of myasthenia gravis. *Journal of*

Neurology, Neurosurgery, and Psychiatry, *76,* 1297-1300.

Logemann, J. A. (1998). *Evaluation and treatment of swallowing disorders* (2nd ed.). Austin, TX: Pro-Ed.

Logemann, J. A., Fisher, H. B., Boshes, B., & Blonsky, E. R. (1978). Frequency and co-occurrence of vocal tract dysfunctions in the speech of a large sample of Parkinson patients. *Journal of Speech and Hearing Disorders, 43,* 47-53.

Mackay, L. E., Morgan, A. S., & Bernstein, B. A. (1999). Factors affecting oral feeding with severe traumatic brain injury. *Journal of Head Trauma Rehabilitation, 14,* 435-447.

Martin, R. E., MacIntosh, B. J., Smith, R. C., Barr, A. M., Stevens, T. K., Gati, J. S., et al. (2004). Cerebral areas processing swallowing and tongue movements are overlapping but distinct: A functional magnetic resonance imaging study. *Journal of Neurophysiology, 92,* 2428-2443.

Martin, R. E., & Sessle, B. J. (1993). The role of the cerebral cortex in swallowing. *Dysphagia, 8,* 195-202.

Martin-Harris, B., Brodsky, M. B., Michel, Y., Ford, C. L., Walters, B., & Heffner, J. (2005). Breathing and swallowing dynamics across the adult life span. *Archives of Otolaryngology-Head and Neck Surgery, 131,* 762-770.

Martin-Harris, B., Brodsky, M. B., Price, C. C., Michel, Y., & Walters, B. (2003). Temporal coordination of pharyngeal and laryngeal dynamics with breathing during swallowing: Single liquid swallows. *Journal of Applied Physiology, 94,* 1735-1743.

Martin-Harris, B., Logemann, J. A., McMahon, S., Schleicher, M., & Sandidge, J. (2000). Clinical utility of the modified barium swallow. *Dysphagia, 15,* 136-141.

Martin-Harris, B., Michel, Y., & Castell, D. O. (2005). Physiologic model of oropharyngeal swallowing revisited. *Otolaryngology-Head and Neck Surgery, 133,* 234-240.

Martino, R., Terrault N., Ezerzer, F., Mikulis, D., & Diamant N. E. (2001). Dysphagia in a patient with lateral medullary syndrome:

Insight into the central control of swallowing. *Gastroenterology, 121,* 420-426.

Mascia, M. M., Valls-Solé, J., Martí, M. J., & Sanz, S. (2005). Chewing pattern in patients with Meige's syndrome. *Movement Disorders, 20,* 26-33.

Meng, N. H., Wang, T. G., & Lien, I. N. (2000). Dysphagia in patients with brainstem stroke: Incidence and outcome. *American Journal of Physical Medicine and Rehabilitation, 79,* 170-175.

Miller, A. J. (1999). *The neuroscientific principles of swallowing and dysphagia.* San Diego, CA: Singular Publishing Group.

Morgan, A., Ward, E., & Murdoch, B. (2004). Clinical progression and outcome of dysphagia following paediatric traumatic brain injury: A prospective study. *Brain Injury, 18,* 359-376.

Morgan, A., Ward, E., Murdoch, B. & Bilbie, K. (2002). Acute characteristics of pediatric dysphagia subsequent to traumatic brain injury: Videofluoroscopic assessment. *Journal of Head Trauma Rehabilitation, 17,* 220-241.

Morgan, A., Ward, E., Murdoch, B., Kennedy, B., & Murison, R. (2003). Incidence, characteristics, and predictive factors for dysphagia after pediatric traumatic brain injury. *Journal of Head Trauma Rehabilitation, 18,* 239-251.

Mosier, K., & Bereznaya, I. (2001). Parallel cortical networks for volitional control of swallowing in humans. *Experimental Brain Research, 140,* 280-289.

Mosier, K. M., Liu, W. C., Maldjian, J. A., Shah, R., & Modi, B. (1999). Lateralization of cortical function and swallowing: A functional MR imaging study. *American Journal of Neuroradiology, 20,* 1520-1526.

Mukand, J. A., Blackinton, D. D., Crincoli, M.G., Lee, J. J., & Santos, B. B. (2001). Incidence of neurologic deficits and rehabilitation of patients with brain tumors. *The American Journal of Physical Medicine and Rehabilitation, 80,* 346-350.

Müller, J., Wenning, G. K., Verny, N., McKee, A., Chaudhuri, K. R., Jellinger, K., et al. (2001).

Progression of dysarthria and dysphagia in postmortem confined parkinsonian disorders. *Archives of Neurology, 58*, 259–264.

Murray, J. & Musson, N. (2005). *Understanding dysphagia* (Version 1.0) [CDROM]. (Available from the North Florida Foundation for Research and Education, Inc., c/o Joy Mitchell, CCRC, CCRA, Executive Director, North Florida/South Georgia Veterans Health System, 1601 SW Archer Rd. (151), Gainesville, FL 32608).

Nagaya, M., Kachi, T., Yamada, T., & Sumi, Y. (2004). Videofluorographic observations on swallowing in patients with dysphagia due to neurodegenerative diseases. *Nagoya Journal of Medical Science, 67*, 17–23.

Newton, H. B., Newton, C., Pearl, D., & Davidson, T. (1994). Swallowing assessment in primary brain tumor patients with dysphagia. *Neurology, 44*, 1927–1932.

Nilsson, H., Ekberg, O., Olsson, R., & Hindfelt, B. (1996). Quantitative assessment of oral and pharyngeal function in Parkinson's disease. *Dysphagia, 11*, 144–150.

Oder, W., Grimm, G., Kollegger, H., Ferenci, P., Schneider, B., & Deecke, L. (1991). Neurological and neuropsychiatric spectrum of Wilson's disease: A prospective study of 45 cases. *Journal of Neurology, 238*, 281–287.

O'Neill, P. A. (2000). Swallowing and prevention of complications. *British Medical Bulletin, 56*(2), 457–465.

Ozsancak, C., Auzou, P., Jan, M., Defebvre, P., Derambure, P., & Destee, A. (2006). The place of perceptual analysis of dysarthria in the differential diagnosis of corticobasal degeneration and Parkinson's disease. *Journal of Neurology, 253*, 92–97.

Parrott, L. C., Selley, W. G., Brooks, W. A., Lethbridge, P. C., Cole, J. J., Flack, F. C., et al. (1992). Dysphagia in cerebral palsy: A comparative study of the Exeter Dysphagia Assessment Technique and a multidisciplinary assessment. *Dysphagia, 7*, 209–219.

Pfeiffer, R. F. (2004). Wilson's disease. In R. L. Watts & W. C. Koller (Eds.), *Movement disorders: Neurologic principles and practice* (pp. 779–797). New York: McGraw-Hill Medical.

Priefer, B. A., & Robbins, J. (1997). Eating changes in mild-stage Alzhemier's disease: A pilot study. *Dysphagia, 12*, 212–221.

Prosiegel, M., Holing, R., Heintze, M., Wagner-Sonntag, E., & Wiseman, K. (2005a). The localization of central pattern generators for swallowing in humans—A clinical-anatomical study on patients with unilateral paresis of the vagal nerve, Avellis' syndrome, Wallenberg's syndrome, posterior fossa tumours and cerebellar hemorrhage. *Acta Neurochirurgica Supplementum, 93*, 85–88.

Prosiegel, M., Holing, R., Heintze, R., Wagner-Sonntag, E., & Wiseman, K. (2005b). Swallowing therapy—A prospective study on patients with neurogenic dysphagia due to unilateral paresis of the vagal nerve, Avellis' syndrome, Wallenberg's syndrome, posterior fossa tumours and cerebellar hemorrhage. *Acta Neurochirurgica Supplementum, 93*, 35–37.

Prosiegel, M., Schelling, A., & Wagner-Sonntag, E. (2004). Dysphagia and multiple sclerosis. *International MS Journal, 11*, 22–31.

Redstone, F., & West, J. F. (2004). The importance of postural control for feeding. *Pediatric Nursing, 30*, 97–100.

Reilly, S., Skuse, D., & Problete, X. (1996). Prevalence of feeding problems and oral motor dysfunction in children with cerebral palsy: A community survey. *Journal of Pediatrics, 129*, 877–882.

Riski, J. E., Horner, J., & Nashold, B. S. (1990). Swallowing function in patients with spasmodic torticollis. *Neurology, 40*, 1443–1445.

Robbins, J., (1987). Swallowing in ALS and motor neuron disorders. *Neurology Clinics, 5*, 213–229.

Robbins, J., & Levine, R. (1993). Swallowing after lateral medullary syndrome plus. *Clinical Communication Disorders, 3*, 45–55.

Robbins, J., Levine R. L., Maser A., Rosenbek J. C., & Kempster, G. B. (1993). Swallowing after unilateral stroke of the cerebral cortex. *Archives of Physical Medicine and Rehabilitation, 74*, 1295–1300.

Robbins, J. A., Loggemann, J. A., & Kirshner, H. S. (1986). Swallowing and speech production in Parkinson's disease. *Annals of Neurology, 19*, 283-287.

Rogers, B., Arvedson, J., Buck, G., Smart, P., & Msall, M. (1994). Characteristics of dysphagia in children with cerebral palsy. *Dysphagia, 9*, 69-73.

Ropper, A. H., & Brown, R. H. (2005). *Adams and Victor's principles of neurology* (8th ed.). New York: McGraw-Hill Medical.

Rosenbek, J. C., Robbins, J. A., Roecker, E. B., Coyle, J. L., & Wood, J. L. (1996). A penetration-aspiration scale. *Dysphagia, 11*, 93-98.

Rub, U., Brunt, E. R., Del Turco, D., de Dos, R. A. I., Gierga, K., Paulson, H., et al. (2003). Guidelines for the pathoanatomical examination of the lower brain stem in ingestive and swallowing disorders and its application to a dysphagic spinocerebellar ataxia type 3 patient. *Neuropathology and Applied Neurobiology, 29*, 1-13.

Scola, R. H., Werneck, L. C., Prevedello, D. M. S., Toderke, E. L., & Iwamoto, F. M. (2000). Diagnosis of dermatomyositis and polymyositis: A study of 102 cases. *Arquivos de Neuro-Psiquiatria, 58*, 789-799.

Selley, W. G., Parrott, L. C., Lethbridge, P. C., Flack, F. C., Ellis, R. E., Johnston, K. J., et al. (2001). Objective measures of dysphagia complexity in children related to suckle feeding histories, gestational ages, and classification of their cerebral palsy. *Dysphagia, 16*, 200-207.

Senner, J. E., Logemann, J., Zecker, S., & Gaebler-Spira, D. (2004). Drooling, saliva production, and swallowing in cerebral palsy. *Developmental Medicine and Child Neurology, 46*, 801-806.

Sharkawi, A. E., Ramig, L., Logemann, J. A., Pauloski, B. R., Rademaker, A. W., Smith, C. H., et al. (2002). Swallowing and voice effects of Lee Silverman Voice Treatment (LSVT[R]): A pilot study. *Journal of Neurology, Neurosurgery, and Psychiatry, 72*, 31-36.

Shulman, L. M., Minagar, A., & Weiner, W. J. (2004). Multiple-system atrophy. In R. L. Watts & W. C. Koller (Eds.), *Movement disorders: Neurologic principles and practice* (pp. 359-369). New York: McGraw-Hill Medical.

Siffert, J., Poussaint, T. Y., Goumnerova, L. C., Scott R. M., LaValley, B., Tarbell, N. J., et al. (2000). Neurological dysfunction associated with postoperative cerebellar mutism. *Journal of Neuro-oncology, 48*, 75-81.

Sonies, B. C. (1997). Evaluation and treatment of speech and swallowing disorders associated with myopathies. *Current Opinion in Rheumatology, 9*, 486-495.

Stover, N. P., Wainer, B. H., & Watts. (2004). Corticobasal degeneration. In R. L. Watts & W. C. Koller (Eds.), *Movement disorders: Neurologic principles and practice* (pp. 763-778). New York: McGraw-Hill Medical.

Strand, E. A., Miller R. M., Yorkston, K. M., & Hillel, A. D. (1996). Management of oral-pharyngeal dysphagia symptoms and amyotrophic lateral sclerosis. *Dysphagia, 11*, 129-139.

Tagliati, M., Golden, A., & Bressman, S. B. (2004). Childhood dystonia. In R.L. Watts & W. C. Koller (Eds.), *Movement disorders: Neurologic principles and practice* (pp. 495-509). New York McGraw-Hill Medical.

Tasko, S. M., Kent, R. D., & Westbury, J. R. (2002). Variability in tongue movement kinematics during normal liquid swallowing. *Dysphagia, 17*, 126-138.

Thomas, C. E., Mayer, S. A., Gungor, Y., Swarup, R., Webster, E. A., Chang, I., et al. (1997). Myasthenic crisis: Clinical features, mortality, complications, and risk factors for prolonged intubation. *Neurology, 48*, 1253-1260.

Thomas, F. J., & Wiles, C. M. (1999). Dysphagia and nutritional status in multiple sclerosis. *Journal of Neurology, 246*, 677-682.

Trejo, A., Tarrats, R. M., Alonso, E., Boll, M.-C., Ochoa, A., & Velásquez, L. (2004). Assessment of the nutrition status of patients with Huntington's disease. *Nutrition, 20*, 192-196.

Volonté, A., Porta, M. & Comi, G. (2002). Clinical assessment of aphasia in early phases of Parkinson's disease. *Neurological Sciences, 23*, S121-S122.

Wang, X.-h., Cheng, F., Zhang, F., Li, X. C., Kong, L. B., Li, G. Q., et al. (2005). Living-related liver transplantation for Wilson's disease. *Transplants International, 18,* 651–656.

Wang., S. J., Lin, W. Y., Hsu, C. Y., Kao, C. H., Chang C. P., & Lau, J. L. (1993). Solid phase radionuclide esophageal motility in polymyositis and dermamyositis. *Kao-Hsiung I Hsueh Ko Hsueh Tsa Chih, 9,* 338–343.

Weisner, W., Wetzel, S.G., Kappos, L., Hoshi, M. M., Witte, U., Radue, E. W., et al. (2002). Swallowing abnormalities in multiple sclerosis: Correlation between subjective symptoms. *European Radiology, 12,* 789–792.

Wesling, M., Brady, S., Jensen, M., Nickell, M., Statkus, D., & Escobar, N. (2003). Dysphagia outcomes in patients with brain tumors undergoing inpatient rehabilitation. *Dysphagia, 18,* 203–210.

Willig, T. M., Paulus, J., Lacau Saint Guily, J., Béon, C., & Navarro, J. (1994). Swallowing problems in neuromuscular disorders. *Archives of Physical Medicine and Rehabilitation, 75,* 1175–1181.

Wilmot, G. R., & Subramony, S. H. (2004). The molecular genetics of the ataxia. In R. L. Watts, & W. C. Koller (Eds.), *Movement disorders: Neurologic principles and practices* (pp. 705–722). New York: McGraw-Hill.

Winstein, C. J. (1983). Neurogenic dysphagia: Frequency, progression, and outcome in adults following head injury. *Physical Therapy, 63,* 1992–1997.

Wszolek, Z. K., Markopoulou, K., & Chase, B. A. (2004). Genetics of Parkinson's disease and parkinsonian disorders. In R. L. Watts & W. C. Koller (Eds.), *Movement disorders: Neurologic principals and practice* (pp. 163–176). New York: McGraw-Hill Medical.

Yorkston, K. M., Miller, R. M., & Strand, E. A. (1995). *Management of speech and swallowing in degenerative diseases,* San Antonio, TX: Communication Skill Builders.

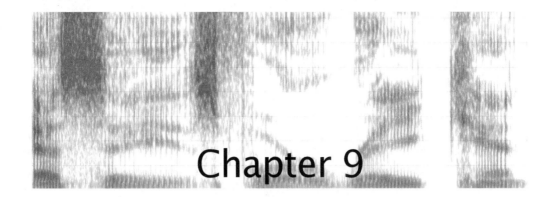

Chapter 9

A CONTINUUM OF INTERVENTIONS FOR INDIVIDUALS WITH DYSARTHRIA

Compensatory and Rehabilitative Treatment Approaches

Katherine C. Hustad and Gary Weismer

As discussed in the preceding chapters, individuals with dysarthria often have difficulty with motor control of the muscles involved in speech, including those associated with the respiratory, phonatory, velopharyngeal, and articulatory subsystems. Differences in the perceptual features of speech are an important consequence of the underlying motor control problems of dysarthria. These differences can range from very mild disturbances in speech production that have little effect on functional communication, to complete anarthria (inability to produce speech).

Because the ultimate purpose for producing speech is to communicate, the construct of intelligibility is very important for speech pathologists working with individuals who have dysarthria. Reduced intelligibility is a common problem for speakers with dysarthria that often results in important social-communicative consequences. One such consequence is a reduced ability to participate fully in the spectrum of life activities involving communication. Indeed, improving intelligibility is often a primary intervention goal for speakers with dysarthria (Ansel & Kent, 1992; Yorkston, Beukelman, Strand, & Bell, 1999). For those individuals with dysarthria who do not have problems with intelligibility, intervention may focus on rehabilitating speech to "normal" by helping speakers sound more natural and speak as efficiently as possible. There are a wide range of intervention approaches for improving speech production and communication abilities. The World Health Organization's International Classification of Functioning, Disability, and Health (ICF) (2002) provides a useful framework for conceptualizing different types of intervention approaches and their goals (Figure 9-1).

The ICF (2002) addresses the impact of a person's health condition or disease/disorder (in this case dysarthria) at three different, yet inter-related, levels. These are: (1) the person's body structures (anatomy) and functions (physiology); (2) the person's ability to engage in activities, and (3) the person's ability to participate in his or her life. Problems at the different levels result in impairment, activity limitations, and participation restrictions, respectively. The ICF model also incorporates the interaction of contextual factors (personal and environmental) with the three levels of functioning and disability. Contextual factors are unique to each person and result in different disability profiles (or lack

thereof) for individual people. In the context of speech, the level of body structures and functions encompasses the anatomy and physiology of the speech subsystems —respiration, phonation, resonaton, and articulation. The activities level encompasses speech intelligibility; and the participation level encompasses communication participation within the broad social context of the person's life. Although the levels of the ICF model are related, the relationships between and among levels are not always linear. That is, impairment does not always lead to activity limitation; and activity limitation does not always lead to participation restriction. For example, a person may have weakness in the muscles of the tongue, which results in articulation that sounds slightly distorted (articulation impairment). However, the person may still be able to produce intelligible speech (although it may not sound perfectly normal) that is functional for communication and does not result in

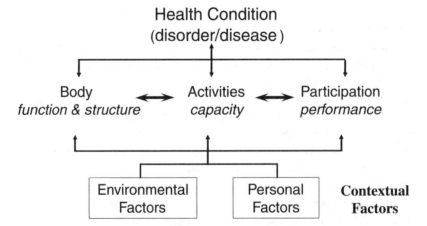

International Classification of Functioning, Disability, and Health

Figure 9–1. A schematic diagram of the World Health Organization's International Classification of Functioning, Disability, and Health (ICF) (2002).

participation restrictions. In this case, the person has an impairment that does not lead to activity or participation restrictions because the person is still able to communicate adequately in his or her life situations.

Treatment for dysarthria can be focused on any level of the ICF model; and the best treatments consider the speaker's performance at all levels of the model. One important consideration regarding any treatment relates to the existence and quality of the research evidence that supports the particular intervention. In recent years, evidence-based practice, or the use of evidence to support clinical decisions, has received increasing attention and has become an important component of the treatment process. Publications outlining practice guidelines are one vehicle for advancing the use of evidence-based practice. Within the area of motor speech disorders, a series of practice guidelines papers pertaining to different treatment approaches has recently been published (see Hanson, Yorkston, & Beukelman, 2004; Spencer, Yorkston, & Duffy, 2003; Yorkston, Spencer, Duffy, Beukelman, Golper, Miller, Strand, & Sullivan, 2001a, 2001b; Yorkston, Spencer, & Duffy, 2003a, 2003b). These papers are referenced throughout this chapter and are a very useful resource for evaluating the strength of the research evidence and the state of the knowledge base regarding the effectiveness of a variety of different interventions.

In this chapter, the focus is on two different, yet often complementary, intervention paths: (1) remediating underlying impairments in the speech subsystems (body structures and functions) and (2) reducing activity limitations and participation restrictions that are imposed by the dysarthria. Interventions that target speech subsystem impairment typically have an indirect impact on speech production in general, and speech intelligibility specifically. The philosophy behind impairment-oriented interventions is that reducing the underlying subsystem impairment ultimately will lead to improvements in speech production, which will enhance intelligibility and, in some situations, normalcy of speech (Rosenbek & LaPointe, 1985). However, these improvements may take protracted periods of time to occur or may not generalize to speech intelligibility at all.

Interventions that aim to reduce activity limitations and participation restrictions typically have a direct impact on functional communication, and often on speech intelligibility. These interventions are focused on compensatory communication strategies that may include behavioral speech compensations and/or use of augmentative and alternative communication (AAC) systems and strategies. The ultimate goal of compensatory approaches is functional communication and active participation in any and all communication situations.

For many speakers, the best intervention package involves a combination of impairment-oriented approaches and participation-oriented approaches. Compensatory strategies are used to enhance functional communication and meet immediate communication needs that cannot be fulfilled without some type of compensation. Impairment-oriented activities are used to try to reduce the underlying impairment for longer term return of function. However, it is critical to note that the etiology of the dysarthria and its course have a direct effect on the kinds of interventions that are appropriate for a given speaker and on expectations, planning, and outcomes for speakers with dysarthria (Yorkston et al., 1999).

Impact of Etiology on Intervention Approaches

Speakers can fall into one of three general groups with regard to the course of dysarthria. These are: (1) improving, (2) degenerating, and (3) chronic/stable. In speakers who have an improving course, it is expected that the underlying impairment will resolve or be rehabilitated to some extent so that the severity of the dysarthria and associated intelligibility reductions will be reduced over time. Common etiologies that are likely to show improvement with recovery include traumatic brain injury, cortical or brainstem stroke, or tumor resection. For individuals with these etiologies, time post-onset is an important factor in the recovery of speech. Most recovery is likely to be seen within the first few years post-onset; after this time, the dysarthria may be more appropriately considered as chronic/stable. Speakers with an improving course are likely to progress through a series of stages that may begin with complete anarthria. Some individuals may make a full recovery to "normal." Others may progress to a point and then plateau with substantial communication limitations remaining. The expected course of improvement will vary based upon individual circumstances. For the former group, compensatory interventions are likely to be short term and impairment-oriented interventions may play an important role in the return of functional speaking ability. For the latter group, compensatory interventions will likely be a long-term solution to communication difficulties.

In speakers who have a degenerating course, it is expected that the underlying impairment will worsen over time so that dysarthria and associated communication problems worsen with the progression of the disease. Common etiologies associated with degenerative dysarthrias include amyotrophic lateral sclerosis (ALS), Huntington's disease, Parkinson's disease, and multiple sclerosis. Speakers with these diseases begin with normal speech and may progress through a series of stages ranging from mildly reduced intelligibility to complete anarthria. The course of the disease including the rate, extent, and limits of deterioration will vary with the specific disease and the individual person. However, for some speakers in this group (particularly those with ALS), return to "normal" may not be a reasonable treatment goal (Yorkston, Miller, & Strand, 2003). For speakers with degenerative dysarthrias, a key aspect of treatment is understanding the expected course of the disease and the host of possible outcomes. Using this information, a series of interventions can be developed and implemented at appropriate junctures where changes in speech are observed. Interventions for speakers with degenerative dysarthrias and reduced intelligibility usually move from being less involved to more involved. For example, a speaker with ALS initially may use behavioral speech compensations; however, as his dysarthria worsens, he may come to need supplemental AAC strategies, and finally a comprehensive voice output AAC system.

In speakers who have a chronic/stable course, it is expected that underlying impairment will be grossly static or unchanging over time. As a result, dysarthria and associated reductions in intelligibility will be relatively consistent. Common etiologies for chronic dysarthria include cerebral palsy, traumatic brain injury, and cortical or brainstem stroke. Again, time post-onset is an important factor for acquired dysarthria. Usually individuals are not considered "chronic" unless dysarthria and communication problems persist beyond a year or two after the initial onset. Because improvements in underlying impairments generally are not expected for speakers with chronic dysarthria, compensatory techniques and strategies are usually intended for long-term use to improve functional communication and participation. Again, interventions can range from simple strategies such as rate reduction to more complex AAC interventions.

Regardless of whether the individual is improving, degenerating, or chronic/stable, the ultimate treatment goal is the same, to improve speech performance and functional communication. Yorkston and Beukelman (2000) suggested that two key problems often hinder the success of communication intervention for speakers with dysarthria. The first is failure to address *current* communication needs; the second is failure to address *future* needs or problems. In an attempt to remedy this, Yorkston and colleagues (Yorkston et al., 1999; Yorkston & Beukelman, 2000) described a staging framework for considering both current and future intervention needs for speakers with dysarthria. The framework consists of five different intervention stages based on the person's level of intelligibility. Moving from least to most involved, these are: (1) no detectable communication disorder; (2) obvious disorder with intelligible speech; (3) reduced intelligibility; (4) residual speech supplemented by augmentative techniques; and (5) no functional speech. Speakers with improving etiologies progress through these stages in reverse sequence (5-1), whereas speakers with degenerating etiologies progress through the stages in forward sequence (1-5). Regardless of the course of the dysarthria, speakers may persist at any stage.

For speakers who are in the "no detectable disorder" stage, intervention may involve consultation and education, particularly if the individual has a degenerative etiology and is expected to develop speech and/or communication problems in the future. For speakers in the obvious disorder with intelligible speech stage, intervention may employ indirect approaches designed to reduce the underlying impairment(s) responsible for the disorder. For speakers who are in the reduced intelligibility stage, residual speech supplemented by augmentative techniques stage, or no functional speech stage, high-quality intervention should always include a compensatory component. Depending on the etiology and expected course of the problem, impairment-oriented approaches may also be appropriate.

Speech Intelligibility

As mentioned previously, speech intelligibility is a critical consideration when developing a treatment plan for individuals with dysarthria. In the simplest sense, intelligibility refers to the extent to which an acoustic signal, generated by a speaker, can be correctly recovered by a listener. Intelligibility is a dyadic phenomenon that is not solely attributable to a speaker or to a listener. Rather, it is a product of the joint efforts of the speaker and the listener as communication *partners*. Intelligibility is a complex and multifaceted construct that is dynamic in nature. It is influenced by a host of variables related to the speaker and his or her impairment(s), the listener and his or her ability to make sense of a distorted speech signal, and contextual factors such as the communicative environment, and shared knowledge between the speaker and the listener. Studies have shown that intelligibility can be markedly affected when different contextual variables are manipulated. For example, research indicates that the semantic predictability of the message (Garcia & Cannito, 1996; Garcia & Dagenais, 1998; Hustad & Garcia, 2002), the length of the message (Miller, Heise, & Lichten, 1951; Sitler, Schiavetti, & Metz, 1983; Yorkston & Beukelman, 1981), and the semantic cohesion of the message(s) (Drager & Reichle, 2001; Hustad & Beukelman, 2002) each affect intelligibility. Other contextual factors that affect intelligibility include the presence of supplemental cues (Crow & Enderby, 1989; Garcia & Dagenais, 1998; Hunter, Pring, & Martin, 1991; Hustad, Jones, & Dailey, 2003), the presence of visual information (Hustad & Cahill, 2003; Hustad & Garcia, 2005), and listener experience with dysarthric speech (Hustad & Cahill, 2003; Spitzer, Liss, Caviness, & Adler, 2000; Tjaden & Liss, 1995).

Because so many variables affect intelligibility, no one measure can accurately and adequately provide a complete index of it. Intelligibility measures, then, are best considered a snapshot of speech adequacy at a moment in time on a particular set of stimuli with a particular set of listeners. To generalize beyond this is dangerous, and likely inaccurate. Nonetheless, clinical intelligibility measures are a longstanding tradition in speech-language pathology and can serve important clinical purposes. For example, intelligibility measures are widely used as an index of functional limitation, as a measure of severity of the speech disorder, and as basis of comparison for documenting and monitoring change in speech performance (Yorkston, et al., 1999). Critical clinical decisions such as whether or not to discontinue intervention sometimes may be made on the basis of intelligibility measures. There are sev-

eral strategies for measuring intelligibility, which can be divided into two groups, subjective measures and objective measures (Yorkston & Beukelman, 1978).

Subjective Measurement of Intelligibility

Subjective measures generally require listeners to quantify their personal perceptions of a speaker's intelligibility by assigning a number to what they heard. One method for this involves the use of equal-appearing interval (EAI) scales (Darley, Aronson, & Brown, 1969; Platt, Andrews, Young, & Quinn, 1980; Subtelny, 1977; Zraick & Liss, 2000). As the name implies, EAI scales require listeners to select a number that best represents a particular speech sample from a discrete linear interval scale, usually ranging from 1 to 5 or 1 to 7 (Schiavetti, 1992). Descriptors are often used to anchor the numeric points on the extreme ends of the scale (i.e., 1 = completely unintelligible; 7 = completely intelligible). The classic research of Darley, Aronson, and Brown (1969) employed EAI scales to characterize intelligibility.

Another subjective measure of intelligibility, primarily used in research applications, is direct magnitude estimation (DME) (Sciavetti, 1992; Schliesser, 1985; Weismer, Jeng, Laures, & Kent, 2001; Weismer & Laures, 2002; Zraick & Liss, 2000). In DME scaling, listeners assign values that reflect proportional differences among speech samples (Schiavetti, 1992), often relative to a standard example or modulus that is assigned a numeric value (Weismer & Laures, 2002). Generally, for both DME and EAI scaling, speakers produce a standard set of speech stimuli, the content of which is given to listeners so that they know what the speaker is saying. Both scaling methods have been used extensively in research involving speech intelligibility as well as other perceptual phenomena that otherwise may be difficult to quantify such as naturalness (Southwood & Weismer, 1993) and voice quality (Zraick & Liss, 2002).

Finally, percentage estimates are another subjective strategy for measuring intelligibility (Carter, Yorkston, Strand, & Hammen, 1996; Yorkston & Beukelman, 1978). Percentage estimates require listeners to estimate the percentage of words understood on an absolute scale, ranging from 0 to 100 (Schiavetti, 1992; Yorkston & Beukelman, 1978). Research suggests that the accuracy of percentage estimates can be variable, relative to transcription intelligibility measures (Hustad, 2006a). Thus, the reliability of this measure is questionable.

Objective Measurement of Intelligibility

Objective measurement of intelligibility most commonly involves orthographic transcription of single words or connected speech by listeners. Again, a standard set of stimuli is produced by a speaker and recorded for playback to listeners. In this paradigm, however, when listeners orthographically transcribe productions, they are naïve to what the speaker actually said. Individual words transcribed by listeners are counted as correct if they match the target word phonemically or incorrect if they do not. The percentage of words identified correctly is calculated by dividing the number of words identified correctly by the number of words possible, multiplied by 100 (Tikofsky & Tikofsky, 1964; Yorkston et al., 1999; Yorkston & Beukelman, 1978; Yorkston & Beukelman,

1980). Such a measure provides information about the integrity of the acoustic signal relative to "normal" speech (Hustad & Beukelman, 2002), which is assumed to be at or near 100% intelligible under comparable recording and listening conditions. Standard clinical tools such as the Sentence Intelligibility Test (SIT) (Yorkston, Beukelman, & Tice, 1996) and the Assessment of Intelligibility of Dysarthric Speech (Yorkston & Beukelman, 1981) employ this type of transcription method. Clinically, transcription intelligibility is considered by some to be the "gold standard" because listeners are forced to commit to paper their perceptions of what a speaker is saying, resulting in a quantitative measure of the integrity of the speech signal. However, there are some limitations to the interpretation of transcription intelligibility scores. For example, some words carry more information than others (i.e., content words vs. functor words), and consequently make a more important contribution to the overall meaning of an utterance. However, this is not reflected in the transcription intelligibility score where each word is weighted equally. Thus, words that carry little meaning (e.g., *a*, *the*, *in*) make the same contribution to the intelligibility score as words that carry important content.

There are several other limitations relevant to all types of intelligibility measures. For example, the underlying production basis for the intelligibility deficit cannot be determined (Kent, Weismer, Kent, & Rosenbek, 1989; Weismer & Martin, 1992), nor can the success or failure of different perceptual strategies employed by listeners. In addition, the extent to which intelligibility scores relate to functional performance in real communicative contexts is completely unknown. However, it is very likely that intelligibility scores underestimate communicative success.

Comprehensibility

Comprehensibility is a slightly different construct that is related to intelligibility. Comprehensibility has been defined as "the extent to which a listener understands a speaker in a communicative context" (Barefoot, Bochner, Johnson, & vom Eigner, 1993, p. 32). In this definition, there are two key components, *understanding* of a message and communicative *context*. Comprehensibility differs from intelligibility in that intelligibility does not provide a direct measure of whether a listener *understands* a message, per se. Rather transcription intelligibility measures provide an index of how well the speech signal can be parsed into the phonetic and lexical units that comprise it, arguably, a lower level precursor to *understanding* or *comprehension*. In addition, intelligibility measures typically do not provide information about the extent to which contextual factors impact results. In fact, context (beyond what is contained within the utterance itself) is deliberately controlled in most clinical intelligibility measures.

Yorkston, Strand, and Kennedy (1996) used the term *comprehensibility* to refer to contextual intelligibility, or intelligibility when contextual information is present in various forms, including semantic cues, syntactic cues, orthographic cues, and gestures. The impact of these cues on intelligibility is reviewed in the section on speech supplementation strategies, below. It is important to note that, in their definition of comprehensibility, Yorkston and colleagues make the implicit assumption that intelligibility is a measure of listener *understanding*. However, recent research (Hustad, 2006b; Hustad & Beukelman, 2002) suggests that these two measures are, in fact, different.

Comprehension or understandability differs from intelligibility in that compre-

hension tasks require listeners not only to decode the acoustic signal, but also to process the linguistic information carried within that signal at a higher cognitive level. Listener comprehension can be evaluated by examining the listener's ability to answer questions about the content of a message or narrative (Hustad, submitted; Hustad & Beukelman, 2002) or by examining the listener's ability to summarize the content of a narrative passage (Higginbotham, Drazek, Kowarsky, Scally, & Segal, 1994) produced by a speaker. Thus, listener comprehension measures deal more directly with the information-bearing capability of the speech signal than transcription intelligibility measures (Hustad & Beukelman, 2002).

One recent study showed that listeners' comprehension of dysarthric speech tended to be better than their ability to transcribe the same samples. (Hustad, 2006b). Because the focus of comprehension measures is the gestalt or overall meaning that cuts across words (rather than the individual words themselves), all constituent words do not necessarily need to be accurately decoded for a listener to comprehend a message. In part, this is because not all words contain informative content and because listeners are able to apply top-down processes that may help them infer the meaning of missed information.

Measures of listener comprehension may provide important and complementary information to traditional intelligibility measures and comprehensibility measures as described by Yorkston et al. (1996). Figure 9–2 provides a schematic illustration of intelligibility and listener comprehension as separate, yet related, measures that are influenced by the same speaker-related and listener-related factors. For individuals with reduced intelligibility, comprehensibility, or listener compre-

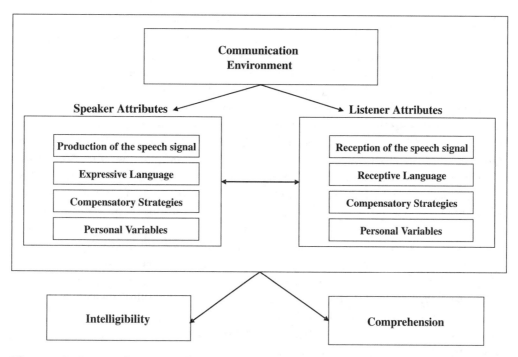

Figure 9–2. A schematic illustration of potential factors that influence both intelligibility and listener comprehension.

hension, compensatory interventions are critical for enhancing functional communication and participation.

Historically, the primary focus of speech therapy for individuals with dysarthria has been on remediating the underlying impairment. However, establishing a means of functional communication is an equally, if not more, important objective. Ideally, these two foci should be considered simultaneously for many individuals with dysarthria. However, it can easily be argued that an essential first step in intervention should be to address functional communication deficits. Thus, approaches oriented toward reducing activity limitations and participation restrictions are described first in this chapter, followed by impairment-oriented approaches in subsequent sections.

Interventions to Reduce Activity Limitations and Participation Restrictions

Interventions to reduce activity limitations and participation restrictions are often compensatory in nature. That is, their primary goal is not to fix underlying problems, but rather to use any and all means possible to compensate for, or work around, impairments. Speakers who require compensatory interventions can vary along a number of dimensions including expected course of the dysarthria and severity of involvement. In general, any speaker who is unable to meet his or her communication needs using speech alone across all partners and contexts is a candidate for compensatory intervention.

Three different groups of intervention strategies that correlate with the later three stages of the Yorkston et al. (1999) staging framework (reduced intelligibility, residual speech supplemented by augmentative techniques, and no functional speech) are discussed in this section. The first group of interventions is for speakers who need minimal compensatory support. These individuals use speech to meet all their communication needs, but have trouble being understood in at least some situations. The second group of interventions is for speakers who require modest supplemental support to enhance the functionality of natural speech. Again, these individuals may be able to use speech successfully in some situations, but they require various types of AAC, implemented in conjunction with speech, to ensure communicative success across all partners and contexts. The third group of interventions is for speakers who require extensive augmentative support because they have limited or no functional speech. This support often takes the form of voice output technology, which can be an alternative to natural speech in some or all situations. For each of these groups, it is critical to remember that the goal is to improve overall communicative function. Specific interventions are discussed in the sections that follow.

Interventions for Speakers Who Need Minimal Support: Behavioral Speech Compensations

Individuals who need minimal compensatory support are able to use natural speech for all communication, but they may have reduced intelligibility that can be im-

proved through global behavioral changes in speech production. For these speakers, then, the goal of intervention is to improve intelligibility by learning to implement different behavioral strategies. In some instances, changes in production may make speech sound more "normal" or "natural." However, the primary objective is improved communicative function. Three different areas of focus are discussed below, prosody, rate control, and clear speech. Although the intervention approaches differ, they have one important thing in common. Each addresses speech in an integrated way that is intended to have a direct impact on intelligibility.

Prosody

Prosody has been defined as changes in intonation, stress, and rhythm of speech (Lehiste, 1970) that are overlaid on speech sounds. Regarded as suprasegmental, prosodic features of speech are interwoven into the acoustic signal and carry information that can aid in the transmission of meaning at multiple levels (e.g., lexical, syntactic, and discourse structure) (Cutler, Dahan, & van Donselaar, 1997). From a perceptual perspective, one prominent feature of dysarthria is monopitch (Darley et al., 1969). Studies designed to quantify prosody, particularly fundamental frequency (F_0), in speakers with dysarthria have been limited primarily to individuals with relatively mild intelligibility impairments. However, these studies have consistently shown that speakers with dysarthria tend to produce smaller variations in F_0 than nondysarthric speakers (Bunton, Kent, & Kent, 2000; Le Dorze, Ouellet, & Ryalls, 1994; Yorkston & Beukelman, 1981). In other experimental studies, flattened F_0 has been associated with reduced intelligibility (Bunton, Kent, Kent, & Duffy, 2001; Laures & Bunton, 2003; Laures & Weismer, 1999).

Compensatory interventions that target prosody have the potential to increase intelligibility as well as speech naturalness in some cases. The first step in providing intervention is obviously to assess the individual's use of prosody and to determine the ways in which prosodic characteristics such as breath group patterns, stress patterns, and F_0 may influence the intelligibility of the speech signal. From this information, intervention targets can be identified. Several intervention approaches for addressing different aspects of prosody have been examined in the literature. For example, Bellaire, Yorkston, and Beukelman (1986) demonstrated clinical changes in F_0 for a speaker with dysarthria whose prosody was affected by unnecessary breathing between each word. In this intervention, Bellaire and colleagues taught the speaker to modify prosody by altering speech breathing, specifically increasing the length of breath groups and pausing without inhaling where possible. In another study, Hartelius, Wising, and Nord (1997) taught speakers to use contrastive stress via a seven-step program that included clinician modeling and extensive speaker practice with signaling stress. Results of Hartelius and colleagues showed that of their speakers who had difficulty signaling stress, two of three made gains following intervention. Other studies have examined modulation of F_0 with or without use of biofeedback and general exaggeration of prosodic contours during speech (Yorkston, Beukelman, Hakel, & Fager, in progress). The specificity of instructions and the specificity of feedback to speakers have varied among intervention studies. In addition, the characteristics of speakers studied

have also varied considerably; consequently, generalizations regarding treatment are difficult to make. Outcome measures from the various interventions have also varied, with some studies examining acoustic changes in speech associated with intervention techniques and others using perceptual ratings. In general, studies to date indicate that treatment for prosody can be effective; however, the exact effects on intelligibility and functional communication are unclear (Yorkston et al., in progress).

Additional work is needed to compare different intervention approaches to determine which one(s) are most effective with speakers who have different kinds of underlying deficits and severity of involvement. In addition, studies are needed that examine the social validity of different intervention approaches and generalization of treatment to real word communication situations (Yorkston et al., in progress).

Speaking Rate

Although reduced rate is a common characteristic of speakers with dysarthria, one seemingly counterintuitive intervention strategy that can increase intelligibility involves reducing rate even further. Studies suggest that the impact of rate reduction on intelligibility is complex and depends, at least in part, on the means by which rate is reduced. For example, studies using *digital manipulation* (e.g., electronically lengthened speaking and/or pause durations), whereby a computer is responsible for reducing rate, have generally shown different results than studies using *behavioral* methods, in which the speaker is responsible for reducing his or her rate (e.g., speaker-implemented pacing techniques). Specifically, studies where habitual speech rate was reduced using computer software that alters the acoustic signal generally have shown no improvement or clinically insignificant changes in intelligibility (Dagenais, Brown, & Moore, 2006; Gutek & Rochet, 1996; Hammen, Yorkston, & Minifie, 1994; Maassen, 1986). However, studies where rate was reduced via speaker-implemented behavioral strategies generally have shown significant intelligibility gains (Hustad & Sassano, 2002; Pilon, McIntosh, & Thaut, 1998; Yorkston, Beukelman, & Traynor, 1990).

Considered collectively, these two types of rate-reduction studies suggest that important *production changes* that occur when speakers implement rate-reduction strategies likely contribute to increases in intelligibility. Duffy (1995) suggested that speakers with dysarthria may achieve vocal tract configurations that more closely approximate those of neurologically intact speakers when they implement behavioral rate-reduction strategies. In addition, Beukelman and Yorkston (1977) suggested that listener-processing related variables may be affected by rate reduction. For example, speaker-implemented rate reduction may serve to increase word segmentation and to provide listeners with increased processing time. Thus, both listener-processing variables and speaker-production variables may contribute to gains in intelligibility associated with behavioral rate reduction.

In a review of evidence concerning the effectiveness of rate-reduction interventions, Yorkston et al. (in progress) identified a range of speaker-implemented behavioral strategies used for reducing rate in research studies. These include pacing boards, delayed auditory feedback, specific verbal instructions to pause between words, general verbal instructions to reduce rate by some proportion, and computerized pacing software. Outcomes from these differ-

ent techniques have varied depending on the severity and etiology of the dysarthria. Consequently, the magnitude of benefit from different techniques is difficult to generalize. However, results are generally positive, demonstrating improved intelligibility when speakers implement behavioral rate-reduction techniques.

Research examining behavioral rate reduction strategies has been primarily experimental in nature. Studies are needed to investigate the effects of rate reduction on communicative success in real environments. In addition, research is needed to examine the specific effects of rate reduction on production characteristics of speech and on listener perceptual strategies to understand the means by which rate reduction strategies improve intelligibility.

Clear Speech

A final, seemingly obvious, behavioral speech compensation to improve intelligibility is the use of clear speech. When a speaker uses clear speech, he or she speaks in a deliberate manner, characterized by exaggerated articulation, reduced rate, and increased loudness relative to habitual speech. Research on acoustic features of clear speech has confirmed that speakers, tend to use slower-than-normal speaking rate, produce better defined acoustic landmark events (such as stop bursts), use a larger acoustic vowel space, and use greater speech intensities for certain segments (Picheny, Durlach, & Braida, 1986). Research has also demonstrated that these acoustic changes are accompanied by increases in intelligibility of approximately 15% when nondisabled speakers produced clear speech for listeners with hearing impairment (Picheny, Durlach, & Braida, 1985).

Studies of speakers with dysarthria have shown that clear speech can have an important effect on intelligibility. For example, Beukelman and colleagues (Beukelman, Fager, Ullman, Hanson, & Logemann, 2002) found that intelligibility increased an average of 8% when speakers with dysarthria of varying severity implement-ed clear speech. Gains in this study ranged from 0 to 29%, for individual speakers. Interestingly, speech rate for the clear speech condition was similar to speech rate for the habitual condition for most speakers. In another study, Kennedy, Strand, and Yorkston (1994) also showed gains in intelligibility when speakers were instructed to use clear speech as a means of verbal repair.

Although there have been few studies examining the use of clear speech with individuals who have dysarthria, this intervention seems to have the potential to improve intelligibility for some speakers. Additional studies are needed to investigate characteristics of good candidates for clear speech, the effects of clear speech on communication success in real contexts, and the acceptance of clear speech by speakers and their partners. Studies are also necessary to describe the production features of clear speech in individuals with dysarthria so that those production changes that have the greatest impact on intelligibility can be emphasized in intervention.

Interventions for Speakers Who Need Modest Support: Integrating AAC with Natural Speech

Individuals who need modest compensatory support are able to use natural speech as their primary mode of communication, but alone it is not sufficient to carry the full load of communication across all partners and contexts. The frequency and extent of communication difficulty may vary for different speakers, with some individuals requiring supplemental augmentative support only in limited situations such as communication breakdowns or with unfamiliar partners. Others may require supplemental augmentative support in most communication situations.

Augmentative and alternative communication (AAC) interventions are broad in scope. In general, AAC is defined as " . . . a set of procedures and processes by which an individual's communication skills (i.e., production as well as comprehension) can be maximized for functional and effective communication" (ASHA, 2002, p. III-2). AAC systems and strategies can be used to supplement or replace natural speech and/or writing through aided or unaided symbols and techniques. AAC interventions encompass a wide range of options that include use of simple gestures, low-tech alphabet or picture communication boards, dedicated voice output devices, and computer-based voice output options. The primary goal of AAC is to enhance the individual's ability to actively participate in his or her daily life by communicating with a diverse range of partners and in a variety of settings (Beukelman & Mirenda, 2005). This philosophy represents an important conceptual shift from improving *speech* to improving *communication*. Any person who has a discrepancy between communication abilities and communication needs, whether temporary or permanent is a candidate for AAC (ASHA, 2002, 2004).

AAC and natural speech are not mutually exclusive communication options. Most individuals are able to produce at least some residual speech or vocal behavior that can be used in a communicative capacity.

Good interventions should consider the primacy of natural speech and make every effort to integrate residual abilities to the greatest extent possible into the individual's communication system. Consequently, interventions should be multimodal, employing any and all modes of communication available to the individual, including speech, gestures, and AAC systems and strategies. In the sections that follow, low tech supplemental AAC strategies are described.

Speech Supplementation Strategies

Speech supplementation strategies are a group of multimodal interventions in which natural speech is supplemented or augmented with AAC. In essence, individuals use speech as a primary mode of communication, while at the same time providing their listeners with different types of explicit augmentative cues that correspond to the spoken message. In some cases, the act of pointing to cues while simultaneously speaking can result in changes in the speech signal that have a positive effect on intelligibility (Beukelman et al., 2002; Hustad et al., 2003; Hustad & Garcia, 2005). Thus, use of supplemental AAC strategies can improve speech production while providing listeners with contextual information related to the spoken message, both of which serve the goal of improving intelligibility. Most often speech supplementation strategies involve low-tech communication boards and books or unaided gestures. However, high-tech voice output communication devices can also be used for speech supplementation. There are several different types of speech supplementation strategies including iconic hand gestures,

topic cues, alphabet cues, and combined cues. Table 9–1 provides a summary of each speech supplementation strategy. These are described in detail below.

Iconic Hand Gestures

Speakers naturally use different types of gestures in conjunction with speech to communicate (Garcia, Cannito, & Dagenais, 2000). Iconic hand gestures are one form of natural hand movement that illustrate or add meaning to content words of the spoken message (Garcia et al., 2000). When a speaker uses iconic hand gestures as a speech supplementation strategy, he or she produces target gestures concurrently with speech. Gestures are generally timed to coincide with production of the target word or phrase to which they refer. Hand gestures are an unaided AAC strategy because their use does not require anything external to the body (Lloyd & Fuller, 1986), unlike the other speech supplementation strategies discussed below. There are certain advantages to this, particularly portability and durability.

Research suggests that scripted iconic hand gestures can increase intelligibility of predictable sentences by an average of about 25% (range = 6–50%) across studies (Garcia & Cannito, 1996; Garcia & Dagenais, 1998; Garcia, Crowe, Redler, & Hustad, 2004; Hustad & Garcia, 2005). It is unclear from existing studies whether iconic hand gestures differentially benefit speakers with more or less severe dysarthria. One important mitigating variable for this strategy is upper extremity control and the quality of the gestures produced. Speakers who produce better gestures are likely to benefit more from this strategy. Studies suggest that implementation of hand gestures can have an effect on production characteristics of speech (Garcia & Cobb, 2000;

Table 9–1. Summary of Speech Supplementation Strategies

Iconic Hand Gestures	Tools:	▪ One or two hands
	Implementation:	▪ Speaker produces gestures for key content words while simultaneously speaking a message
	Effects on Speech Production:	▪ Reduced rate in some speakers (Hustad & Garcia, 2005) ▪ Changes to phrasing of messages so that content associated with gestures is "chunked" together during production (Garcia & Cobb, 2000)
	Effects on Intelligibility:	▪ Increases in sentence intelligibility of approximately 25% (range 6–50%) across studies.
Topic Cues	Tools:	▪ Communication display containing topics
	Implementation:	▪ Speaker indicates the topic via some type of direct selection, then produces the target message
	Effects on Speech Production:	▪ None identified to date
	Effects on Intelligibility:	▪ Increases in sentence intelligibility of approximately 10% (range 0–52%) (Hanson, Yorkston, & Beukelman, 2004)
Alphabet Cues	Tools:	▪ Communication display containing the alphabet.
	Implementation:	▪ Speaker direct selects the first letter of each word of his/her message while simultaneously producing the word
	Effects on Speech Production:	▪ Rate of speech is reduced by up to 70% when speakers implement alphabet cues (Hustad, Jones, & Daily, 2003)
	Effects on Intelligibility:	▪ Increases in sentence intelligibility of approximately 25% (range 5%–69%) (Hanson et al., 2004)
Combined Topic and Alphabet Cues	Tools:	▪ Communication display containing topics and the alphabet
	Implementation:	▪ Speaker indicates the topic of each word of his/her message while simultaneously producing the word.
	Effects on Speech Production:	▪ Reductions in rate of speech similar to those observed for alphabet cues (Hustad, Jones, & Dailey, 2003)
	Effects on Intelligibility:	▪ Increases in sentence intelligibility of approximately 40% (range 28–50%) (Hustad, Jones, & Dailey, 2003; Hustad, Auker, et al., 2003)

Source: Adapted with permission from Hustad, K. C. (2005). Effects of speech supplementation strategies on intelligibility and listener attitudes for a speaker with mild dysarthria. *Augmentative and Alternative Communication, 21,* 256–263.

Hustad & Garcia, 2005). In particular, some individuals may reduce their speaking rate when implementing iconic hand gestures (Hustad & Garcia, 2005). In addition, some speakers may tend to change the phrasing of their speech so that content linked to the gestures is chunked together (Garcia & Cobb, 2000). Studies are needed to examine how implementation of gestures impacts other production variables beyond rate and pause behavior.

Candidacy requirements for use of iconic hand gestures as a speech supplementation strategy have not been systematically studied. However, there are several basic requirements to use the strategy. Speakers should: (1) be able to produce speech, (2) have adequate motor control in at least one arm to produce gestures, and (3) have the motor and cognitive skills to time the production of gestures with specific words and phrases in the spoken message.

With the exception of one study (Garcia et al., 2004), all research examining gestures as a speech supplementation strategy for individuals with dysarthria has been highly controlled and experimental in nature. Particularly important is that studies have examined only the influence of a core of scripted gestures that corresponded to a set of controlled experimental sentences. In these studies, speakers practiced producing the target gestures and sentences; and optimal productions were recorded and shown to listeners. The effectiveness of spontaneously produced unscripted iconic gestures in conjunction with spontaneous speech is an important avenue for future study. One limitation of iconic hand gestures is that they are paralinguistic in nature, thus their meaning is not universal and is open for interpretation (Hustad & Garcia, 2005). Also, some words and ideas are not easily gestured, so iconic gestures cannot necessarily be provided for all messages. In spite of these limitations, iconic hand gestures are a promising speech supplementation strategy with the potential to have an important effect on intelligibility.

Topic Supplementation

Topic supplementation combines the use of natural speech along with a communication book, board, or device that is used to provide topical words, phrases, or pictures to the communication partner. To implement topic supplementation, a speaker would first indicate the topic of his or her message and then say the message using natural speech (Yorkston et al, 1999). For example if the speaker wanted to say the message "It was hot and sunny today," she or he would first point to the topic cue "weather" on a communication board, and then say the message. This strategy is useful because the top-down contextual information provided by the cues serves as a frame of reference for the listener. In essence, topic cues prepare the listener for the forthcoming message and narrow the possible range of options to which the message might pertain (Hustad & Beukelman, 2001).

Studies investigating topic supplementation indicate that topic cues result in modest improvements in intelligibility. A small body of research suggests that broad topic cues can increase sentence intelligibility by an average of about 10% (range = 0–52%) across studies for individuals with dysarthria (Beukelman et al., 2002; Carter et al., 1996; Dongilli, 1994; Hustad, Auker, Natale, & Carlson, 2003; Hustad & Beukelman, 2001; Hustad et al., 2003). Research suggests that topic cues have similar effects for speakers across the severity range. However, because speech is clearly the primary communication modality with this strategy, topic cues are probably most beneficial for individuals whose residual speech is relatively functional. Existing studies suggest that there are exceptions to this generalization, with individual differences among speakers sometimes being very unpredictable (Hanson et al., 2004).

Candidacy requirements for this strategy have not been systematically studied; however, the following skills would likely be important if a speaker is to implement topic cues. In general candidates for topic cues should: (1) be able to produce speech, (2) have the motor skills to make topic choices, ideally through direct selection (although use of scanning on a high-tech AAC device may be a possibility for some speakers), (3) have adequate vision to see topic choices, (4) be able to read or recognize picture communication symbols that represent topics; and (5) have the motor and cognitive skills to indicate a topic and then speak.

All research investigating topic supplementation has been highly controlled and experimental in nature. Studies involving spontaneous use of topic supplementation have not been conducted, so the effectiveness of the strategy in real situations is unknown. In addition, acceptance by speakers and partners is also unknown. Other important issues that have not been investigated relating to topic supplementation include the impact of topic cue specificity and cue frequency on intelligibility. All published research has employed relatively broad topic cues that were delivered for individual sentences. Narrower or more focused cues that are delivered less frequently may have a different impact

on intelligibility. Additionally, in situations where there is richer contextual information inherent in the communicative act, topic cues may be more or less helpful than experimental studies suggest. In the form described here, topic cues are a preventive strategy, designed to reduce the occurrence of communication breakdowns. However, they can also be used as a communication repair strategy so that if a speaker and partner experience a misunderstanding or breakdown, topic cues could be used for clarification.

Alphabet Supplementation

Alphabet supplementation combines natural speech with alphabet cues representing the first letter of each constituent word of spoken messages. To implement alphabet supplementation, a speaker would say each word of his or her message while simultaneously pointing to word-initial graphemes on an alphabet board. For example, if the speaker wanted to say the message "I want ice cream," he or she would point to the letter "I" while saying the word "I," point to the letter "w" while saying the word "want," point to the letter "i" while saying the word "ice," point to the letter "c" while saying "cream." A sample alphabet board is provided in Figure 9–3.

Studies investigating alphabet supplementation have consistently shown positive results. In general, research suggests that alphabet cues can improve intelligibility by an average of about 25% (range = 5–69%) (Beukelman et al., 2002; Beukelman & Yorkston, 1977; Crow & Enderby, 1989; Hustad & Beukelman, 2001; Hustad et al., 2003; Hustad & Garcia, 2002, 2005). All studies are marked by individual differences among speakers and their listeners regarding the magnitude of benefit from alphabet

A	B	C	D	E	F
G	H	I	J	K	L
M	N	O	P	Q	R
S	T	U	V	W	X
Y	Z	space		delete	

0 1 2 3 4 5 6 7 8 9

You misunderstood

Wait a minute

I'll say it again

I'll spell it

• **I will point to the first letter of each word that I'm saying.**

• **Please repeat each word after I say it so I know you understood me.**

Figure 9–3. A sample alphabet board for use with alphabet supplementation.

supplementation. However, speakers with more severe impairment have tended to show greater benefit from alphabet supplementation than less severely involved speakers (Hanson et al., 2004).

Research suggests that alphabet supplementation affects speech intelligibility in three different ways. First, when speakers implement alphabet cues, rate of speech is reduced (Beukelman et al., 2002; Hustad et al., 2003; Hustad & Garcia, 2005) and intelligibility is increased, even when listeners cannot see the alphabet cues (Beukelman & Yorkston, 1977; Crow & Enderby, 1989; Hustad & Garcia, 2005). Preliminary research suggests that one

production change involves use of longer and more frequently occurring interword pauses (Hustad et al., 2003; Hustad & Garcia, 2005). Prosody also seems to be affected by alphabet supplementation. For example, speech tends to sound monotone with equal stress on individual words when speakers implement the strategy. However, prosodic and other spectral production changes have not been systematically studied to date, so the nature and extent of potential changes are unknown. The second way that alphabet cues seem to improve intelligibility is through the linguistic information provided by the letters themselves. Studies where alphabet cues are superimposed on habitual speech via digital technology have demonstrated that the cues alone have an independent effect on intelligibility (Beliveau, Hodge, & Hagler, 1995; Hustad & Beukelman, 2001), even when concomitant production changes are not present. Hustad and Beukelman speculated that the linguistic information from alphabet cues may help reduce lexical ambiguity so that only those word candidates beginning with the target letter are viable options. The third way that alphabet cues seem to affect intelligibility is through the interactive influence of the letter cues and the changes in speech production associated with implementing the strategy. When speech production changes and letter cues are present, they appear to have a combined impact on intelligibility that may be additive or perhaps even multiplicative. However, the independent and overlapping contributions of the various factors have not been studied in ways that permit definitive attribution of effects.

Candidacy requirements for use of alphabet supplementation have not been systematically studied. However, the following skills would seem to be important in order to implement alphabet cues. Speakers should: (1) be able to produce speech, even if intelligibility is markedly reduced; (2) have the motor skills to directly select letters from an alphabet display; (3) have adequate vision to see letter choices; (4) have functional literacy skills that permit accurate first letter identification for spoken words; and (5) be able to coordinate simultaneous speech movements with body movements (usually upper extremities).

It is important to note that, like the other speech supplementation strategies, all studies examining alphabet sup-

plementation have been highly controlled and experimental in nature. Although the strategy is simple in concept, successful use of alphabet supplementation is somewhat more complex, involving simultaneous coordinated movement of the speech mechanism and the body. In addition, there is a cognitive load associated with formulating a message and then identifying and selecting first letters. The impact of motor coordination, timing, and cognitive variables on intelligibility and acceptance (by speakers and partners) in spontaneous contexts is unknown. This is an important direction for future research.

Combined Topic and Alphabet Supplementation

As the name suggests, combined supplementation involves use of both topic and alphabet cues as described above. To implement this strategy, a speaker would first indicate the topic of his or her message and then provide alphabet cues for the first letter of each word while simultaneously speaking. As a result, the listener receives broad topical information and narrow word-specific information, both pertaining to the content of the speaker's message.

Few studies have investigated the effects of combined cues on intelligibility. However, results appear promising, especially for speakers with more severe dysarthria. Average gains associated with combined cues across all studies have been about 36% (range = 29–50%) (Hustad & Beukelman, 2001; Hustad et al., 2003). In these studies, without exception, all speakers showed an increase in intelligibility associated with combined cues. For some speakers, this gain was similar to that observed for alphabet cues alone. Therefore, it is important to evaluate in individual speakers whether there is added benefit associated with combined alphabet and topic cues relative to alphabet cues alone, and whether the benefit is worth the extra effort required to implement both types of cues.

Again, studies have not been conducted to determine the characteristics of ideal candidates for this strategy. However, candidacy requirements for combined cues would be similar to those outlined for alphabet cues. Existing studies on combined cues have been experimental in nature. Clinical studies in which speakers implement combined cues in real contexts are necessary to further evaluate the effectiveness of this strategy for improving intelligibility.

In general, speech supplementation strategies are an inexpensive and cost-effective intervention that can be implemented easily and without special equipment. Anecdotal reports from experimental studies of the different supplementation techniques suggest that the strategies are easy for speakers to learn, with a high level of accuracy reached in 10 minutes of learning time. Consequently, there is little to lose by trying speech supplementation interventions with individuals who have reduced intelligibility but prefer to use natural speech as a primary mode of communication.

Although speech supplementation strategies as described above often involve low-tech AAC, high-tech options can also be used to supplement speech. For example, high-tech devices could be used to deliver alphabet or topic cues. Regardless of the tools used, the critical outcome of AAC strategies to supplement speech should be improved communicative success.

Interventions for Individuals Who Need Extensive Support: Comprehensive AAC Systems

For individuals who are more severely involved and require extensive communication support, comprehensive AAC systems are an important avenue for enhancing functional communication and participation. Individuals who require comprehensive AAC systems can vary in their capability to produce speech. Some may be able to use speech as a primary mode of communication, but may require voice output AAC for particular situations where they experience difficulty, such as the telephone, communicating urgent or time-sensitive messages, or communicating with particular partners or in particular communication environments. Other individuals may have extremely limited speech and require AAC for all communication. The common thread across individuals is the need for an AAC system that is versatile and can stand alone, independent of residual natural speech, if necessary.

Individuals who require comprehensive AAC systems may present with a range of issues that make thorough, high-quality AAC assessment and intervention very complex. These include, but are not limited to, physical access problems, cognitive and language problems, and sensory problems. Each of these variables and the extent of its presence can have a critically important impact on the AAC options that are most appropriate for a given individual. In addition, whether the underlying problem is expected to be stable, degenerative, or improving also has an important impact on AAC options.

AAC systems can range from very simple to very complicated. Although the technology is an important tool, the focus of AAC assessment and intervention should always be on the *person* and his or her ability to communicate successfully. It is critical to remember that the technology is simply a tool to bridge the gap between the person's capabilities and communication needs. Technology alone is only part of the solution. Accordingly, the main aim of AAC assessment is first to identify the individual's physical, perceptual, language, and cognitive capabilities, and his or her communication needs and then to identify technology that is consistent with the person's profile of needs and capabilities. To accomplish this, thorough assessment of the person, and knowledge of and access to current technology is necessary. A complete review of AAC assessment processes for individuals with dysarthria is beyond the scope of this chapter. However, there are several excellent and recent resources that deal specifically with AAC applications for individuals with neurogenic communication disorders (see Beukelman, Garrett, & Yorkston, in press; Beukelman & Mirenda, 2005; Beukelman, Yorkston, & Reichle, 1999).

A Brief Overview of the Tools: AAC Technology

A wide, and ever changing, array of technology is available to enable individuals to communicate who have a broad range of capabilities and needs. AAC systems can be divided into five general groups based on their level of complexity. These are (1) low tech systems, (2) simple digitized systems, (3) dynamic digitized systems, (4) dedicated text-to-speech voice output systems, and (5) personal computer-based text-to-speech voice output systems. In addition, many individuals have difficulty

or are unable to access a communication device using their hands. For these individuals, an array of highly specialized switches and other peripheral equipment is available to facilitate access.

Low-tech systems include, but are not limited to, paper-based communication books and boards, remnant books (e.g., photo albums, scrap books, and tangible remnants from important activities), calendar or day-planner books, and gestures or manual systems. These systems are simple, inexpensive, and often easily replaceable. It is frequently the case that a therapist or family member uses computer technology to *create* low-tech systems, but actual implementation of the system by the individual does not incorporate technology. Low-tech systems can vary markedly in complexity. For example, in its simplest form, a low-tech communication system could consist of a limited array of individual symbols or written messages, or basic communication boards. On other end of the continuum, a low-tech communication system could consist of an elaborate, carefully organized, and multipurpose notebook of messages expressing wants and needs, small talk, conversational scripts, personal narratives, maps, photographs, and so forth. Low-tech backup systems are important for all individuals who use higher-tech devices as there are always situations where use of technology is not practical or feasible.

Simple digitized systems are those that contain a limited number of messages on a static display. In these systems, spoken messages are associated with symbols (orthographic or picture-based) via digital recording of individual messages by a person who is highly intelligible. Simple digitized systems, by their nature, tend to have limited generative capability, so the user can only express messages that are preprogrammed in the system. This type of device tends to be relatively inexpensive, but is also somewhat limiting with regard to capacity. Most simple digitized systems can hold fewer than 50 messages on one display; and some systems can hold only one message. Although some systems have the capability to store additional messages on different "levels" of the device, accessing those levels usually requires that a new overlay be manually placed in the display. This can be physically difficult for individuals with motor impairment and cumbersome to do during a communication exchange if the desired message is stored on a different level. However, simple digitized systems can be very useful for individuals with limited voice output needs or limited new learning capability. In spite of the limitations of simple digitized systems, they can provide a very powerful means of enhancing social participation.

Dynamic digitized systems are generally more complex than simple digitized systems. Devices in this group are similar to those in the simple digitized group in that they require messages to be digitally recorded by an intelligible speaker. Dynamic digitized systems are generally not generative in nature, so the individual user's ability to create unique messages is typically limited to what has been preprogrammed in the device. One advantage of digitized output (on dynamic or simple digitized systems) is that speakers with degenerative diseases, such as ALS, can begin planning for future AAC needs by recording messages in their own voice on any type of analog or digital recorder. These messages can later be transferred to a voice output AAC system with digitized message capability when the person's intelligibility becomes sufficiently compromised that voice output technology is needed.

Dynamic digitized systems differ from simple digitized systems in that they have a dynamic display, which enables users to change the array of visible message options dynamically, without the need for manually changing the static overlay. Most of these systems have the capability to store a large number of pages that are linked together and appear with the simple touch of a button. As a result, the potential complexity of such a system is significant. Issues related to vocabulary and message selection, as well as systematic organization of messages so that they are easy for the user to find, are paramount to the success of this type of system, which may contain a large number of pages with an even larger number of prestored messages.

Dedicated text-to-speech AAC systems can range from very complex to relatively simple. The common feature among these systems is text-to-speech voice output capability via synthesized speech. Text-to-speech voice output enables the device to say anything that the user can generate via spelling or symbol selection. There are a variety of different high-quality speech synthesizers that are built into the different AAC devices. Although there are differences in how the various synthesizers work and how they sound, all are highly intelligible. The primary weakness of synthesizers used in AAC devices relates to limitations in suprasegmental characteristics, particularly intonation. Consequently, synthesized speech does not sound as natural as speech produced by humans. Text-to-speech voice output systems that are *dedicated* are special electronic devices that were developed for the exclusive purpose of AAC. Because their primary function is to serve as a communication aid, their relevance to the everyday consumer who does not need AAC is very limited or nil. A large variety of these systems are available, with each offering slightly different features. Many systems have dynamic displays and large preprogrammed dictionaries. Other devices consist of a small simple keyboard and LCD display used for typing and then speaking messages. Because these devices are highly specialized, they are very costly. Considerable expertise is necessary to match the capabilities and needs of the individual with the features of the various devices. Evaluations are often a lengthy and ongoing process involving trials with multiple devices before a final recommendation is made as to which one is best for a given individual. There are many important considerations in the assessment process in addition to the person's capabilities and needs. A few of these include the personal investment of significant others, the individual's own motivation, his or her life experiences (e.g., previous computer competence), his or her desire to use the telephone, and his or her ability to use multimodal communication. Intervention to integrate the device into the person's life is critical to successful use.

Computer-based text-to-speech systems can also range from very complex to relatively simple. Like dedicated systems, most computer-based systems also feature text-to-speech capability and are, therefore, generative in nature. Dedicated and computer-based systems differ in that computer-based systems operate on personal computers. Accordingly, these systems also offer personal computer functions such as word processing, money management, and Web browsing in addition to their function as a communication device. Computer-based AAC software is often used on portable computers, and there are several companies that make special laptop computers that are built to be more durable than regular mass-market machines. These types of computers are attractive to some users who may be more active. There are a variety of AAC software programs that can be used on personal computers. As with dedicated AAC devices, computer-based AAC systems range in complexity from very simple to very complex. For the most part, the same features and capabilities are available on both dedicated systems and computer-based systems. In fact, some companies even sell personal-computer software that is the same or very similar to what is available on dedicated AAC devices. Again, considerable expertise is necessary to match capabilities and needs with features of particular AAC software; and, again, ongoing intervention to integrate the system into the individual's life is critical to success.

Switches and other peripherals are often necessary to facilitate physical access to the different types of devices. These include a wide range of different microswitches, headmice, trackpads/balls, alternative keyboards, optical pointers, and mounting devices for the AAC system. Assessment of access needs is a highly specialized component of AAC. Usually this is done by an occupational or physical therapist with expertise in human factors and assistive technology. Examples of specific AAC devices and access peripherals consistent with the general groups discussed above are provided in Table 9–2.

Role of the Speech Language Pathologist in AAC Assessment and Intervention

Because those who require AAC often have complex issues, it is essential that a team of professionals, minimally composed of individuals with expertise in seating and

Table 9–2. Examples of Specific AAC Devices Organized by General Category

Device Category	Examples of Devices*
Low tech	Communication wallets Communication books Communication boards
Simple digitized	Big Mac (Ablenet) Message mate (Words +) TechScan (AMDi) Supertalker progressive communicator (Ablenet)
Dynamic digitized	Mighty Mo (Dynavox) Springboard (Prentke Romich) Leo (Assistive Technology)
Text-to-speech dedicated	Lightwriter (Zygo) MT4 (Dynavox) Pathfinder (Prentke Romich) Linkplus (Assistive Technology)
Text-to-speech computer-based	EZ-Keys (software) (Words +) Talking Screen (software) (Words +) Speaking Dynamically Pro (software) (Mayer Johnson) Mercury (hardware & software) (Assistive Technology) Panasonic Toughbook (hardware) (Panasonic) Say It Sam Tablet XP (hardware & software) (Words +) Tufftalker Plus (hardware & software) (Words +)
Access-related peripheral devices	Pneumatic switch (Prentke Romich) Tongue switch (Prentke Romich) Cyberlink (Words +) Intellikeys (Intellitools) Headmouse (Words +)

*Manufacturer or vendor is provided in parentheses.

positioning, access (upper extremity control, head control, identification of switch site), and vision be involved in AAC assessment and intervention, along with the speech-language pathologist (SLP). In most situations, the SLP will lead the assessment team, although this can depend on the dynamics of the team and the requirements of the agency that is funding the assessment and the AAC system.

Speech-language pathologists (SLP) can play a variety of roles in working with individuals who require AAC. The level of expertise including training (knowledge and skills) and experience, along with access to current technologies all have a direct impact on the role that an SLP may play in AAC assessment and intervention. Three broad roles are described below.

SLPs who have *highly specialized AAC knowledge and skills* and expertise in assessment and intervention play a critical role in working with those who need AAC. These SLPs typically have completed advanced coursework or extensive continuing education in AAC and have significant clinical experience with AAC assessment and intervention. SLPs who are AAC experts often work in highly specialized settings, such as hospitals or clinics that offer comprehensive AAC services including multidisciplinary expertise. AAC experts have competence with the full range of AAC technologies and usually will have access to a variety of AAC devices. These SLPs are able to provide the full range of AAC services such as assessment, intervention, consultation, and follow-up. They also are knowledgeable about funding sources, and usually generate the assessment report and recommendations required to secure funding for the AAC system. Because AAC assessment services are highly specialized, AAC specialists often work with individuals and their families intensively for a short period of time and then perform periodic follow-up and consultation as necessary. As a result, day-to-day intervention after an AAC system has been acquired or initially established may ultimately fall on SLPs who provide a more general range of services n outpatient or community-based settings.

SLPs who have *general AAC knowledge and skills* and basic clinical competence in AAC play a different, but important, role in AAC assessment and intervention. Many of these therapists have experience in AAC, but limited access to and/or knowledge of current AAC technology. The important characteristic of SLPs with general knowledge and skills is that they have fundamental clinical competence in the area of AAC. They may be able to develop a comprehensive low-tech AAC system, and they may even have access to a small number of AAC devices. However, SLPS with general knowledge and skills will usually need to refer patients who require more complex voice output technology and/or have access concerns to AAC specialists. In many situations, SLPs with general knowledge and skills are key contributors and team members in the AAC assessment process. They may inform the assessment process in a critical way by providing information related to the individual's capabilities and needs. SLPs with general knowledge and skills often are the primary service providers for AAC intervention after the assessment with AAC experts has been completed and equipment obtained.

SLPs who have *limited AAC knowledge and skills* may primarily play the role of identifying individuals who need AAC and referring them to a service provider with appropriate expertise. These SLPs have awareness of AAC and its potential to enhance communication, but do not have sufficient knowledge and skills to provide a comprehensive AAC assessment. Therapists in this group may be able to implement speech supplementation strategies and also to develop very basic low-tech AAC systems. However, they likely would have difficulty with more complex multipurpose low-tech systems.

SLPs can play a variety of roles in AAC assessment and intervention, ranging from being a referral source, to a partner in the assessment and intervention process, to a specialist. Which role a therapist plays depends on a number of factors, most importantly knowledge, skills, and experience in AAC. Also important is whether the SLP has access to and expertise with current technology. Effective in 2005, the American Speech-Language and Hearing Association's standards for the certificate of clinical competence require all new applicants to demonstrate knowledge of, among other things, communication modalities (including oral, manual, augmentative, alternative communication techniques, and assistive technologies) (ASHA, 2005). Thus, new SLPs in most cases will have good working knowledge of AAC assessment and intervention through their graduate education, which will enable them, at a minimum, to have general knowledge and skills and basic clinical competence in AAC.

At the same time that compensatory interventions to enhance intelligibility and participation are being implemented, consideration should be given to remediating the underlying impairment where appropriate. In many cases, treatment can and should focus simultaneously on compensatory management and reducing the underlying subsystem impairment, especially for those with an improving course who have some residual speech. See Figure 9–4 for a flow chart of treatment options based on level of speech intelligibility. However, in some situations impairment-oriented interventions may be contraindicated. For example, in speakers with the degenerative condition ALS, impairment-oriented interventions may induce fatigue which in turn may result in reduced functional ability for a period of time. In the sections that follow specific impairment-oriented approaches are discussed in detail.

Interventions to Remediate the Underlying Impairment

Interventions to remediate the underlying impairment are typically focused on rehabilitation of the resonation subsystems—respiration, phonation, velopharyngeal function, and articulation. Although the ultimate goal is to improve speech function, this is most often targeted indirectly. Speakers who are candidates for impairment-oriented interventions may fit within any of the Yorkston et al. (1999) intervention stages (no detectable disorder, obvious disorder with intelligible speech, reduced intelligibility, residual speech supplemented by augmentative techniques, and no functional speech). Clearly, speaker characteristics can vary greatly. For example, some speakers may be very mildly impaired, requiring fine tuning to make speech sound more natural or normal. Other speakers may be completely unable to speak, but show potential for recovery that warrants basic impairment-oriented intervention to reestablish support for speech. Again, etiology and expected course are critical variables in determining candidacy for impairment-oriented interventions.

Traditionally, impairment-oriented interventions approaches have been the mainstay of speech-language pathology. Therapies of this type often involve rote drill and practice at various activities in a one-on-one treatment context. There are a wide variety of such interventions, and the evidence supporting their use is variable. However, one point is clear; generalization of impairment-oriented activities to production of intelligible speech should not be taken for granted. In this section, three different groups of impairment-

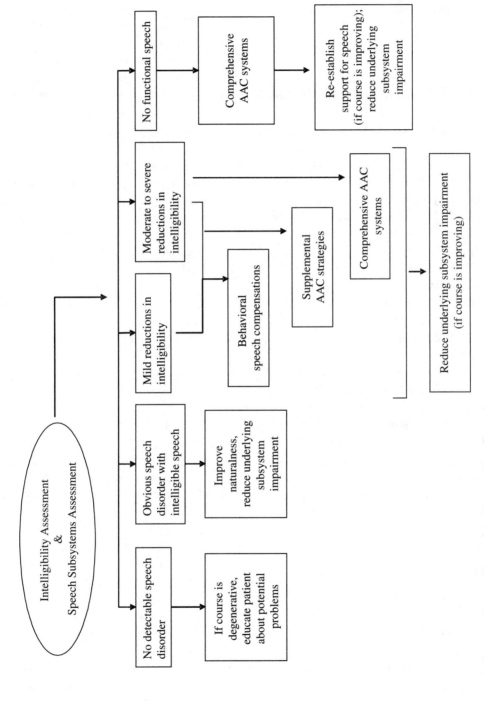

Figure 9–4. Clinical intervention flowchart.

oriented interventions are discussed. The first is speech mechanism exercises that are related to all speech subsystems. The second is subsystem-specific intervention. The third is pharmacologic and surgical intervention.

Speech Mechanism Exercises

Individuals with dysarthria often have weakness and reduced motor control of structures of the speech mechanism, relative to healthy individuals. Nonspeech deficits involving the lips, jaw, tongue, and even the respiratory system have been well documented in speakers with dysarthria (see Weismer, 2006a). Although weakness is the most obvious problem, deficits have also been demonstrated for several other oral motor tasks. For example, speakers with dysarthria can have difficulty holding a muscle contraction at a steady level even when the level is not at maximal strength. They can have difficulty rapidly and accurately achieving a strength target. Speakers with dysarthria also can experience fatigue such that they have reduced ability to hold a given strength level for an extended period of time. Finally, speakers with dysarthria can have reduced ability to create an accurate pattern of movement (such as creating a sinusoidal pattern by movement of the lips, jaw, or tongue).

The kinds of deficit described above are not surprising for a group of speech disorders in which the underlying neuropathology produces muscle weakness, instability, and in some cases discoordination. One interpretation of oromotor and respiratory deficits might be that their presence contributes to difficulty with *speech*. Based on this interpretation, it follows that management of oromotor deficits

might serve to improve speech performance and, subsequently, the larger and most important clinical issue of functional communication ability.

For the purposes of this section, the term "speech mechanism exercises" will be used to cover any type of therapeutic focus where the motor performance of the lips, jaw, tongue, soft palate, laryngeal muscles, and/or respiratory structures is practiced for improvement of a particular variable or variables. These variables may include strength, speed of movement or contraction, accuracy, coordination, and/or stability. The important point is that speech mechanism exercises do not involve *speech*, although they do involve structures of the *speech mechanism*. The theory behind use of speech mechanism exercises is that improvement in the non-speech performance of speech mechanism structures will transfer to speech production skills and, therefore, to speech intelligibility. Presumably, these sorts of exercises may be part of the physiologic support that has been discussed as a prerequisite to speech improvement in therapy (Rosenbek & LaPointe, 1985).

According to Weismer (2006a), studies have not established a meaningful relationship between oromotor, nonspeech performance, and speech production performance. That is, measures such as tongue strength, fatigue, or stability do not seem to provide much information about an individual's speech production abilities, most typically measured by a speech intelligibility score. Weismer (2006a) argues that the lack of a meaningful relationship between the two kinds of performance is not surprising because the two tasks—for example, creating a maximum strength effort by pressing the tongue blade against a rubber bulb compared to creating an intelligible string of speech sounds—are so different that they would likely have very different styles of central nervous system control. This view is consistent with that of Ziegler (2003) who reports cases of neurologic disease in which speech is affected, but not oromotor, nonspeech functions (such as swallowing), and cases in which the opposite occurs (e.g., impaired swallowing but not impaired speech). These *double dissociations*, according to Ziegler (2003), argue for control of speech mechanism structures that is *task specific*, not *structure specific*. A structure specific view would suggest that neurologic damage to orofacial, laryngeal, and/or respiratory structures would affect the performance of the structures regardless of the task. As stated above, the evidence does not support this. Moreover, fields such as physical therapy are moving away from a rehabilitative approach that emphasizes strengthening and general accuracy to one of functional task performance (see for example, Mathiowetz & Bass Haugen, 1994).

Nevertheless, speech-language clinicians often use speech mechanism exercises as a prominent component of their therapy plans for individuals with dysarthria. Indeed, the interested student can find therapeutic recommendations for nonspeech training of speech mechanism structures in several textbooks (e.g., Johns, 1985; McNeil, 1997). Most notable among these texts is Dworkin (1991), which provides detailed diagnostic and management procedures for nonspeech activities that are expected to enhance speech production capabilities. In addition, it has been urged that the use of these nonspeech tasks as therapeutic activities should be structured as motor learning tasks, taking advantage of known principles of skill acquisition (McNeil, Robin, & Schmidt, 1997). If a decision is made to incorporate speech mechanism exercises into the treat-

ment plan, these sources provide information regarding the various ways in which speech mechanism exercises can be pursued, measured, and interpreted.

From the perspective of evidence-based practice, however, there are very few studies that have assessed the therapeutic effect of speech mechanism exercises on speech production skills. Moreoever, the few existing studies (e.g., Dworkin, Abkarian, & Johns, 1988; Solomon, 2004) have not demonstrated effects that would support the use of oromotor, nonspeech activities to improve speech production skills. It is important to understand the distinction made here. Clearly, such exercises may result in improvement in the nonspeech behavior being trained (see, for example, Lazarus, Logemann, Huang, & Rademaker, 2003) but that does not mean that the improvement transfers to speech production skills. Additional research is necessary to examine the relationship between specific speech mechanism exercises and functional speech outcomes.

Speech Subsystem Interventions

In this section, an overview of approaches for managing impairments in the respiratory, phonatory, velopharyngeal, and articulatory subsystems in speakers with dysarthria is provided. In general, subsystems intervention is best addressed using a bottom-up approach. This means that deficits involving respiration and then phonation should be addressed first because they are the driving force behind speech. Then, after respiratory and phonatory issues have been managed, intervention should address resonation and articulation, which serve to filter or shape the sounds of the language. The focus in this section is on a broad orientation to management strategies for each subsystem, rather than detailed information about specific techniques. Students should see Yorkston et al. (1999) for additional information, including descriptions of treatment sequences for each subsystem.

Respiratory Subsystem

Individuals with dysarthria often have difficulty with speech breathing. The consequences of respiratory impairment can have a critical impact on speech production. Common consequences include short phrases, low vocal intensity, and inability to produce phonation, all of which can interfere with intelligibility. The evaluation of speech breathing problems in individuals with dysarthria is discussed in detail in Chapter 4. Treatments for speech breathing problems are most often directed toward three main issues: (1) modification of tracheal pressures and inappropriate lung volume for speech, (2) modification of inappropriate coordination between components of the chest wall, and (3) modification of breath group size and content. It is often the case that treatment directed at any one of these modifications may not be independent of the others. For example, modification of tracheal pressures may result from changes in lung volume range for speech, or modification of the lung volume range for speech may promote a higher tracheal pressure. Similarly, the speaker who is having problems coordinating the rib cage and abdomen during speech may have low tracheal pressures because these two parts of the chest wall are not contributing to compression of the lungs. Moreover, it is important to realize that it is difficult to separate the effects of treatment of speech breathing from treatment of the larynx; both may be

affected by therapy that is assumed to be directed independently at either level of the speech mechanism.

The interdependencies among these issues related to speech breathing, and between treatment of speech breathing and laryngeal function for speech, is reflected in a review published by Yorkston, Spencer, and Duffy (2003a, 2003b). These authors summarized the available literature on treatment effects for respiratory and phonatory dysfunction in dysarthria, and concluded that clear and consistent effects had yet to be established. However, it is apparent from their review that for selected speakers, treatment of speech breathing problems can produce positive results (see also Solomon, Makashay, Kessler, & Sullivan, 2004). Treatment approaches for each of the potential problems listed above are summarized here; also Chapter 4 provides specific details of speech breathing physiology and its effects on speech production.

Modification of Tracheal Pressure and Inappropriate Lung Volume.
When treatment is directed at speech breathing only, with no explicit focus on laryngeal mechanisms, the most likely way to get increased tracheal pressure in speakers with inadequate voice loudness is to modify the starting lung volume. As reviewed in Chapter 4, efficient speech breathing takes advantage of the non-muscular, recoil pressures generated by stretched respiratory structures. These recoil pressures are best suited for normal speech loudness levels when the speaker produces utterances between 60 to 35% vital capacity (VC). If an individual is initiating speech at low lung volumes—a common observation in those with dysarthria—the clinician should treat the problem by first estimating the starting lung vol-

ume using the noninstrumental approach described in Chapter 4, and then shaping a higher and more efficient starting lung volume by instructing the speaker to inhale from around resting expiratory level (REL) before initiating utterances.

Relatedly, some speakers with dysarthria will inhale to a reasonable starting lung volume but will then exhale a sizable volume of air before initiating speech (e.g., Murdoch, Theodoros, Stokes, & Chenery, 1993). The effect of this behavior is the same as beginning speech at a low lung volume and it should be watched carefully during the lung-volume shaping process. A simple approach to teach speakers to initiate phonation at the onset of expiration (using a reasonable lung volume) might be to begin with a sustained vowel. After the speaker learns to initiate phonation without exhaling beforehand, intervention should incorporate actual speech.

It is important to remember that an inefficient lung volume for speech will not only result in reduced loudness and the obvious effects on speech intelligibility, but will also likely make speech production much more effortful for the speaker. This is because the reduced lung volume will require the speaker to exert much more muscular effort to generate tracheal pressures than would be required in the 60 to 35% VC range.

Modifications of Coordination Between Components of the Chest Wall. As summarized in Chapter 4 (see Table 4–2), during speech the rib cage and abdomen should both be getting smaller and, therefore, contributing to compression of the lungs to maintain a relatively constant tracheal pressure. Speakers who produce paradoxic breathing during speech, however, will have one part of the chest wall moving in the inspiratory

direction while the other part moves in the expiratory direction. When this is a chronic behavior, it is very inefficient and will certainly compromise an individual's ability to produce efficient and adequate tracheal pressures for speech.

With the correct instruments, it is possible to monitor the motions of these two parts of the chest wall and attempt to use biofeedback to train the speaker to coordinate the rib cage and abdomen for speech, so both parts are moving in the expiratory direction. However, this requires specialized equipment (such as a Respitrace) and even then may be a difficult cognitive task for the speaker. In those with abdominal weakness or paralysis, paradoxic motions of the abdomen can be observed or felt as an outward motion of the abdominal surface during speech. In these cases, it is possible that temporary abdominal binding can substitute for the weakened or paralyzed muscles, and allow the speaker to generate better tracheal pressures. There is some evidence (Simpson, Till, & Goff, 1988) that abdominal binding can improve tracheal pressures (see also Hixon & Hoit, 2005, pp. 400–406). However, medical approval is necessary for use of abdominal binding as this technique may potentially interfere with inspiration in some speakers.

Modification of Breath Group Size and Content. Breath group structure, including length and content, may have a profound effect on the way in which speech is perceived. Variables such as naturalness of speech and even intelligibility can be affected by the packaging of speech information (see Chapter 7). Bellaire et al. (1986) reported a case in which they successfully changed the duration of breath groups in speakers with brain injury. The modification of what these authors called "breath patterning" seemed to result in a favorable change in perceived naturalness of speech. There are likely a number of ways in which breath groups and their boundaries—pauses—can be trained for greater duration and possible content (e.g., terminating breath groups at major grammatical boundaries), including rate control strategies, external pacing devices, and simple instruction relating to current and desired behaviors.

Clearly, the duration and structure of breath groups may be dependent on lung volume usage for speech. A low and inefficient starting lung volume for speech will likely result in shorter breath groups as the speaker will avoid expending too much muscular effort to extend an utterance. The clinician should be aware of the potential interactions between all aspects of speech breathing treatment.

Phonatory Subsystem

As described previously, many interventions for respiration also have an effect on phonation, and vice versa. In this section, one particular voice treatment is highlighted, the Lee Silverman Voice Treatment (LSVT). In LSVT, the primary focus is phonation, but the treatment also has an effect on respiratory support for speech. LSVT has been the focus of considerable research and has gained extensive popularity for the treatment of individuals with Parkinson's disease (PD). For information about other voice interventions, both behavioral and surgical, readers are referred to Ramage, Morrison, and Nichol (2001) and relevant chapters in Rubin, Sataloff, and Korovin (2003). Efficacy of behavioral voice treatments is reviewed by Verdolini and Ramig (1998).

For many speakers, reduced loudness may result in compromised intelligibility.

Although problems with loudness can affect individuals with different types of dysarthria, those with hypokinetic characteristics, especially individuals with PD, seem to be most frequently affected. LSVT focuses on behavioral modification to increase effort and magnitude of motor movement for speakers with PD (Ramig, Pawless, & Countryman, 1995). Speakers are taught to "think big" and "think loud," using a variety of intervention activities that teach them how to do this. The goals of LSVT are to increase respiratory support, increase vocal fold adduction, and increase phonatory effort, with the ultimate goal to return and/or maintain functional and in many cases normal speaking abilities.

The goal of increasing phonatory effort is key to the application of the LSVT in individuals with PD because the therapy is based on the assumption that one result of the disease is an altered calibration of the relationship between perceived effort and vocal output. The speaker may have an abnormally low vocal loudness that affects speech intelligibility, but may deny feeling that his or her vocal effort should be greater. Similarly, when the speaker is prompted to produce a normal vocal loudness he or she may tell the clinician that it feels as if he or she is shouting. The adjustment of this miscalibration is a central goal of LSVT, which strives to teach the individual the correct match between effort and output, the latter being vocal loudness.

LSVT intervention is intensive and includes subsystem-related activities such as sustained phonation and vocal glides to increase respiratory support for speech and laryngeal flexibility, respectively. In addition, the LSVT approach also includes use of meaningful utterances and spontaneous speech. LSVT is a carefully controlled treatment protocol that has been well studied. LSVT is unique in that the role of the clinician goes well past the knowledge and skills gained in clinical training and on-the-job experience. LSVT clinicians are urged to present themselves to patients with "high enthusiasm and high energy." The presumption is that the clinician's energy level and enthusiasm will contribute to the speaker's efforts to generate the kind of respiratory and laryngeal control required for normal vocal loudness. Therapists must complete intensive workshop training in order to be certified to provide LSVT.

A number of studies have evaluated the effectiveness of LSVT. Yorkston and colleagues (in progress) summarized the results of those studies in a review of the evidence concerning the effectives of treatment for loudness. Outcome measures for LSVT have included acoustic, physiologic, perceptual, and psychosocial. In addition, articulatory variables have also been examined, even though the LSVT is directed exclusively to laryngeal mechanisms of vocal loudness (adduction of the vocal folds). One claim of LSVT is that treatment effects spread to other parts of the speech mechanism and, therefore, have an effect on communication ability that goes past adjustments of vocal loudness. The spreading effects notion of speech therapy, where a treatment aimed at a basic level of the speech production process produces beneficial effects in other, nontreated parts of the mechanism, was first described in detail by Rosenbek and LaPointe (1985).

In general, LSVT studies seem to indicate that this is a promising and effective approach to improving loudness, among other things, in speakers with Parkinson's disease. However, long-term outcome studies examining effects of treatment across settings and over time are necessary. In addition, the effectiveness of LSVT for pop-ulations of speakers besides those with PD is unclear; this is an important direction for future research.

Velopharyngeal Subsystem

Velopharyngeal impairment is common in dysarthria, and may refer to several different problems that can affect communication. In general, when a speaker is diagnosed with velopharyngeal impairment, he or she has some problem with the opening and closing gestures of the velopharyngeal port. If the diagnosis is based on imaging or direct viewing studies (e.g., a nasoendoscopic study, or x-ray motion pictures) or aerodynamic observations (e.g., nasal flow), the physiologic problem can be identified more or less directly. More commonly, the physiologic problem is inferred from acoustic or perceptual observations.

Some speakers may have the problem of a chronically open velopharyngeal port, which will affect speech in several ways. First, the speaker will be perceived as having a chronic hypernasal quality during speech. Second, the speaker is likely to be perceived as having reduced loudness because a chronically open velopharyngeal port causes sound energy to be absorbed in the nasal cavities which results in an overall reduction in the acoustic energy radiating from the vocal tract. And third, the speaker will have problems producing sounds that require pressure inside the mouth to be greater than the pressure outside the mouth (e.g., stops and fricatives). This pressure, typically called *intraoral air pressure*, can only be developed and maintained when the velopharyngeal port is closed completely, in effect sealing the vocal tract at one end. The other "seal-off" point will be located in the vocal tract where the articulators make the closure for the consonant (e.g., at the lips for stops like /p/ and/b/, between the tongue tip and alveolar ridge for /s/ and /z/, and so forth). Clearly, the combination of these problems will not only have an effect on speech intelligibility, but it is also likely to produce a negative social reaction to the speaker (e.g., Blood & Hyman, 1977; Lallh & Rochet, 2000). In other words, chronic hypernasality is likely to have social consequences for a speaker that extend past her or his problem in transmitting an intelligible message.

Some speakers may have more episodic problems with velopharyngeal impairment, perhaps best described as a coordination problem. Speakers with this kind of problem may be able to close the velopharyngeal port but may experience timing problems. For example, a speaker may open and/or close the port at inappropriate times relative to the prevailing phonetic requirements. Such speakers are less likely to have the problem of chronic hypernasality, and relatively more likely to experience speech intelligibility problems related directly to the mistimed velopharyngeal gesture (e.g., such as opening the port during the articulation of a stop consonant).

The treatment options for velopharyngeal impairment are fairly straightforward, and a solid body of research suggests what does and does not work. Typically, nonspeech exercises such as blowing or any other form of palatal exercise do not seem to work because the velopharyngeal gestures exercised in these tasks are not like those used during speech. This has been known for some time in the cleft palate literature (see, for example, Ruscello, 1982, and Golding-Kushner, 1995) and is also the conclusion reached by Yorkston et al. (2001b) in their review of treatment options for velopharyngeal impairment

in dysarthria. What does seem to work for many speakers with dysarthria and velopharyngeal impairment is the use of a speech appliance such as a palatal lift. Palatal lifts are devices that are secured to the teeth and have an acrylic shelf that maintains the soft palate in an elevated position. As summarized by Yorkston et al. (2001b), palatal lifts seem to improve speech intelligibility, chronic hypernasality, and articulation of individual sounds. Decisions concerning which speakers are the best candidates for a palatal lift are complicated. In general, it seems that good candidates have flaccid dysarthria, intact dentition, and good movement of the lateral pharyngeal walls (an essential part of velopharyngeal closure in many speakers). Moreover, the design, fitting, and evaluation of an effective palatal lift require the services of an experienced prosthodontist. Yorkston et al. (1999, 2001b) provide additional information regarding palatal lifts for speakers with dysarthria. Also, the extensive cleft palate literature is an important source for more information on treatment options for velopharyngeal impairment.

Articulatory Subsystem

Treatment of the articulatory subsystem, for the purposes of this section, involves treatment of the vocal tract gestures that create the different sounds of a language. The velopharyngeal system can certainly be included in this definition, but that has been covered above; in this section, the rest of the sound-shaping structures are considered.

As reviewed earlier and in the section on the velopharyngeal system, the use of oromotor exercises to facilitate articulatory behavior in speech is not supported by experimental evidence. Even though such exercises are often used by speech-language pathologists, at the current time they do not meet the standards of evidence-based practice.

Under the assumption that the best way to deal with a speech production problem is to work on speech production skills, there are two general clinical approaches, one that is direct and the other indirect.

Direct Approaches. Direct approaches involve therapies where the articulatory gesture(s) for a particular sound are trained. This is often accomlished by manual placement of an articulator (at first, usually clinician-assisted) with subsequent instruction for what kind of gesture is to be produced, or possibly simply by description of what the articulators should be doing. A necessary precursor to this kind of therapy is some knowledge on the part of the speaker concerning speech production. One strategy is to provide the patient with one or two lessons in articulatory phonetics, using diagrams, demonstrations, and other materials (we are indebted to J. C. Rosenbek for this notion of educating patients as the first step in therapy). When the point is reached where instructions are being given and placements are being attempted, the lessons will guarantee a common vocabulary between the clinician and patient.

Direct approaches to articulation therapy have little firm supporting evidence, and there are limitations to their application. For example, it is easy to imagine clinician-assisted articulatory placements for bilabial stops, even lingua-alveolar stops. It is even possible to imagine a straightforward explanation of an opening gesture of the vocal tract from consonant to vowel.

But placements of dorsal consonants (/k/ and /g/) and assistance with tongue shaping for fricatives are harder to envision. The clinician should be aware, therefore, that direct approaches may have some fairly severe restrictions in application.

Indirect Approaches. As noted previously in this chapter and in Chapter 6, there are some manipulations that have been shown to change articulatory behavior in ways that might be useful for the patient with dysarthria. Specifically, slowing of speaking rate, stressing a syllable, and speaking with greater voice intensity have all been associated with larger displacements of articulators, and in some cases faster movements of the articulators. Many speakers with dysarthria have reduced articulatory movements, which seem to have a direct bearing on their speech intelligibility (Weismer, 2006b). The theory behind treatment of the articulatory subsystem is, therefore, to provide a means to expand the "articulatory working space," that is, to increase articulatory displacements generally with the result that important phonetic contrasts will be better defined and, therefore, more intelligible. Slowing of speaking rate, stress on the syllable carrying targeted sounds, and increased loudness all have the potential to produce this effect. Each of these approaches has some potential drawbacks: slowed speaking rate can sound unnatural; excessively loud speech is socially undesirable; and unusual degrees of stress on individual syllables may have an odd perceptual effect. But it is possible to imagine using these manipulations and then attempting to shape more natural-sounding speech if segmental success is achieved.

Neuoropharmacologic and Neurosurgical Approaches to Speech Improvement

For some speakers, medical management involves surgical and pharmacologic intervention. Usually, such interventions target limb and other functions, but nonetheless can have an impact on speech production. Parkinson's disease is one disease for which surgical and pharmacologic treatments have proliferated. Neuropharmacologic treatments in Parkinson's disease are aimed primarily at the loss of dopamine concentrations in the striatum. Decades of clinical experience have shown that levodopa (administered as various drugs) improves the classical symptoms of Parkinson's disease (bradykinesia, rigidity, tremor), but the literature on co-occurring speech effects is much more ambiguous. Several recent reviews of drug effects on hypokinetic dysarthria show highly variable and sometimes negative effects of levodopa on speech production characteristics (Goberman & Coelho, 2002; Pinto et al., 2004; Schulz, 2002). At this point in time, it is prudent to conclude that levodopa does not have predictable effects on hypokinetic dysarthria, although some individuals may experience improvements in certain aspects of speech production when the drug is at peak effect.

Much the same conclusion can be reached about the effect of neurosurgical approaches to Parkinson's disease. Neurosurgical approaches may include the creation of lesions or the implantation of an electrode for deep-brain stimulation (DBS). Within the cortical-basal nuclei motor loop described in Chapter 3, parts of the globus pallidus, thalamus, and subthalamic nucleus have been the target of lesion and/or stimulation therapy for the symptoms of

Parkinson's disease. As reviewed by Pinto et al. (2004), both approaches have shown positive effects on limb symptoms but very mixed effects on speech, including some markedly negative outcomes. Among the structures targeted for lesions or DBS, unilateral lesions or DBS of the subthalamic nucleus seem to have had the most success (but still very mixed) in lessening the severity of hypokinetic dysarthria; bilateral lesions or stimulation of the subthalamic nucleus seem to have a clear, negative effect on speech symptoms.

Other types of drug therapy may also have an effect on dysarthria. For example, baclofen is an antispasticity drug that reduces hypertonia in individuals with cerebral palsy. A very limited number of case reports suggest that when baclofen is administered intrathecally, or in the cerebrospinal fluid surrounding the spinal cord, improvements in dysarthria may be measurable (e.g., Leary, Giplin, Lockley, Rodriguez, Jarrett, & Stevenson, 2006).

As part of a health care team, the SLP should know the existing evidence for the effects of neuropharmacologic and neurosurgical treatments on speech production characteristics. Knowledge of the potential effects of such treatments on behavioral modification of dysarthria symptoms is very desirable. An SLP who is planning a course of therapy for the patient with dysarthria should consider how current and previous drug and surgical treatments might impact the success of speech treatment. Unfortunately, this latter kind of information—the influence of drug and surgical treatments on traditional speech therapy—is not currently available. Is the individual receiving unilateral DBS of the subthalamic nucleus a better candidate for speech therapy than an individual who is not? Is the teenager with cerebral palsy and severe dysarthria likely to show more progress in speech therapy if she is being treated with baclofen? These are questions that have not been addressed yet, and practicing SLPs should be able to represent the state of knowledge in our field to other members of the health care team.

Summary

Improving speech intelligibility is often a primary goal of treatment for individuals with dysarthria. This chapter has presented a continuum of intervention approaches ranging from compensatory treatments aimed at reducing activity limitations and participation restrictions to speech subsystem treatments aimed at reducing the underlying impairment. Our primary premise has been twofold: functional communication should be addressed immediately when working with a speaker who has dysarthria and speech itself should be used to improve speech. Etiology and expected course of the dysarthria are important considerations in designing treatment; and it is critical that clinicians consider both current and future abilities and needs when developing intervention packages. In the past, compensatory interventions and impairment-oriented interventions have been viewed as mutually exclusive options. However, we have advocated for a two-pronged approach to intervention where both functional communication and remediation of underlying impairment (where appropriate) are addressed simultaneously. As Daniel Webster once said, "Communication is the essence of human life." The ultimate goal of the SLP is to enable individuals with dysarthria to communicate as effectively, efficiently, and naturally as possible through any and all means available.

References

American Speech-Language-Hearing Association. (2002). Augmentative and alternative communication: Knowledge and skills for service delivery. *ASHA Supplement, 22,* 97–106.

American Speech-Language-Hearing Association. (2004). Roles and responsibilities of speech-language pathologists with respect to augmentative and alternative communication: Technical report. *ASHA Supplement, 24,* 1–18.

American Speech-Language and Hearing Association. (2005*). Membership and certification handbook*. Retrieved July 14, 2006 from http://www.asha.org/about/membership-certification/handbooks/slp/slp_standards.htm

Ansel, B. M., & Kent, R. D. (1992). Acoustic-phonetic contrasts and intelligibility in the dysarthria associated with mixed cerebral palsy. *Journal of Speech and Hearing Research, 35,* 296–308.

Barefoot, S. M., Bochner, J. G., Johnson, B. A., & vom Eigner, B. A. (1993). Rating deaf speakers' comprehensibility: An exploratory investigation. *American Journal of Speech-Language Pathology, 2,* 31–35.

Beliveau, C., Hodge, M., & Hagler, P. (1995). Effect of supplemental linguistic cues on the intelligibility of severely dysarthric speakers. *Augmentative and Alternative Communication, 11,* 176–186.

Bellaire, K., Yorkston, K. M., & Beukelman, D. R. (1986). Modification of breath patterning to increase naturalness of a mildly dysarthric speaker. *Journal of Communication Disorders, 19,* 271–280.

Beukelman, D. R., Fager, S., Ullman, C., Hanson, E., & Logemann, J. (2002). The impact of speech supplementation and clear speech on the intelligibility and speaking rate of people with traumatic brain injury. *Journal of Medical Speech Language Pathology, 10*, 237-242.

Beukelman, D. R., Garrett, K. L., & Yorkston, K. M. (Eds.). (in press). *AAC intervention for adults in medical settings: Integrated assessment and treatment protocols.* Baltimore: Paul H. Brookes.

Beukelman, D. R., & Mirenda, P. (2005). *Augmentative and alternative communication: Supporting children and adults with complex communication needs* (3rd ed.). Baltimore: Paul H. Brookes

Beukelman, D., & Yorkston, K. (1977). A communication system for the severely dysarthric speaker with an intact language system. *Journal of Speech and Hearing Disorders, 42*, 265-270.

Beukelman, D. R., Yorkston, K., & Reichle J. (2000). *Augmentative communication for adults with acquired neurologic disabilities.* Baltimore: Paul H. Brookes.

Blood, G., & Hyman, M. (1977). Children's perception of nasal resonance. *Journal of Speech and Hearing Disorders, 42*, 446-448.

Bunton K., Kent R., & Kent, J. (2000). Perceptuo-acoustic assessment of prosodic impairment in dysarthria. *Clinical Linguistics and Phonetics, 14*, 13-24.

Bunton K., Kent R., Kent J., & Duffy J. (2001). The effects of flattening fundamental frequency contours on sentence intelligibility in speakers with dysarthria. *Clinical Linguistics and Phonetics, 15*, 181-193.

Carter, C., Yorkston, K., Strand, E., & Hammen, V. (1996). Effects of semantic and syntactic context on actual and estimated sentence intelligibility of dysarthric speakers. In D. Robin, K. Yorkston, & D. Beukelman (Eds.), *Disorders of motor speech: Assessment, treatment, and clinical characterization* (pp. 67-87). Baltimore: Paul H. Brookes.

Crow, E., & Enderby, P. (1989). The effects of an alphabet chart on the speaking rate and intelligibility of speakers with dysarthria. In K. Yorkston & D. Beukelman (Eds.), *Recent advances in clinical dysarthria* (pp. 100-108). Boston: College-Hill Press.

Cutler, A., Dahan, D., & van Donselaar, W. (1997) Prosody in the comprehension of spoken language: A literature review. *Language and Speech, 40*, 141-201.

Dagenais, P. A., Brown, G. R., & Moore, R. E. (2006). Speech rate effects upon intelligibility and acceptability of dysarthric speech. *Clinical Linguistic and Phonetics, 20*, 141-148.

Darley, F., Aronson, A., & Brown, J. (1969). Clusters of deviant speech dimensions in the dysarthrias. *Journal of Speech and Hearing Research, 12*, 462-496.

Dongilli, P. (1994). Semantic context and speech intelligibility. In J. Till, K. Yorkston, & D. Beukelman (Eds.), *Motor speech disorders: Advance in assessment and treatment* (pp. 175-191). Baltimore: Paul H. Brookes.

Drager, K. D. R., & Reichle, J. E. (2001). Effects of discourse context on the intelligibility of synthesized speech for young adult and older adult listeners: Applications for AAC. *Journal of Speech, Language, and Hearing Research, 44*, 1052-1057.

Duffy, J. (1995). *Motor speech disorders: Substrates, differential diagnosis, and management.* St. Louis, MO: Mosby.

Dworkin, J. P. (1991). *Motor speech disorders: A treatment guide.* St. Louis, MO: Mosby.

Dworkin, J. P., Abkarian, G. G., & Johns, D. F. (1988). Apraxia of speech: The effectiveness of a treatment regimen. *Journal of Speech and Hearing Disorders, 53*, 280-294.

Garcia, J., & Cannito, M. (1996). Influence of verbal and nonverbal contexts on the sentence intelligibility of a speaker with dysarthria. *Journal of Speech and Hearing Research, 39*, 750-760.

Garcia, J. M., Cannito, M. P., & Dagenais, P. A. (2000). Hand gestures: Perspectives and preliminary implications for adults with acquired dysarthria. *American Journal of Speech-Language Pathology, 9*, 107-115.

Garcia, J. M., & Cobb, D. S. (2000). The effects of gesturing on speech intelligibility and rate in ALS dysarthria: A case study. *Journal of Medical Speech-Language Pathology, 8*, 353-357.

Garcia, J. M., Crowe, L. K., Redler, D., & Hustad, K. C. (2004). Effects of spontaneous gestures on comprehension and intelligibility of dysarthric speech: A case report. *Journal of Medical Speech-Language Pathology, 12*(4), 145–148.

Garcia, J. M., & Dagenais, P. A. (1998). Dysarthric sentence intelligibility: Contribution of iconic gestures and message predictiveness. *Journal of Speech, Language, and Hearing Research, 41*, 1282–1293.

Goberman, A., & Coelho, C. (2002). Acoustic analysis of Parkinsonian speech: I. Speech characteristics and L-Dopa therapy. *Neuro-Rehabilitation, 17*, 237–246.

Golding-Kushner, K. J. (1995). Treatment of articulation and resonance disorders associated with cleft palate and VPI. In R. J. Shprintzen & J. Bardach (Eds.), *Cleft palate speech management: A multidisciplinary approach* (pp. 327–551). St. Louis, MO: Mosby.

Gutek, J., & Rochet, A. (1996). Effects of insertion of interword pauses on the intelligibility of dysarthric speech. In D. Robin, K. Yorkston & D. Beukelman (Eds.), *Disorders of motor speech: Assessment, treatment, and clinical characterization* (pp. 105–120). Baltimore: Paul H. Brookes.

Hammen, V. L., Yorkston, K. M., & Minifie, F. D. (1994). Effects of temporal alterations on speech intelligibility in parkinsonian dysarthria. *Journal of Speech and Hearing Research, 37*, 244–253.

Hanson, E. K., Yorkston, K. M., & Beukelman, D. R. (2004). Speech supplementation techniques for dysarthria: A systematic review. *Journal of Medical Speech-Language Pathology, 12*(2), ix–xxix.

Hartelius, L., Wising, C., & Nord, L. (1997). Speech modification in dysarthria associated with multiple sclerosis: An intervention based on vocal efficiency, contrastive stress, and verbal repair strategies. *Journal of Medical Speech-Language Pathology, 5*, 113–140.

Higginbotham, D. J., Drazek, A. L., Kowarsky, K., Scally, C., & Segal, E. (1994). Discourse comprehension of synthetic speech delivered at normal and slow presentation rates. *Augmentative and Alternative Communication, 10*(3), 191–202.

Hixon, T. J., & Hoit, J. D. (2005). *Evaluation and management of speech breathing disorders: Principles and methods.* Tucson, AZ: Redington Brown.

Hunter, L., Pring, T., & Martin, S. (1991). The use of strategies to increase speech intelligibility in cerebral palsy: An experimental evaluation. *British Journal of Disorders of Communication, 26*, 163–174.

Hustad, K. C., (2006a). Estimating the intelligibility of speakers with dysarthria. *Folia Phoniatrica et Logopaedica, 58*, 217–228.

Hustad, K. C. (2006b). *Describing the functionality of dysarthric speech: Are intelligibility scores reflective of listener comprehension?* Manuscript submitted for publication.

Hustad, K. C., Auker, J., Natale, N., & Carlson, R. (2003). Improving intelligibility of speakers with profound dysarthria and cerebral palsy. *Augmentative and Alternative Communication, 19*, 187–198.

Hustad, K. C., & Beukelman, D. R. (2001). Effects of linguistic cues and stimulus cohesion on intelligibility of severely dysarthric speech. *Journal of Speech, Language, and Hearing Research, 44*, 497–510.

Hustad, K. C., & Beukelman, D. R. (2002). Listener comprehension of severely dysarthric speech: Effects of linguistic cues and stimulus cohesion. *Journal of Speech, Language, and Hearing Research, 45*, 545–558.

Hustad, K. C., & Cahill, M. A. (2003). Effects of presentation mode and repeated familiarization on intelligibility of dysarthric speech. *American Journal of Speech-Language Pathology, 12*, 1–11.

Hustad, K. C., & Garcia, J. (2002). The influences of alphabet supplementation, iconic gestures, and predictive messages on intelligibility of a speaker with cerebral palsy. *Journal of Medical Speech-Language Pathology, 10*(4), 279–285.

Hustad, K. C., & Garcia, J. M. (2005). Aided and unaided speech supplementation strategies: Effect of alphabet cues and iconic hand gestures on dysarthric speech. *Journal of Speech, Language, and Hearing Research, 48,* 996-1012.

Hustad, K. C., Jones, T., & Dailey, S. (2003). Implementing speech supplementation strategies: Effects on intelligibility and speech rate of individuals with chronic severe dysarthria. *Journal of Speech, Language, and Hearing Research, 46,* 462-474.

Hustad, K. C., & Sassano, K. (2002). Effects of rate reduction on severe spastic dysarthria in cerebral palsy. *Journal of Medical Speech-Language Pathology, 10,* 287-292.

Johns, D. F. (1985). *Clinical management of neurogenic communicative disorders* (2nd ed.). Boston: Little, Brown.

Kennedy, M. R. T., Strand, E. A., & Yorkston, K. M.(1994). Selected acoustic changes in the verbal repairs of dysarthric speakers. *Journal of Medical Speech Language Pathology, 2,* 263-279.

Kent, R., Weismer, G., Kent, J., & Rosenbek, J. (1989). Toward phonetic intelligibility testing in dysarthria. *Journal of Speech and Hearing Disorders, 54,* 482-499.

Lallh, A. K., & Rochet, A. P. (2000). The effect of information on listeners' attitude towards speakers with voice and resonance disorders. *Journal of Speech, Language, and Hearing Research, 43,* 782-795.

Laures, J. S., & Bunton, K. (2003). Perceptual effects of a flattened fundamental frequency at the sentence level under different listening conditions. *Journal of Communication Disorders, 36,* 449-464.

Laures J. S., & Weismer G. (1999). The effects of a flattened fundamental frequency on intelligibility at the sentence level. *Journal of Speech, Language, and Hearing Research, 42,* 1148-1156.

Lazarus, C., Logemann, J. A., Huang, C. F., & Rademaker, A. W. (2003). Effects of two types of tongue strengthening exercises in young normals. *Folia Phoniatrica et Logopaedica, 55,* 199-205.

Leary, S. M., Giplin, P., Lockley, L., Rodriguez, L., Jarrett, L., & Stevenson, P. L. (2006). Intrathecal Baclofen therapy improves functional intelligibility of speech in cerebral palsy. *Clinical Rehabilitation, 20,* 228-231.

LeDorze, G., Ouellet, L., & Ryalls, J. (1994). Intonation and speech rate in dysarthric speech. *Journal of Communication Disorders, 27,* 1-18.

Lehiste, I. (1970). *Suprasegmentals.* Cambridge, MA: MIT Press.

Lloyd, L., & Fuller, D. (1986). Toward an augmentative and alternative communication symbol taxonomy: A proposed superordinate classification. *Augmentative and Alternative Communication, 2,* 165-171.

Maassen, B. (1986). Marking word boundaries to improve the intelligibility of the speech of the deaf. *Journal of Speech and Hearing Research, 29,* 227-230.

Mathiowetz, V., & Bass Haugen, J. (1994). Motor behavior research: Implications for therapeutic approaches to central nervous system dysfunction. *American Journal of Occupational Therapy, 48,* 733-745.

McNeil. M. R. (1997). *Clinical management of sensorimotor speech disorders.* New York: Thieme.

McNeil, M. R., Robin, D. A., & Schmidt, R. A. (1997). Apraxia of speech: Definition, differentiation, and treatment. In M. R. McNeil (Ed.), *Clinical management of sensorimotor speech disorders* (pp. 311-344). New York: Thieme.

Miller, G. A., Heise, G. A., & Lichten, W. (1951). The intelligibility of speech as a function of the context of the test materials. *Journal of Experimental Psychology, 41,* 329-335.

Murdoch, B. E., Theodoros, D. G., Stokes, P. E., & Chenery, H. J. (1993). Abnormal patterns of speech breathing in dysarthric speakers following severe closed head injury. *Brain Injury, 7*(4), 295-308.

Picheny, M., Durlach, N., & Braida, L. (1985). Speaking clearly for he hard of hearing I: Intelligibility differences between clear and conversational speech. *Journal of Speech,*

Language, and Hearing Research, 28, 96-103.

Picheny, M., Durlach, N., & Braida, L. (1986). Speaking clearly for the hard of hearing II: Acoustic characteristics of clear and conversational speech. *Journal of Speech, Language, and Hearing Research, 29,* 434-446.

Pilon, M. A., McIntosh, K. W., & Thaut, M. H. (1998). Auditory vs. visual speech timing cue as external rate control to enhance verbal intelligibility in mixed spastic-ataxic dysarthric speakers: A pilot study. *Brain Injury, 12,* 793-803.

Pinto, S., Ozsancak, C., Tripoliti, E., Thobois, S., Limousin-Dousey, P., & Auzou, P. (2004). Treatments for dysarthria in Parkinson's disease. *The Lancet: Neurology, 3,* 547-546.

Platt, L. J., Andrews, G., Young, M., & Quinn, P. T. (1980). Dysarthria of adult cerebral palsy: I. Intelligibility and articulatory impairment. *Journal of Speech and Hearing Research, 22,* 28-40.

Ramage, L., Morrison, M., & Nichol, H. (2001). *Management of the voice and its disorders* (2nd ed.). San Diego, CA: Singular Publishing Group.

Ramig, L.O., Pawlas, A.A., & Countryman, S. (1995). *The Lee Silverman voice treatment: A practical guide for treating the voice and speech disorders in Parkinson disease.* Denver, CO: National Center for Voice and Speech.

Rosenbek, J. C., & LaPointe, L. L. (1985). The dysarthrias: Description, diagnosis, and treatment. In D. F. Johns (Ed.), *Clinical management of neurogenic communicative disorders* (2nd ed., pp. 97-152). Boston: Little, Brown and Co.

Rubin, J. S., Sataloff, R. T., & Korovin, G. S. (Eds.) (2003). *Diagnosis and treatment of voice disorders* (2nd ed.). Clifton Park, NY: Delmar Learning.

Ruscello, D.M. (1982). A selected review of palatal training procedures. *Cleft Palate Journal, 18,* 181-193.

Schiavetti, N. (1992). Scaling procedures for the measurement of speech intelligibility. In R. Kent (Ed.), *Intelligibility in speech disorders: Theory, measurement, and management.* (pp. 11-34). Amsterdam: John Benjamins.

Schliesser, H. F. (1985). Psychological scaling of speech by students in training compared to that by experienced speech-language pathologists. *Perceptual and Motor Skills, 61,* 1299-1302.

Schulz, G. M. (2002). The effects of speech therapy and pharmacological treatments on voice and speech in Parkinson's disease: A review of the literature. *Journal of Current Medicinal Chemistry, 9,* 1241-1253.

Simpson, M. B., Till, J. A., & Goff, A. M. (1988). Long-term treatment of severe dysarthria: A case study. *Journal of Speech and Hearing Research, 53,* 433-440.

Sitler, R. W., Schiavetti, N., & Metz, D. E. (1983). Contextual effects in the measurement of hearing-impaired speakers' intelligibility. *Journal of Communication Disorders, 11,* 22-30.

Solomon, N. P. (2004). Assessment of tongue weakness and fatigue. *International Journal of Orofacial Myology, 30,* 8-19.

Solomon, N. P., Makashay, M. J., Kessler, L. S., & Sullivan, K. W. (2004). Speech-breathing treatment and LSVT for a patient with hypokinetic-spastic dysarthria after TBI. *Journal of Medical Speech-Language Pathology, 12,* 213-219.

Southwood, H. M., & Weismer, G. (1993). Listener judgments of the bizarreness, acceptability, naturalness, and normalcy of the dysarthria associated with amyotrophic lateral sclerosis. *Journal of Medical Speech-Language Pathology, 1*(3), 151-161.

Spencer, K., Yorkston, K. M., & Duffy, J. R. (2003). Behavioral management of respiratory/phonatory dysfunction from dysarthria: A flowchart for guidance in clinical decision making. *Journal of Medical Speech-Language Pathology, 11*(2), x1-1xi.

Spitzer, S. M., Liss, J. M., Caviness, J. N., & Adler, C. (2000). An exploration of familiarization effects in the perception of hypokinetic and ataxic dysarthric speech. *Journal of Medical Speech-Language Pathology, 8,* 285-293.

Subtelney, J. (1977). Assessment of speech with implications for training. In F. Bess (Ed.), *Childhood deafness* (pp. 183-194), New York: Grune & Stratton.

Tikofsky, R. S., & Tikofsky, R. P. (1964). Intelligibility as a measure of dysarthric speech. *Journal of Speech and Hearing Research*, 7, 325-333.

Tjaden, K. K., & Liss, J. M. (1995). The role of listener familiarity in the perception of dysarthric speech. *Clinical Linguistics and Phonetics*, 9(2), 139-154.

Verdolini, K., & Ramig, L.O. (1998). Treatment efficacy: Voice disorders. *Journal of Speech, Language, and Hearing Research*, 41, S101-S116.

Weismer, G. (2006a). Philosophy of research in motor speech disorders. *Clinical Linguistics and Phonetics*, 20, 315-349.

Weismer, G. (2006b, June). *Classification in motor speech disorders: What are the issues?* Invited keynote address to the 5th International Conference on Speech Motor Control, Nijmegen, Holland.

Weismer, G., Jeng, J., Laures, J. S., & Kent, R. D. (2001). Acoustic and intelligibility characteristics of sentence production in neurogenic speech disorders. *Folia Phoniatrica et Logopaedica*, 53, 1-18.

Weismer, G., & Laures, J. S. (2002). Direct magnitude estimates of speech intelligibility in dysarthria: effects of a chosen standard. *Journal of Speech, Language, and Hearing Research*, 45, 421-433.

Weismer, G., & Martin, R. (1992). Acoustic and perceptual approaches to the study of intelligibility. In R. Kent (Ed.), *Intelligibility in speech disorders* (pp. 67-118). Philadelphia: John Benjamins.

World Health Organization. (2002). *International classification of functioning, disability, and health*. Retrieved June 1, 2006 from http://www3.who.int/icf/

Yorkston, K., & Beukelman, D. (1978). A comparison of techniques for measuring intelligibility of dysarthric speech. *Journal of Communication Disorders*, 11, 499-512.

Yorkston, K., & Beukelman, D. (1980). A clinician-judged technique for quantifying dysarthric speech based on single-word intelligibility. *Journal of Communication Disorders*, 13, 15-31.

Yorkston, K., & Beukelman, D. (1981). Communication efficiency of dysarthirc speakers as measured by sentence intelligibility and speaking rate. *Journal of Speech and Hearing Disorders*, 46, 296-301.

Yorkston, K., & Beukelman, D. (2000). Decision making in AAC intervention. In D. R. Beukelman, K. Yorkston, & J. Reichle (Eds.). *Augmentative communication for adults with acquired neurologic disabilities*, (pp. 55-82). Baltimore: Paul H. Brookes.

Yorkston, K. M., Beukelman, D. R., Hakel, M., & Fager, S. (in progress). Practice guidelines for dysarthria: Evidence for the treatment of rate, loudness, or prosody (ANCDS Technical Report). Minneapolis, MN: Academy of Neurologic Communication Disorders and Sciences.

Yorkston, K. M., Beukelman, D. R., Strand, E., & Bell, K. (1999). *Management of motor speech disorders in children and adults* (2nd ed., pp. 483-541). Austin, TX: Pro-Ed.

Yorkston, K., Beukelman, D., & Tice, R. (1996). *Sentence Intelligibility Test for Macintosh*. Lincoln, NE: Communication Disorders Software. Distributed by Tice Technology Services, Lincoln, NE.

Yorkston, K. M., Beukelman, D. R., & Traynor, C. D. (1990). The effect of rate control on the intelligibility and naturalness of dysarthric speech. *Journal of Speech and Hearing Disorders*, 55, 550-560.

Yorkston, K., Miller, R., & Strand, E. (2003). *Management of speech and swallowing in degenerative diseases* (2nd ed.). St. Louis, MO: Mosby.

Yorkston, K. M., Spencer, K. A., & Duffy, J. R. (2003a). Behavioral management of respiratory/phonatory dysfunction from dysarthria: A systematic review of the evidence. *Journal of Medical Speech-Language Pathology*, 11, 13-38.

Yorkston, K. M., Spencer, K. A., & Duffy, J. R. (2003b). Behavioral management of respiratory/phonatory dysfunction from dysarthria: A flowchart for guidance in clinical decision making. *Journal of Medical Speech-Language Pathology*, *11*, 39–61.

Yorkston, K. M., Spencer, K. A., Duffy, J. R., Beukelman, D. R., Golper, L. A., Miller, R. M., et al. (2001a). Evidence-based medicine and practice guidelines: Application to the field of speech-language pathology. *Journal of Medical Speech-Language Pathology*, *9*, 243–256.

Yorkston, K. M., Spencer, K. A., Duffy, J. R., Beukelman, D. R., Golper, L. A., Miller, R. M., et al. (2001b). Evidence-based practice guidelines for dysarthria: Management of velopharyngeal function. *Journal of Medical Speech-Language Pathology*, *9*, 257–273.

Yorkston, K., Strand, E., & Kennedy, M. (1996). Comprehensibility of dysarthric speech: Implications for assessment and treatment planning. *American Journal of Speech-Language Pathology*, *5*, 55–66.

Ziegler, W. (2003). Speech motor control is task-specific: Evidence from dysarthria and apraxia of speech. *Aphasiology*, *17*, 3–36.

Zraik, R. I., & Liss, J. M. (2000). A comparison of equal-appearing interval scaling and direct magnitude estimation of nasal voice quality. *Journal of Speech, Language, and Hearing Research*, *43*, 979–988.

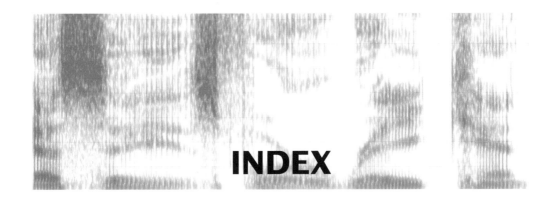

INDEX